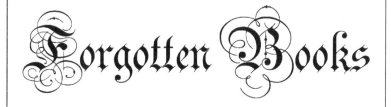

ISBN 978-1-5283-2936-1
PIBN 10941176

1 MONTH OF
FREE
READING

at

www.ForgottenBooks.com

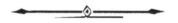

By purchasing this book you are eligible for one month membership to ForgottenBooks.com, giving you unlimited access to our entire collection of over 1,000,000 titles via our web site and mobile apps.

To claim your free month visit:

www.forgottenbooks.com/free941176

English
Français
Deutsche
Italiano
Español
Português

www.forgottenbooks.com

Mythology Photography **Fiction**
Fishing Christianity **Art** Cooking
Essays Buddhism Freemasonry
Medicine **Biology** Music **Ancient**
Egypt Evolution Carpentry Physics
Dance Geology **Mathematics** Fitness
Shakespeare **Folklore** Yoga Marketing
Confidence Immortality Biographies
Poetry **Psychology** Witchcraft
Electronics Chemistry History **Law**
Accounting **Philosophy** Anthropology
Alchemy Drama Quantum Mechanics
Atheism Sexual Health **Ancient History**
Entrepreneurship Languages Sport
Paleontology Needlework Islam
Metaphysics Investment Archaeology
Parenting Statistics Criminology
Motivational

TRANSACTIONS

OF THE

NEW YORK STATE MEDICAL ASSOCIATION.

COMMITTEE ON PUBLICATIONS.

E. D. FERGUSON, M. D., of Rensselaer County, CHAIRMAN AND EDITOR OF THE TRANSACTIONS.

J. C. BENHAM, M. D., of Columbia County.

J. B. HARVIE, M. D., of Rensselaer County.

PRINTED BY
REPUBLICAN PRESS ASSOCIATION,
CONCORD, N. H.

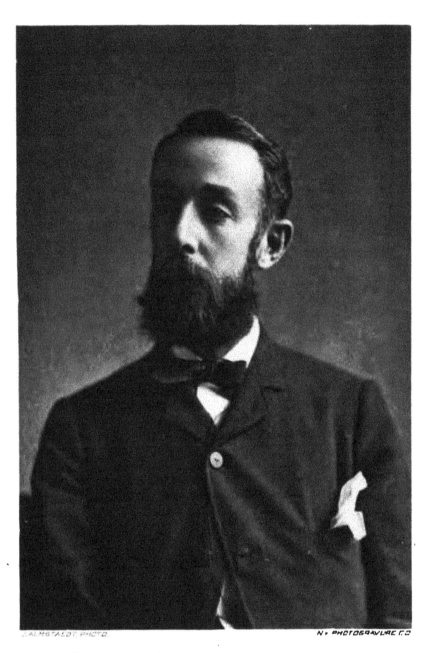

Alfred Ludlow Carroll, M.D.

TRANSACTIONS

OF

THE NEW YORK STATE MEDICAL ASSOCIATION,

FOR THE YEAR 1893,

VOLUME X.

EDITED FOR THE ASSOCIATION

By E. D. FERGUSON, M. D.,

OF RENSSELAER COUNTY.

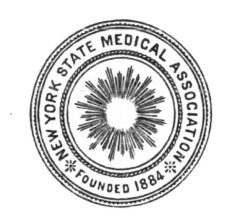

PUBLISHED BY THE ASSOCIATION:
· 64 MADISON AVENUE,
NEW YORK CITY.

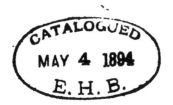

COPYRIGHT, 1894,
BY THE NEW YORK STATE MEDICAL ASSOCIATION.

CONTENTS.

OFFICERS AND COUNCIL FOR 1892-'93.

PRESIDENT.

S. B. W. McLEOD, M. D., New York County, Fifth District.

VICE-PRESIDENTS.

FIRST DISTRICT, R. N. COOLEY, M. D., Oswego County.
SECOND DISTRICT, J. C. HANNAN, M. D., Rensselaer County.
THIRD DISTRICT, N. JACOBSON, M. D., Onondaga County.
FOURTH DISTRICT, Z. J LUSK, M. D., Wyoming County.

SECRETARY AND TREASURER.

E. D. FERGUSON, M. D., Rensselaer County.

CHAIRMAN OF THE LIBRARY COMMITTEE.

J. W. S. GOULEY, M. D., New York County.

MEMBER OF THE COUNCIL AT LARGE.

JOHN SHRADY, M. D., New York County.

ELECTED MEMBERS OF THE COUNCIL.

FIRST DISTRICT, E. T. RULISON, M. D., Montgomery County.
"   "   A. P. DODGE, M. D., Oneida County.
SECOND DISTRICT, THOMAS WILSON, M. D., Columbia County.
"   "   J. B. HARVIE, M. D., Rensselaer County.
THIRD DISTRICT, H. O. JEWETT, M. D., Cortland County.
"   "   M. CAVANA, M. D., Madison County.
FOURTH DISTRICT, THOMAS D. STRONG, M. D., Chautauqua County.
"   "   F. H. MOYER, M. D., Livingston County.
FIFTH DISTRICT, JOHN D. TRUAX, M. D., New York County.
"   "   A. L. CARROLL, M. D., New York County.
    2

COMMITTEE OF ARRANGEMENTS FOR 1892–'93.

S. B. WYLIE McLEOD, President.
E. D. FERGUSON, Secretary.
Ex-officio Members of the Committee.

JOHN G. TRUAX, *Chairman.*
CHARLES E. DENISON, *Secretary.*

F. A. BALDWIN.	OGDEN C. LUDLOW.
C. G. CAMPBELL.	JAMES C. MACKENZIE.
ALFRED L. CARROLL.	WILLIAM McCOLLOM.
ELLERY DENISON.	JOHNSTON McLEOD.
A. PALMER DUDLEY.	VALENTINE MOTT.
JOHN F. ERDMANN.	A. D. RUGGLES.
JOHN W. S. GOULEY.	JOHN SHRADY.
GEORGE T. HARRISON.	STEPHEN SMITH.
CHARLES A. LEALE.	E. H. SQUIBB.

OFFICERS AND COUNCIL FOR 1893–'94.

The Eleventh Annual Meeting will be held at the Mott Memorial Library, in New York City, on October 9, 10, and 11, 1894.

PRESIDENT.

THOMAS D. STRONG, M. D., Westfield, Chautauqua County.

VICE-PRESIDENTS.

FIRST DISTRICT, ISAAC DE ZOUCHE, M. D.,
Gloversville, Fulton County.
SECOND DISTRICT, J. C. BENHAM, M. D., Hudson, Columbia County.
THIRD DISTRICT, H. O. JEWETT, M. D., Cortland, Cortland County.
FIFTH DISTRICT, J. D. RUSHMORE, M. D., Brooklyn, Kings County.

SECRETARY AND TREASURER.

E. D. FERGUSON, M. D., Troy, Rensselaer County.

CHAIRMAN OF THE LIBRARY COMMITTEE.

J. W. S. GOULEY, M. D., 324 Madison Ave.,
New York, New York County.

MEMBER OF THE COUNCIL AT LARGE.

C. E. DENISON, M. D., 124 W. 18th St., New York City.

ELECTED MEMBERS OF THE COUNCIL.

FIRST DISTRICT, A. P. DODGE, M. D.,
Oneida Castle, Oneida County ; term expires 1894.
"   C. H. GLIDDEN, M. D.,
Little Falls, Herkimer County ; term expires 1895.

SECOND DISTRICT, J. B. HARVIE, M. D.,
　　　　　Troy, Rensselaer County; term expires 1894.
　　"　　THOMAS WILSON, M. D.,
　　　　　Claverack, Columbia County; term expires 1895.
THIRD DISTRICT, M. CAVANA, M. D.,
　　　　　Oneida, Madison County; term expires 1894.
　　"　　F. G. SEAMAN, M. D.,
　　　　　Seneca Falls, Seneca County; term expires 1895.
FOURTH DISTRICT, F. H. MOYER, M. D.,
　　　　　Moscow, Livingston County; term expires 1894.
　　"　　GEORGE W. GOLER, M. D.,
　　　　　Rochester, Monroe County; term expires 1895.
FIFTH DISTRICT, A. L. CARROLL, M. D.,
　　　30 W. 59th St., New York, New York County; term expires 1894.
　"　DISTRICT, JOHN D. TRUAX, M. D.,
　　17 E. 127th St., New York, New York County; term expires 1895.

OFFICERS OF THE BRANCH ASSOCIATIONS FOR 1894.

FIRST OR NORTHERN BRANCH.

The Tenth Annual Meeting will be held at Amsterdam, as appointed by the President and Secretary.

OFFICERS.

PRESIDENT, ISAAC DE ZOUCHE, M. D., Gloversville, Fulton County.
SECRETARY, EZRA GRAVES, M. D., Amsterdam, Montgomery County.

EXECUTIVE COMMITTEE.

WILLIAM GILLIS, M. D., Fort Covington, Franklin County.
ISAAC DE ZOUCHE, M. D., Gloversville, Fulton County.
THOMAS McGANN, M. D., Wells, Hamilton County.
W. D. GARLOCH, M. D., Little Falls, Herkimer County.
J. MORTIMER CRAWE, M. D., Watertown, Jefferson County.
ALBEBT A. JOSLIN, M. D., Martinsburg, Lewis County.
E. T. RULISON, M. D., Amsterdam, Montgomery County.
G. ALDER BLUMER, M. D., Utica, Oneida County.
E. F. MARSH, M. D., Fulton, Oswego County.
GUY REUBEN COOK, M. D., Louisville, St. Lawrence County.

SECOND OR EASTERN BRANCH.

The Tenth Annual Meeting will be held at Troy, Rensselaer County, on the fourth Thursday in June, 1894.

OFFICERS.

PRESIDENT, J. C. BENHAM, M. D., Hudson, Columbia County.
SECRETARY, JOSEPH E. BAYNES, M. D., Troy, Rensselaer County.

EXECUTIVE COMMITTEE.

L. B. RULISON, M. D., West Troy, Albany County.
O. W. HOLCOMB, M. D., Plattsburgh, Clinton County.
J. W. LOCKWOOD, M. D., Philmont, Columbia County.
C. A. CHURCH, M. D., Bloomingdale, Essex County.
GEORGE CONKLING, M. D., Durham, Greene County.
W. H. NICHOLS, M. D., West Sand Lake, Rensselaer County.
C. S. GRANT, M. D., Saratoga Springs, Saratoga County.
CHARLES HAMMER, M. D., Schenectady, Schenectady County.
H. F. KINGSLEY, M. D., Schoharie, Schoharie County.
D. J. FITZGERALD, M. D., Glens Falls, Warren County.
JOHN LAMBERT, M. D., Salem, Washington County.

THIRD OR CENTRAL BRANCH.

The Tenth Annual Meeting will be held at Syracuse, Onondaga County, on the third Thursday in May, 1894.

OFFICERS.

PRESIDENT, H. O. JEWETT, M. D., Cortland, Cortland County.
SECRETARY, F. H. STEPHENSON, M. D.,
                101 Warren St., Syracuse, Onondaga County.

EXECUTIVE COMMITTEE.

J. H. CHITTENDEN, M. D., Binghamton, Broome County.
W. R. LAIRD, M. D., Auburn, Cayuga County.
F. W. ROSS, M. D., Elmira, Chemung County.
H. C. LYMAN, M. D., Sherburne, Chenango County.
F. W. HIGGINS, M. D., Cortland, Cortland County.
W. B. MORROW, M. D., Walton, Delaware County.
M. CAVANA, M. D., Oneida, Madison County.
H. D. DIDAMA, M. D., Syracuse, Onondaga County.
J. K. LEANING, Cooperstown, Otsego County.
B. T. SMELZER, M. D., Havana, Schuyler County.
ELIAS LESTER, M. D., Seneca Falls, Seneca County.
W. L. AYER, M. D., Owego, Tioga County.
WILLIAM FITCH, M. D., Dryden, Tompkins County.

FOURTH OR WESTERN BRANCH.

The Tenth Annual Meeting will be held at Buffalo, Erie County, on the second Tuesday in May, 1894.

OFFICERS.

PRESIDENT, T. D. STRONG, M. D., Westfield, Chautauqua County.
SECRETARY, WM. H. THORNTON, M. D.,
570 Niagara St., Buffalo, Erie County.

EXECUTIVE COMMITTEE.

J. A. STEPHENSON, M. D., Scio, Alleghany County.
S. J. MUDGE, M. D., Olean, Cattaraugus County.
R. T. ROLPH, M. D., Fredonia, Chautauqua County.
A. H. BRIGGS, M. D., Buffalo, Erie County.
A. P. JACKSON, M. D., Oakfield, Genesee County.
G. H. JONES, M. D., Fowlerville, Livingston County.
G. W. GOLER, M. D., Rochester, Monroe County.
W. Q. HUGGINS, M. D., Lockport, Niagara County.
J. H. ALLEN, M. D., Gorham, Ontario County.
JOHN H. TAYLOR, M. D., Holley, Orleans County.
D. J. CHITTENDEN, M. D , Addison, Steuben County.
DARWIN COLVIN, M. D., Clyde, Wayne County.
A. G. ELLINWOOD, M. D., Attica, Wyoming County.
WILLIAM OLIVER, M. D., Penn Yan, Yates County.

FIFTH OR SOUTHERN BRANCH.

The Tenth Annual Meeting will be held in Brooklyn, Kings County, on the fourth Tuesday in May, 1894.

OFFICERS.

PRESIDENT, J. D. RUSHMORE, M. D.,
129 Montague St., Brooklyn, Kings County.
SECRETARY, E. H. SQUIBB, M. D.,
P. O. Box 760, Brooklyn, Kings County.

Executive Committee.

I. D. Le ROY, M. D., Pleasant Valley, Dutchess County.
J. D. RUSHMORE, M. D., Brooklyn, Kings County.
ROBERT NEWMAN, M. D., New York, New York County.
M. C. CONNER, M. D., Middletown, Orange County.
G. W. MURDOCK, M. D., Cold Spring, Putnam County.
E. G. RAVE, M. D., Hicksville, Queens County.
F. E. MARTINDALE, M. D., Port Richmond, Richmond County.
WILLIAM GOVAN, M. D., Stony Point, Rockland County.
WALTER LINDSAY, M. D., Huntington, Suffolk County.
C. W. PIPER, M. D., Wurtsborough, Sullivan County.
H. VAN HOEVENBERG, M. D., Kingston, Ulster County.
H. E. SCHMID, M. D., Tarrytown, Westchester County.

LIST OF PRESIDENTS AND VICE-PRESIDENTS FROM THE FOUNDING OF THE ASSOCIATION.

1884.

PRESIDENT.

HENRY D. DIDAMA, M. D., Onondaga County, Third District.

VICE-PRESIDENTS.

FIRST DISTRICT, J. MORTIMER CRAWE, M. D., Jefferson County.
SECOND DISTRICT, TABOR B. REYNOLDS, M. D., Saratoga County.
FOURTH DISTRICT, B. L. HOVEY, M. D., Monroe County.
FIFTH DISTRICT, NATH'L C. HUSTED, M. D., Westchester County.

1885.

PRESIDENT.

*JOHN P. GRAY, M. D., Oneida County, First District.

VICE-PRESIDENTS.

SECOND DISTRICT, WILLIAM H. ROBB, M. D., Montgomery County.
THIRD DISTRICT, JOHN G. ORTON, M. D., Broome County.
FOURTH DISTRICT, JOSEPH C. GREENE, M. D., Erie County.
FIFTH DISTRICT, *JOSEPH C. HUTCHINSON, M. D., Kings County.

1886.

PRESIDENT.

E. M. MOORE, M. D., Monroe County, Fourth District.

* Deceased.

VICE-PRESIDENTS.

FIRST DISTRICT, WILLIAM GILLIS, M. D., Franklin County.
SECOND DISTRICT, H. C. VAN ZANDT, M. D., Schenectady County.
THIRD DISTRICT, *FREDERICK HYDE, M. D., Cortland County.
FIFTH DISTRICT, J. G. PORTEOUS, M. D., Dutchess County.

1887.

PRESIDENT.

*ISAAC E. TAYLOR, M. D., New York County, Fifth District.

VICE-PRESIDENTS.

FIRST DISTRICT, JOHN P. SHARER, M. D., Herkimer County.
SECOND DISTRICT, L. C. DODGE, M. D., Clinton County.
THIRD DISTRICT, *GEORGE W. AVERY, M. D., Chenango County.
FOURTH DISTRICT, DARWIN COLVIN, M. D., Wayne County.

1888.

PRESIDENT.

JOHN CRONYN, M. D., Erie County, Fourth District.

VICE-PRESIDENTS.

FIRST DISTRICT, BYRON DE WITT, M. D., Oswego County.
SECOND DISTRICT, ROBERT SELDEN, M. D., Greene County.
THIRD DISTRICT, CHARLES W. BROWN, M. D., Chemung County.
FIFTH DISTRICT, EDWIN BARNES, M. D., Dutchess County.

1889.

PRESIDENT.

WILLIAM T. LUSK, M. D., New York County, Fifth District.

* Deceased.

VICE-PRESIDENTS.

FIRST DISTRICT, S. H. FRENCH, M. D., Montgomery County.
SECOND DISTRICT, R. C. McEWEN, M. D., Saratoga County.
THIRD DISTRICT, ELIAS LESTER, M. D., Seneca County.
FOURTH DISTRICT, THOMAS D. STRONG, M. D., Chautauqua County.

———

1890.

PRESIDENT.

JOHN G. ORTON, M. D., Broome County, Third District.

VICE-PRESIDENTS.

FIRST DISTRICT, DOUGLAS AYRES, M. D., Montgomery County.
SECOND DISTRICT, M. H. BURTON, M. D., Rensselaer County.
FOURTH DISTRICT, E. M. MOORE, JR., M. D., Monroe County.
FIFTH DISTRICT, WILLIAM McCOLLOM, M. D. (vice WILLIAM B.
    EAGER, M. D., deceased), Kings County.

———

1891.

PRESIDENT.

STEPHEN SMITH, M. D., New York County, Fifth District.

VICE-PRESIDENTS.

FIRST DISTRICT, DOUGLAS AYRES, M. D., Montgomery County.
SECOND DISTRICT, A. T. VAN VRANKEN, M. D., Albany County.
THIRD DISTRICT, J. D. TRIPP, M. D., Cayuga County.
FOURTH DISTRICT, ROBERT J. MENZIE, M. D., Livingston County.

———

1892.

PRESIDENT.

JUDSON B. ANDREWS, M. D., Erie County, Fourth District.

VICE-PRESIDENTS.

FIRST DISTRICT, W. D. GARLOCK, M. D., Herkimer County.
SECOND DISTRICT, GEO. E. McDONALD, M. D., Schenectady County.
THIRD DISTRICT, LEROY J. BROOKS, M. D., Chenango County.
FIFTH DISTRICT, HENRY VAN HOEVENBERG, M. D., Ulster County.

1893.

PRESIDENT.

S. B. W. McLEOD, M. D., New York County, Fifth District.

VICE-PRESIDENTS.

FIRST DISTRICT, R. N. COOLEY, M. D., Oswego County.
SECOND DISTRICT, J. C. HANNAN, M. D., Rensselaer County.
THIRD DISTRICT, N. JACOBSON, M. D., Onondaga County.
FOURTH DISTRICT, Z. J. LUSK, M. D., Wyoming County.

LIST OF FELLOWS REGISTERED AT THE TENTH ANNUAL MEETING IN NEW YORK CITY.

Held October 9, 10, 11, and 12, 1893.

FIRST DISTRICT.

MONTGOMERY COUNTY.

Ayres, Douglas, Fort Plain.

Johnson, Richard G., Amsterdam.

Robb, William H., Amsterdam.

ONEIDA COUNTY.

Dodge, A. P., Oneida Castle.

SECOND DISTRICT.

ALBANY COUNTY.

Rulison, L. B., West Troy.

COLUMBIA COUNTY.

Smith, H. Lyle, Hudson.

Vedder, George W., Philmont.

Wilson, Thomas, Claverack.

RENSSELAER COUNTY.

Bontecou, R. B., Troy.

Burbeck, C. B., Troy.

Cahill, John T., Hoosick Falls.

Ferguson, E. D., Troy.

Finder, William, Jr., Troy.

Hannan, J. C., Hoosick Falls.

Hull, W. H., Poestenkill.

Marsh, James P., Troy.

Phelan, M. F., Troy.

SCHENECTADY COUNTY.

Van Zandt, H. C., Schenectady.

THIRD DISTRICT.

BROOME COUNTY.

Dudley, Dwight, Maine.

Greene, C. W., Chenango Forks.

CAYUGA COUNTY.

Tripp, John D., Auburn.

CHENANGO COUNTY.

Brooks, Leroy J., Norwich.   Douglas, George, Oxford.

CORTLAND COUNTY.

Bradford, George D., Homer.   Jewett, Homer O., Cortland.

MADISON COUNTY.

Cavana, Martin, Oneida.   Carpenter, Henry W., Oneida.

ONONDAGA COUNTY.

Van de Warker, Ely, Syracuse.

OTSEGO COUNTY.

Leaning, John K., Cooperstown.   Martin, John H., Otego.

SENECA COUNTY.

Bellows, George A., Waterloo.   Lester, Elias, Seneca Falls.

TIOGA COUNTY.

Ayer, W. L., Owego.

FOURTH DISTRICT.

CHAUTAUQUA COUNTY.

Dean, II. J., Brockton.   Strong, T. D., Westfield.

ERIE COUNTY.

Cronyn, John, Buffalo.   Thornton, W. H., Buffalo.

GENESEE COUNTY.

Jackson, Albert P., Oakfield.

MONROE COUNTY.

Hovey, B. L., Rochester.

ONTARIO COUNTY.

Vanderhoof, F. D., Phelps.

WAYNE COUNTY.

Colvin, Darwin, Clyde.

FIFTH DISTRICT.

DUTCHESS COUNTY.

Barnes, Edwin, Pleasant Plains.
Bayley, Guy Carleton, Poughkeepsie.
Le Roy, Irving D., Pleasant Valley.
Porteous, J. G., Poughkeepsie.
Pultz, Monroe T., Stanfordville.

KINGS COUNTY.

Alleman, L. A. W., Brooklyn.
Baker, Frank R., Brooklyn.
Baker, George W., Brooklyn.
Bierwirth, Julius C., Brooklyn.
Coffin, Lawrence, Brooklyn.
Feeley, James F., Brooklyn.
Hicks, Edward E., Brooklyn.
Leighton, N. W., Brooklyn.
McCollom, William, Brooklyn.
Minard, E. J. C., Brooklyn.
North, Nelson L., Brooklyn.
Raynor, F. C., Brooklyn.
Risch, H. F. W., Brooklyn.
Squibb, Edward H., Brooklyn.
Squibb, Edward R., Brooklyn.
Steinke, C. O. H., Brooklyn.
Sullivan, J. D., Brooklyn.
Wieber, George, Brooklyn.
Williams, Wm. H., Brooklyn.
Wyckoff, Richard M., Brooklyn.

NEW YORK COUNTY.

Arnold, Glover C., New York.
Baldwin, F. A., New York.
Bozeman, Nathan, New York.
Bozeman, Nathan G., New York.
Bryant, J. D., New York.
Burchard, Thomas H., New York.
Carroll, Alfred Ludlow, New York.
Carter, H. Skelton, New York.
Chauveau, J. F., New York.
Cook, Almon H., New York.
Curry, Walker, New York.
Dallas, Alexander, New York.
Davis, R. C., New York.
Denison, C. E., New York.
Denison, Ellery, New York.
Dennis, F. S., New York.
Dudley, A. Palmer, New York.
Eastman, Robert W., New York.
Einhorn, Max, New York.
Eliot, Ellsworth, New York.
Farrington, Joseph O., New York.
Flint, Austin, New York.
Flint, Austin, Jr., New York.
Flint, William H., New York.
Goldthwaite, Henry, New York.
Gouley, J. W. S., New York.
Hepburn, Neil J., New York.
Hodgman, Abbott, New York.
Holmes, M. C., New York.
Hubbard, S. T., New York.
Jackson, Charles W., New York.
Janvrin, J. E., New York.
Judson, A. B., New York.
Kemp, William M., New York.
Leale, Charles A., New York.
Lockwood, C. E., New York.
Ludlow, O. C., New York.
Lukens, Anna, New York.
Lusk, W. T., New York.
MacGregor, J. R., New York.
Mackenzie, J. C., New York.
Manley, Thomas H., New York.
McGillicuddy, T. J., New York.
McIlroy, Samuel H., New York.

McLeod, Johnston, New York.
McLeod, S. B. W., New York.
Milliken, S. E., New York.
O'Meagher, Wm., New York.
Oppenheimer, H. S., New York.
Parsons, John, New York.
Pryor, William R., New York.
Purple, Samuel S., New York.
Ruggles, A. D., New York.

Sayre, Lewis A., New York.
Sayre, Reginald A., New York.
Seaman, Lewis L., New York.
Shrady, John, New York.
Silver, Henry M., New York.
Truax, John G., New York.
Wallach, Joseph G., New York.
White, J. Blake, New York.
Wyeth, John A., New York.

ORANGE COUNTY.

Conner, Milton C., Middletown.
Townsend, C. E., Middletown.

Vanderveer, J. R., Monroe.

PUTNAM COUNTY.

Murdoch, G. W., Cold Spring.

RICHMOND COUNTY.

Johnston, H. C., New Brighton.

SUFFOLK COUNTY.

Hamill, Edward H. (Newark, N. J.).

ULSTER COUNTY.

Van Hoevenberg, Henry, Kingston.

WESTCHESTER COUNTY.

Schmid, H. Ernst, White Plains.

NON-RESIDENT FELLOWS.

Dandridge, N. P., Cincinnati, O.   Maclean, Donald, Detroit, Mich.

SUMMARY BY DISTRICTS OF FELLOWS IN ATTENDANCE.

First District, ...	4
Second District, ...	14
Third District, ...	15
Fourth District, ...	8
Fifth District, ...	95
Non-resident, ...	2
Total, ...	188

DELEGATES FROM OTHER MEDICAL ORGANISATIONS AND INVITED GUESTS IN ATTENDANCE.

CANADA.

SIR JAMES A. GRANT, M. D., K. C. M. G., 150 ELGIN
ST., OTTAWA, ... Invited Guest.

CONNECTICUT.

GUSTAVUS ELIOT, M. D., NEW HAVEN, . . . Delegate.

MASSACHUSETTS.

JOHN M. HARLOW, M. D., WOBURN, . . . Delegate.
GEORGE B. SHATTUCK, M. D., 183 BEACON ST.,
BOSTON, ... Delegate.

VERMONT.

C. E. CHANDLER, M. D., MONTPELIER, . . . Delegate.

FRANCE.

EMILE POUSSIÉ, D. M. P., 2 RUE DE VALOIS, PARIS, Invited Guest.

ADDRESS OF WELCOME AND REPORT OF THE COMMITTEE OF ARRANGEMENTS.

By J. G. TRUAX, M. D., of New York County, Chairman of the Committee.

GENTLEMEN: We bid you welcome to this the tenth annual meeting of the New York State Medical Association.

It gives your Committee of Arrangements great pleasure to be able to inform you that they have provided for your entertainment this year something in addition to hard work. Many members of the Association have contributed liberally of their means that we might be able to celebrate this our decennial meeting in a proper manner. .

Your committee has provided a banquet, a lunch, an excursion and lunch on board of the boat. It is our desire that all who register will contribute towards the expense. Unless each one does his share, it will be a burden to the few, which ought not to be placed upon them. We meet this year to have a good time as well as to do good work.

One of our members, a Fellow who has laboured with us ever since the organisation of the Association, one whom we all love and respect, is about to pass away. I have known him so long, and always found him so kind, gentle, and thoughtful for others' good, that the thought of his leaving us has deprived me of much of the pleasure anticipated from this meeting. I refer to Dr. A. L. Carroll. It seems to me not to be out of place to speak of his illness at this time.

There being so much to do this evening, I will not detain you longer than is necessary to outline the programme.

There are to be four addresses. One by the president, S. B. Wylie McLeod, M. D., of New York county; one by John Shrady, M. D., of New York county, on the "Medical Work of the Association during its First Decade;" one by Stephen Smith, M. D., of New York county, on the "Surgical Work of the Association during its First Decade;" and one by George Tucker Harrison, M. D., of New York county, on the "Obstetrical and Gynaecological Work of the Association during its First Decade." There are to be two discussions, one on "Lesions of the Pleura," which will be opened by John Shrady, M. D., of New York county. The other will be upon the "Treatment of Appendicitis." This discussion will be opened by Frederic S. Dennis, M. D., of New York county.

Altogether there are twenty-two subjects to be considered by forty-four speakers. The contributions come from the five districts of the state, and from other states, in the following proportions:

The First District	3
Second "	3
Third "	3
Fourth "	5
.Fifth "	26
State of Michigan	1
State of Connecticut	1
State of Ohio	1
Canada	1

In the five districts, Fellows of the Association from thirteen counties contribute essays in the following proportion:

First District,	Montgomery county	. . . .	2
" "	Oswego "	. . . .	1
Second "	Rensselaer "	. . . .	3
Third "	Broome	. . . .	1
" "	Onondaga "	. . . .	1
" "	Chemung	. . . .	1
Fourth "	Wyoming "	. . . .	2
" "	Erie	. . . .	2
" "	Wayne	. . . .	1
Fifth "	New York "	. . . .	19
" "	Kings	. . . .	3
" "	Westchester "	. . . .	3
" "	Dutchess	. . . .	1

If all the time be fully occupied, and the discussions confined to the ten minutes allowed to each person, your committee is of the opinion that two evening, three morning, and two afternoon sessions will be sufficient. Taking the second evening and one afternoon from scientific work we hope will not detract from the interest, instruction, or pleasure all hope to derive from this meeting. The morning sessions will be opened at 9 o'clock, the afternoon sessions at 1 o'clock, the evening sessions at 7:30 o'clock.

THE PRESIDENT'S ADDRESS.

A DECENNIAL REVIEW OF THE AFFAIRS OF THE ASSOCIATION.

By S. B. WYLIE McLEOD, M. D., of New York County.

October 9, 1893.

GENTLEMEN AND FELLOWS: Honoured by my election to the Presidency of the Association, permit me to express to you my sincere thanks for the distinction conferred, and my high appreciation of the honour of presiding over your deliberations at this decennial meeting.

Ten years of existence and ten years after death are indeed determining periods in life and life's results. In human existence each decade has its characteristics, and what is true of the individual may also be affirmed of the life of a nation, of a cause, of a party, and of any association of men. At the suggestion of the Committee of Arrangements, by whom you have been so cordially welcomed, the subject of this address will be " A Review of the Affairs of the Association up to This—the End of the First Ten Years of Its Maintenance."

In common with most organisations, our annual meetings are opened with an address by the presiding officer. It is the right of a president to be acquainted with all the departments of the society over which he presides, being informed of its financial, scientific, ethical, and fellowship affairs. If he has given that time and attention to its duties which the needs and responsibilities of the office demand, he should be in condition to give its members a reliable and practical statement of its proceedings, and make such recommendations as his experience has indicated would contribute to its usefulness in the future. From these considerations, it

would seem proper to pass in review the various subjects on
which you were addressed by the Presidents whom you have
elected since the founding of our Association.

In 1884, the address of the first President, Dr. Didama,
consisted of suggestions upon, and illustrations of, this sentiment,—"In medicine much is worthy of conservation. Not
a little is still moot. Research is very active and confident,
and vast fields await exploration."

In 1885, Dr. Gray chose as his subject, "Relations between
the Science of Medicine and the State of New York." His
words and statements in that address have become the more
valuable, because we can hear his voice no more : he is the
first of the presidents of our Association whose career has
been terminated by death. The pleasing memories of him
retained by his successors may now prompt a description of
his own relations to the "science of medicine," as that of
one of its most eminent devotees, and to the "state of New
York," as that of a useful and distinguished citizen.

In 1886, Dr. Moore briefly reviewed the history of previous years, and as a result, announced the declaration, "The
work is good, and the fellowship complete," and he then continued with a scientific address.

In 1887, Dr. Taylor reviewed very briefly the proceedings
of former years, in proof of his chosen theme, "The Medical
Profession One and Continuous." After this, he, too, gave
more time to the presentation of a scientific dissertation.
While he lived, he did much to unify the profession and to
preserve its continuity. Since his death, October 30, 1889,
pleasant memories are retained of his intercourse and fellowship, and we recognise, that though dead, his works and
former deeds are still useful in our affairs.

In 1888, Dr. Cronyn delivered the address on "The Medical Profession and the Public."

In 1889, Dr. Lusk's address was entirely scientific, viz., on
"Tubal Pregnancy." No better opportunity than this could
have been afforded to hear a scientific paper from a well
known author, and the choice of the writer on this occasion,

in departing from usual custom in pronouncing an address exclusively scientific, met the hearty approval of his hearers.

In 1890, Dr. Orton spoke on the theme, " The Medical Profession is a Public Trust."

In 1891, Dr. Stephen Smith selected as his subject, " The Art of Teaching Medicine."

In 1892, Dr. Andrews addressed us on " The Relation of the Alienist to the General Practitioner."

In 1893, I shall be content to leave the plane of originality, and, finding so much that is profitable in the addresses of my predecessors, seek to be the exhibitor of their foresight and genius. If I attempt a paraphrase, with quotations and illustrations, it will be to show that during the closing decade you have had a clear and comprehensive description of the medical profession and a just delineation of some required improvements or reforms.

"The spontaneous growth of science left untrammelled will undoubtedly advance human interest far more rapidly and surely than if put under governmental supervision." " The establishment of voluntary relations among our members, and the pursuit of scientific inquiries through an independent voluntary association, have been found to be more successful than the influence of state control, often malign, or the regulation of our affairs by statute." " The rejection of exclusive dogmas, the acceptance of the accumulated experience of the profession, the constant interchange of thought found in the reading of the journals and discussions in Association meetings, the more careful selection of medical students and their education in all the departments of our science, are unifying the profession and providing for its continuity." " The dealings of medical men are more with individuals than with masses, and the relations of the physician to the public will ever be a matter of speculation." The ethics prescribes, with sufficient exactness, what the duty of the profession to the public is, but the public value the doctor only " for the relief they receive from him, and do not appreciate otherwise his valuable services." " The crowning glory of the medical profession is its opportunities for the prevention of disease and the prolongation of human life—herein is consummated the responsible trust committed to us, and the profession honours the trust confided to its keeping." " There is, indeed, a vein of chivalry in the medical profession. It heeds the cry of suffering poor and lowly, and no pestilence-smitten city has ever made an appeal for aid without meeting with a quick response." " It has no secrets, no patents, but always holds its gifts of healing in trust for the public good."

In every consideration of the science and art of medicine, education must form an important part. If the very ancient method is a " lost art," but was better than that prevailing now, then " let the lost art be restored." " The student of to-day appreciates as never before the constant widening of the fields of medical knowledge, and realises the impossibility of becoming equally proficient in all the various departments which have been developed during recent years." " Much of the real progress in medicine is due to the zeal and patient research of the skilled specialist." " Specialties should not be divorced from the general field of medicine of which they are an outgrowth, nor should they be brought in conflict."

Such is an epitome, or rather a paraphrase, of the presidential addresses of the closing decade.

As a second part of this address, let us briefly pass in review the scientific work during our first ten years. Of 476 papers and dissertations read at our meetings since organisation, 181 have been on surgery, 153 on medicine, 72 on obstetrics and gynaecology, 24 on pathology, 15 on materia medica, 10 on insanity, 8 on ophthalmology, 6 on state medicine, 4 on hygiene, 2 on physiology, and 1 on toxicology. This includes the programme of the present year. These figures would indicate great disproportion among the various subjects, and the apparent estimate of the profession of their comparative importance. It should be remembered in classifying, that many cases of surgery are of brain surgery or thoracic surgery or abdominal surgery, and not in their usual sense originally surgical cases. The surgeon is called to relieve diseases in those regions, as for instance an aploplectic clot, pulmonary tuberculosis, or certain conditions of the appendix vermiformis. Classify them by the disease and they are medical, while by the treatment they are surgical. Some cases classified as obstetrical might be arranged under the heading of medical, as for instance, mitral disease associated with pregnancy, or of physiological when maternal impressions and their effect on the embryo is the subject of consideration.

Ophthalmology and insanity are so much in the hands of specialists as to render it unnecessary for the general practitioner to have so many and constant references to these departments, and hence the number of papers is comparatively small. The papers on physiology, hygiene, state medicine, pathology, and toxicology are all valuable and practical, and each one merits a careful perusal. However desirable it would be to review them, it may be said that being elementary and incidental to other departments in which their. usefulness will be found, they will, as separate subjects, be omitted here.

Wisely and well the Committee of Arrangements has designated certain expert Fellows of the Association to make reviews of special subjects, as announced on the programme. Thus there will be an address on the medical work of the Association during its first decade, one on the surgical work of the Association during the same period, and a third on the obstetrical and gynaecological work. These will secure a complete review of these subjects, which constitute the great bulk of the scientific work performed. They make 406 of the number of papers referred to, and leave, with the omissions just announced, 33 papers divided among ophthalmology, materia medica, and insanity. Entirely passing by surgery, practice of medicine, and obstetrics, which are otherwise provided for, a brief reference to ophthalmology, materia medica, and insanity will complete this review.

Insanity.—Papers on the following subjects have been presented and discussed: "Prevention of Insanity;"

"Shadow-Line of Insanity;" "Causation;" "Heredity and Environment;" "The Examination and Commitment of the Insane;" "Mental Symptoms of Fatigue;" "Limits of Re sponsibility in the Insane;" "The Alienist and the General Practitioner;" "The Voluntary Commitment of the Insane to Hospitals;"—the last of which is appointed to be read at the present meeting. The burden of all these discussions seems to be the importance of prevention and extending relief in the earlier stages of the disease. Many ways are pointed out by which this could be accomplished. By proper care and treatment a favorable prognosis could be given, when under adverse circumstances the case would soon become hopeless. There is a general agreement among all the writers on this subject, that much depends on the general practitioner. The logic of events is constantly showing, that were he better informed, and were there friendly and coöperative relations between him and the specialist, much might be done by the family physician in the way of prevention, and by early attention an arrest of the progress of the disease might be effected. This has been the subject of ten papers and accompanying discussions. In one of these, especially, is a strong advocacy of introducing the subject of insanity, both by lectures and clinical instruction, and requiring it as a part of the curriculum of every medical college.

Dr. Judson B. Andrews quotes from the report of the Association of Medical Superintendents of American Institutions for the Insane the following resolutions in regard to instruction in the colleges, viz. :

Resolved, That lectures should be delivered before all the students attending these schools, and that no one should be allowed to graduate without as thorough an examination on this subject as on the other branches taught.

Resolved, That in connection with these lectures there should be clinical instruction, etc.

He then closed his address thus,—"We would enforce the plea for making the study of psychological medicine obligatory upon all students, and would urge upon our schools the necessity of adding the theoretical and clinical study of insanity to their curriculum. It is done in Great Britain, why should it not be done in America?" In many schools it has never been taught at all. Much more attention has been given to the subject during the last decade than at any time before.

Diseases of the Eye.—This subject has been presented in about eight papers. Among them are "Errors of Refraction;" "Early Recognition of These Errors;" "Remarkable Case of Pyaemia After Operation for Strabismus;" "Exudative Conjunctivitis;" "Tumors of the Orbit;" "Extraction of Foreign Bodies from the Eye;" "Treatment of Cataract," and "Cocaine as a Local Anaesthetic in Ophthalmic Surgery." It may be safe to say that no subject has been more thoroughly cared for than diseases of the eye. In hospitals, general and special, the skilled specialist has brought the treatment of the eye high towards a mark of perfection. It has been taught in the colleges and illustrated in the clinics. It is of course largely in the hands of the specialist, but the importance of detecting and treating certain forms at an early stage has led the general practitioner and family physician to give it attention. We have reason to believe that a kindly feeling prevails between these practitioners, and that the general opinion of the profession now is that the attending physician should early in the case seek the counsel of the specialist in the best interest of the patient whom he serves.

Materia Medica.—This subject has been presented in fifteen special papers. The titles of some of these are,—"Modern Progress in Materia Medica and Therapeutics;" "Chlorate of Potassa;" "Commercial Prescriptions;" "Theory of the Chlorides;" "Ergot;" "Saratoga Mineral Waters;" "Medicine and Pharmacy Abroad;" "Relations of Physicians to their Medical Supplies;" and three papers, in the form of annuals for 1891, 1892, and 1893, styled "Comments on the Materia Medica" for those years. It is probably true that there is no department of the practice of medicine in which the doctor exercises his right of selection more than in the choice of his articles of the materia medica. One of the most recent writers on the subject says that during the last four years the changes that have taken place in pathology, materia medica, and therapeutics have been so great as to be almost "startling in their magnitude." Of course this knowledge is scattered through periodical medical literature, and would require great care in selecting the most important and lasting materials. Believing that these papers in our various Transactions are valuable contributions, I would not hesitate to suggest, that could they be taken from their places in the several volumes and published together in one, it would make a valuable text-book and a good example of modern materia medica.

From the epitome presented, and the analysis of scientific work performed, it must appear that at least a moderate degree of success has attended our efforts during the closing decade. Conservatism is very influential, holding by truths long since adopted, and displaying a willingness to restore old principles and forms of practice; and yet this conservatism is well guarded against in any of its malign influences by the spirit of research and confidence in the result of entirely new experiments, which never was so active as now. More certainty is being every day secured. Moot points have been determined and are no longer matters of speculation, and additional fields are constantly being exposed for exploration. Illustrations of these things are so well known that to this audience it would be supererogation to make special reference to them. We look with special favour on the idea that the medical profession is a public trust, and see the useful citizen, the respected neighbour, and the publicly recognised benefactor of mankind in him who realises it and lives in conformity with its powerful suggestions.

Every one at all acquainted with the subject will acknowledge that medical education has been greatly improved during the last few years, and this does not seem strange when we reflect that we are living in an age of improvements; but when we reflect, again, that the improvement consists in gradation of studies and divisions in small sections of the classes and bringing the students by recitations immediately under the supervision of the professor or tutor, and that all this is the most ancient method, practised in the time of Hippocrates, as we heard from one of the addresses, it does not seem strange that we are willing to restore, as a lost art, this very ancient way of teaching, not because it is old or new, but because it is the best and most likely to make good scholars. The method now long pursued, and therefore old, which consists in constant lecturing to students whom the lecturer never sees except in the amphitheatre, tends to develop and exalt the professor. But the method of the ancients, as restored and now new, brings the young men in small classes and by graded courses under the professor's immediate pupilage, and tends to develop and increase their mental powers. It is for the medical students that the colleges are built and the professors provided, and as our successors come forward we must look to them to keep up the continuity of the profession we have been trying to build.

Kindly feelings between the specialist and general practitioner should be preserved. To do this let all specialists study general medicine, and all family physicians a part at least of the various specialties. Reference to this has been already made, and improvement in this respect has been one of the notable advancements of the closing decade.

Our relation to the state has been a matter of much difference of opinion. That as individuals all are of course amenable as other citizens are, and that there must be some kind of dependence on the state, is acknowledged, but the other opinion has been fully announced in the preceding summary. Believing that medical manners and medical ethics are " necessary to success of the better kind," we hail with satisfaction the disposition that exists to have these taught in our medical schools and a knowledge of them required as a condition of securing the degree of doctor of medicine.

Notwithstanding that the scientific work is the main object of the Association, it is but proper that reasonable time and attention should be given to business and to our legal and other relations. The Council will first consider these, and I shall recommend that whatever is required shall be introduced early in the session, that due attention may be given thereto.

This Association was organised February 4, 1884. From a much smaller number our membership has increased until it has now reached eight hundred. At the first meeting of the Association (November 19, 1884) it was resolved to establish a library, to be called " The Library of the New York Medical Association," and that this library should be placed in the city of New York. By the careful and efficient management of the committee having it in charge, it is now a large and valuable collection, and is open for the use of members. It contains 9,045 volumes.

And now, Fellows of the Association, let us close our books on the termination of the first decade, and open others for the commencement of the second. We have secured prosperity : let us strive for still greater success.

THE MEDICAL WORK OF THE ASSOCIATION DURING ITS FIRST DECADE.

By JOHN SHRADY, M. D., of New York County.

October 10, 1893.

To every individual, community, and nation there comes a period when a review is in order; to the recluse it shapes itself as the act of contemplation, when conscience sternly balances accounts, while with the hero it summarises results and perhaps, with spectral intensity, magnifies errors; with the community, it condones rather than censures; and last of all, as regards the nation in its aggregation of forces, it forgets all in the glare of that glory to which the mass has alone contributed. With advance in the scale, there is an advance in the responsibilities. There cannot, therefore, be much room for individualisation where so many motives, such minute division of labour, and such fierce conflicts for excellence are involved. But let us reflect that the world itself is made up of atoms—welded, coalesced, and defying hasty analysis,—and each constituent element, fulfilling its mission almost automatically, merges itself into a grand consummation.

So has it been with medicine, our own ennobling pursuit—let us not call it a science, for it has not yet attained a knowledge deserving of that name; its logic is faulty, because its examples are not yet fully multiplied, and the brevity of time has crippled its work. Many of its delvers have fallen just over the thin crust of its treasures, and have died without a chance of revealing the splendour of their discoveries,—with half-finished sentences on their lips. But thus it is with all that is mundane: the show is fleeting, and the actors but mortal.

To speak in a humbler strain, this, our Association, has not completed the fulness of its work, nor attained the summit of its hopes. Although its endeavours have been honest, the fruition of its ambition cannot, and probably never will, be enjoyed; but what, has been asked, is the object of its being? Why, in the midst of other and various organisations of similar aims, should this, the latest born, add its infant wail to the family cry? We, its members, answer, The world has room enough even for *its* growth. The excuse for our being is rooted in humility, in kindred ambition, and good fellowship; we love to work together as mates in a shop, to join in the emulation of attainment, to criticise each other's ideals, to sit in judgment and compare results; to indulge in friendly tilts and laugh at each other's hobbies, to enjoy our grand delusions, and to put our own little comedy upon the stage none too soon after the downward plunge of the orchestral bow.

All of which our friends expect us to do without collusion, and without a betrayal of that vanity which lies at the root of most human actions. But what is to be our compensation? Simply that our motives be unsuspected, our schemes undetected, and that we be allowed to pose as the greatest of reformers, with a wisdom larger than that of our competitors. This may seem to be raillery, but please accept it as a recital of our creed, and take away with yourselves, without a confession each to his neighbour, that every member secretly esteems himself as the superior of his "Fellow."

But in sober earnest, with the trust that our egotism may masquerade as enthusiasm, let us proceed to our accounting. First of all, we are ten years old, and have earned the boys' privilege of staying up a little later of nights and interjecting remarks at the family table. Let us hope, however, that our exuberance may not pass the limits of decorum, and that as we are too young to be very wicked, we are also not old enough to forecast uncanny dooms.

We claim not to class everything that savours of the past as effete, nor to plume ourselves on being nihilists in destroying without substituting; nor have we ever proposed to pur-

4

sue the narrow methods of any special division of scientific labour, but rather to apply what powers of ratiocination we may have to the elucidation of such problems as may involve the broader questions of the hour. We are aware that we are still in the process of evolution, that there are many startling discoveries far in the van, that as members of the profession nearest of kin to man, we are interpreters of phenomena as yet within range of a vision subject to many errors of refraction. Nevertheless, we can lay claim to the privilege of working with ardour, in a spirit of honesty, to the right of questioning before accepting, and above all, to that blessing of an advanced civilisation, the undisturbed enjoyment of a defensible opinion.

As an Association whose aim is to advance science, we may live as peaceably in the most despotic of countries as in "Freest America," save only that those not in harmony with our pursuits might look askance and tap their foreheads as they pass us by. But after all, this last is a harmless ceremonial, much in vogue although unconfessed. May we not take to our bosoms the consoling compensation that our lofty critics, not we, are the Pharisees whose nudity requires the covering of broad phylacteries? No doubt, as our years roll on, we shall plume ourselves upon the possession of a tolerant spirit, and ransack biographies for luminous comparisons, in order to satisfy ourselves that we occupy a plane of no despicable altitude. And so with us, after our complaisant toil, at the end of days, few or many, let us hope that there shall come, with the wisdom of Solomon, the rollicking merriment of Democritus, as we ejaculate, "Vanity of vanities! All is vanity!"

Of course we have published Transactions, of which reviewers, so far as has come to our knowledge, have said nothing ; but, nevertheless, their "get-up" is superb, their papers bristling with good sense, unimpeachable grammar, and uncontrovertible logic, carrying conviction in their every line ! In fact, we are ready to say more of them than our worst enemies desire, and so we think, with much more propriety, that they are in reality substantial contributions,—not too hide-bound in their conservatism, nor too iconoclastic in their aggressiveness, and that as a rule they have been philosophical as well as judicial. After all these smirks of self-laudation, who knows but that time may mellow their crudities, and cause them to blossom out from many unsuspected germs! Who knows but that some "Looking Backward" savant may prove that all these mysteries were solved by the Ancients! Who knows what name may then become phosphorescent!

Conceding, therefore, the possession in fee simple of just a modicum of vain-glory, as the prerogative of our callow years, let us enjoy together our retrospect, with a subdued sorrow for those workers, who, as well graced actors, have left the scene.

This, our proposed retrospect, with its many short-comings of effort, has much to encourage us in the way of future endeavour, even with the sacrifice of those more compensating pursuits to which the world yields up honour, glory, and position. Let us say we are merely physicians, some of us surgeons—"only this, nothing more." As with all knowledge, there are many sides to be viewed, many modes of presentation, and many plans of divided topics, so, especially in this, our present review, is there much embarrassment of riches, destined in this necessarily abbreviated evening session to tantalise with merely a running commentary.

Omitting to mention some of the contributions, suggestive as they are and in the best vein of their several authors, we are compelled with the remainder to summarise, to clumsily condense, and perchance to nonchalantly dismiss. But in the bewilderment of the hastily accepted responsibility of a task beyond his ability, is there to be no extenuation of the folly, and no pity for your culprit, who hoped to escape in a mad rush for liberty? From all of which you may readily infer, my good friends, that this self-same culprit, now your burnt-offering, would have much preferred to have been auditor or critic, one or both.

DISCUSSIONS AND ADDRESSES.

A marked feature of the work of this Association has been the prepared discussions, first adopted by the British Medical Association, and styled by them "Collective Investigation." This plan of presenting topics in a series of questions intended to bring out the salient points of interest, has encouraged future continuance, in fact has been copied by some of the most conservative societies of the land. They have been prepared with much economy of verbiage, and will it be too much to say that some of them are models of idiomatic, vigourous English? Should there arise, however, a creeping suspicion that your essayist is somewhat extravagant in his laudations, there is yet left for the "Committee with Power" the right of a personal canvass of opinion among the authors themselves. Their unprejudiced verdict certainly none will have the temerity to gainsay.

Omitting by prearrangement the discussion of the surgical subjects, as being beyond the writer's scope of duty, the "Discussion on Pneumonia" challenges our notice, as the introduction to the series. The idea of the chosen subject emanated from the late Dr. Flint, who presented it in his masterful manner, without a wasted word. The different divisions of the subject were debated by Drs. H. D. Didama, F. W. Ross, E. G. Janeway, W. H. Robb, H. M. Biggs, Thos. F. Rochester, Ely Van de Warker, S. T. Clark, C. S. Wood, John Shrady, E. D. Ferguson, G. Griswold, C. G. Stockton, W. J. Fuller, and J. G. Orton. The last mentioned gentleman alluded to Dr. Flint in the following words: "I can but compliment our distinguished co-worker for the pleasure afforded in thus directing to so delightful a field of investigation. For myself, I owe him much, and I know that in saying this I but voice the sentiments of every member of this body of physicians. In my researches I have been edified, and I am conscious also of a gain in the precision of my own knowledge; and this reward I trust my brethren have likewise shared."

Dr. Gouley's "Address on Human Nosography" opened up a subject to which the writer has given his enthusiastic attention, and which he amplified into a volume. The many forms of nomenclature introduced, the erudition displayed, and the quaint philological references, made of the matter the most readable of discourses. This effort of our colleague originated in the succeeding year the "Discussion on Nosography," in which were engaged Drs. A. L. Carroll, N. L. Britton, S. T. Clark, E. G. Janeway, E. D. Ferguson, Elwyn Waller, and Nelson B. Sizer.

After these items there comes in natural sequence the "Address on Pathology," by Dr. E. G. Janeway, of New York county. The author summarises the advances in this department by newer modes of investigation, by which "the different diseases are rendering up the secret of their ultimate existence." This paper abounds in condensed statement and well put suggestions, cautions against hasty conclusions, and advises still further investigations before the numerous moot questions are decided.

"Address on Some of the Relations of Physiology to the Practice of Medicine," by Dr. Austin. Flint, of New York county. Like the well known Fothergill of London, our distinguished colleague lays much stress upon physiological research, as constituting the keystone of the medical arch. He analyzes the heat-producing factors of the human body, gives heat-unit scales as ascertained by observations of his own personal phenomena, and "in the grand evolution of science, with its new methods of investigation," he forecasts the future in these memorable words, "that the so called physiological ferments, such as the active principles of the digestive fluids, may not be found to contain minute organisms, upon the multiplication of which the peculiar properties of those substances are dependent."

Dr. John Cronyn, of Erie county, also delivered many addresses, the general tenor of which was the higher education, the utilisation of the mosaic knowledge growing out of the course thus adopted, and the pursuit of an ideal which shall bring a sense of an awful responsibility. Dr. H. D. Didama, likewise, in many short contributions, taught the same ethics in a vein most happily satirical and instructive. Dr. Simeon T. Clark, also, should not be ignored in his address on "Medical Jurisprudence," for his hints upon the functions of the medical expert; nor should Dr. M. Cavana, of Madison county, in his voluntary paper on "The Physician as a Witness" be overlooked, since he spurred up a spirited discussion, the drift of which was that in certain doubtful suits for damages a medical examination should be permitted.

All of these enrichments of the Transactions may have been the out-growth of Dr. Ely Van de Warker's paper on "The Medico-Legal Bearing of Pelvic Injuries in Women," wherein the jury decisions in certain of the cases were undoubtedly based upon the testimony of incompetent pretenders, who legally have, what cannot be prevented, "a standing in court."

. Among the other addresses delivered were "Some Classical Allusions to Medicine and Surgery," by Judge Charles G. Truax, which was a happy blending of humor, raillery, and genial philosophy; also that of Rev. Dr. W. C. Bitting on "Biblical Medicine," delivered on a similar evening occasion, and welcomed as an addition to the value of the Transactions, so far as research, erudition, and text references were concerned.

The "Discussion on Typhoid Fever," by Drs. A. L. Carroll, E. G. Janeway, H. M. Biggs, D. E. Salmon, C. A. Leale, E. D. Ferguson, and E. G. Stockton, displayed to advantage the accomplishments of the various participants. The questions of aetiology, simulation, transmission, and sanitation were so thoroughly exhausted that no thesis on the subject could well be prepared without at least a reference to this discussion.

"Discussion on Pulmonary Tuberculosis," introductory remarks by Dr. H. D. Didama, in which the entire field was gone over, *e. g.*, the questions of heredity, bacillary origin, climate, occupations, habits, therapeutic measures, prophylaxis, etc. All these questions were methodically and more or less exhaustively discussed by Drs. J. Cronyn, H. M. Biggs, H. L. Elsner, W. H. Flint, and J. Shrady. The impossibility of proper summarisation precludes even elliptical quotations.

The discussion just mentioned was suggested by Dr. H. D. Didama's paper of a previous year, entitled "Tubercular Consumption, Is It Ever Inherited?" Our colleague argued in the negative, placing the responsibilities upon surroundings, claiming that " two conditions are almost indispensable : abundance of bacilli, with an inviting asylum furnished by an inherited or acquired cellular vincibility." This paper was somewhat hotly debated in an extemporaneous manner.

The discussion on the "New Hypnotics" by Drs. Wm. H. Flint, C. G. Stockton, J. G. Truax, Chas. Rice, E. R. Squibb, and A. L. Carroll, exhausted the literature of the subject to date.

BACTERIOLOGY.

Bacteriology, as one of the newer departments of medicine, also received its share of attention, and was discussed under cover of many of the papers upon various subjects. Dr. F. S. Dennis, of New York county, in the second volume of the Transactions, discussed it in its relations to surgery, along with many wood-cuts. This Dr. N. B. Sizer, of Kings county, ably supplemented with another on " The Rôle of Microbes in Disease," both of which are undisappointing authorities on the present status of our knowledge. Among the Fellows of the Association there is not altogether a perfect accord as regards the significance of the appearing microbe, some holding the view that peculiar forms give rise to peculiar manifestations, while others maintain that they are tests of susceptibility, and are results rather than factors.

Aside from these divergent views, as a semi-sceptical protest, Dr. E. F. Brush, of Westchester county, in his plea against hasty decisions, bearing the title of "The Mimicry of Animal Tuberculosis in Vegetable Forms," maintains that "there is more to be known of human tuberculosis than merely that a germ is present in a mass of morbid material."

"A Case of Poisoning by Two Grains of Strychnia, Treatment by Chloral Hydrate and Coffee," by Dr. William Fitch, of Tompkins county.   Here one hundred and forty grains of chloral hydrate, administered within four hours, produced the most gratifying results.   As regards the dose in this venenous antagonism, there seems to be thus far, according to cited cases, no limitation.   " Chronic Mercurial Poisoning," by Dr. Charles Buckley, of Monroe county, traceable to hard red rubber dental plates, being those in which a preparation of mercury is used for the colouring.   "A Case of Lead Poisoning," by Dr. R. H. Sabin, of Albany county, where, in the absence of an autopsy, coma was accounted for by a rapid effusion on the brain and final affecting of the circulatory centres, as demonstrated by the pulse-beats.

"Alcoholism as a Vice, and as a Result of Inherited or Acquired Brain Diseases," by Dr. Isaac de Zouche, of Fulton county; "Some Personal Observations and Reflections upon Alcoholism, the Effects of Alcoholic Abuse upon Posterity, and the Treatment of Alcoholism," by Dr. H. E. Schmid, of Westchester county, and "Alcoholic Paralysis," by Dr. T. D. Crothers, of Hartford county, as inferred from the titles, fully reflect the views of their authors.   Dr. Crothers, in particular, claims that the ordinary inebriate exhibits the entire line of dissolution, from the quickened brain circulation to the organic paralysis that ends in death.   The alcoholic paralytic shows the same dissolution, only it moves slowly along an organised path and in reverse order to the brain and nerve developments.

PATHOLOGY, MATERIA MEDICA, AND THERAPEUTICS.

The contributions in the department of Therapeutics and Materia Medica have been particularly valuable and suggestive. The subjects have ranged from the expectant method to the opposite verge of over-weening confidence. " Modern Progress in Materia Medica and Therapeutics," "Brief Comments on the Materia Medica," and many other contributions under various titles, have been made by Drs. E. R. and E. H. Squibb, of Kings county, and are still continued, more or less in the shape of reports.

"Recovery versus Cure," by Dr. A. L. Carroll, of Richmond county. The accomplished ex-editor of the Transactions deplores the inroads made on the department by the much advertised virtues of glazed parvules, attractive elixirs, and the hasty endorsements of empirical formulas by reputable physicians.

" Medical and Non-Medical Therapeutics," by the late Dr. Austin Flint, of New York county; "The Proper Attitude of Therapeutics," by Dr. Chas. G. Stockton, of Erie county. Both of these authors conclude that the sphere of therapeutics lies in accepting the laws of the physiologist, when these do not violate the inexplicable results of observation. " The square, the compass, and the theodolite have no place in therapeutics."

"Commercial Prescriptions," by Dr. H. C. Van Zandt, of Schenectady county, treats of the effects upon the physician, the patient, and the community by the use of the ready-made medicine, since the physician becomes careless, inaccurate, and unreliable; the patient, deprived of his right of due consideration, is tempted to ascribe the glory, if there be any, to the manufacturer, and, in the case of the community, self-prescribing of the most indiscriminate character is encouraged.

"Prophylaxis," by Dr. Isaac de Zouche, of Fulton county, discourses upon inherited diatheses as unavoidable influences, showing the value of preventive measures in contagious diseases. Drs. Smith, Baker, Kneeland, and Thornton enhanced the value of this paper by many corroborations. " Nutrition in Lithaemia," by Dr. Charles G. Stockton, of Erie county, enters largely upon the discussion of physiological problems, and gives many valuable dietetic hints. "Common-Sense versus Hypothetical Medication," by Dr. Jonathan S. Kneeland, of Onondaga county, advocates good air, good food, etc., and not placebos or high-sounding nostrums, pushed by commercial travellers.

"The Dietetic Treatment of Dyspepsia," by the late Dr. Austin Flint, of New York county. The writer dwells upon the fallacies of so called dietetic idiosyncrasies and inflexible rules in the choice of food. He especially deprecates "watchful study," "personal experience," "theoretical notions," and "scientific principles."

"Some Observations on the Use of Mineral Waters of Saratoga," by Dr. R. C. McEwen, of Saratoga county. Dr. McEwen claims that our mineral waters are in their infancy of use, and are passing through various phases of ignorant eulogy and reckless experiment. He claims that the waters of Saratoga are possessed of marked medicinal properties, but that restriction is needed in the imbibing and hap-hazard mingling of the same, particularly without judicious advice. "False Albuminuria," by Dr. Gasper Griswold, of New York county. The determination of small quantities of albumen is arrived at by the "cold nitric acid test," otherwise known as Heller's. A drachm of pure nitric acid poured into a test tube of small calibre, and a drachm of the suspected urine allowed to trickle drop by drop upon the acid, constitute the test, and a sharp white band at point of contact the verification. "The Origin and Medical Treatment of Uric Acid Calculi of the Kidney," by Dr. W. D. Garlock, of Herkimer county. This author very justly maintains that treatment should not be conducted on the basis of the laboratory, but that the system should be led into those habits which may induce it to do its work smoothly, to the end that it may easily free itself of its effete material.

"Hiccough, with Notes on Treatment," by Dr. F. W. Putnam, of Broome county, deals in the main with the hysterical form, for the relief of which many modes and medicaments have been proposed. The author, out of the confusion, selects no panacea, but practically recommends a search for the cause. "Recent Experience in the Treatment of Exophthalmic Goitre," by Dr. E. D. Ferguson, of Rensselaer county. This paper may be best summarised by the reviewing remarks of Drs. Cronyn and Carroll. The former believed that digitalis was indicated only in a weak, irritable heart with a valvular lesion. He had, in common with Dr. Ferguson, tried strophanthus in the condition set forth by his paper, with good results; he also remembered the remark of a French academician who pinned his faith on strophanthin as the reliable salt, although his colleagues were divided as regards the value of the strophanthus itself. Dr. Carroll, and the latter gentleman believed that much that was sold for strophanthus was inert. He remembered that after having obtained a freshly imported tincture from a reliable apothecary he found the sphygmographic tracing changed from a wavy line to a nearly normal pulse-trace.

"Medicinal and Dietetic Therapeutics of the Common Forms of Chronic Intestinal Catarrh," by Dr. John S. Jamison, of Steuben county. Discussed by Drs. J. P. Garrish, C. G. Pomeroy, Darwin Colvin, Wm. Gillis, and Isaac G. Collins. "Acute Pleurisy," by Dr. Frank S. Parsons, of Northampton, Mass., dwelt at length upon diagnostic points, advocated thoracentesis with aseptic precautions, etc. Subsequently, Drs. F. W. Higgins, H. D. Didama, and John Cronyn gave their views upon aspiration, venesection, and other remedial measures, including electricity as a promoter of absorption.

"Cold as a Therapeutic Agent," by Dr. B. L. Hovey, of Monroe county. Cases of prostration from heat were cited in which the cold bath acted as a restorative. Dr. Hovey concluded in effect that the rule should be to reduce temperature down to the normal as nearly as possible, thereby preventing waste of tissue and impairment of the vital forces. He attributed the cause of fever to some septic agent which renders the vasomotor nervous system unable to control the heat-regulating forces. Dr. J. Cronyn, in his remarks, noted the distinction between sun-stroke and heat-stroke, and the difference in their therapeutical management. "Methods of Applying Cold," by Dr. H. D. Didama, of Onondaga county. In this paper, Dr. Didama described a plan of his own, by an arrangement of wet sheets, comfortable, agreeable, and efficient.

"Is Erysipelas Ever a Strictly Local Disease? If not, What Should Be Its Rational Treatment?" by Dr. Fred Hyde, of Cortland county. In the discussion upon this valuable paper, Dr. Gouley regarded ordinary erysipelas as an acute lymphangitis, and its graver form as a super-acute lymphangitis. He advocated chloride of iron in large, often repeated doses, and not much reliance on local applications. Drs. Ferguson, Cronyn, and E. M. Moore followed with remarks regarding local applications. Dr. Moore, in view of the alkaline reaction of erysipelas, had been led to use with effect a mild dilution of vinegar. "Membranous Croup, Diphtheritic Croup, True Croup," by Dr. J. Lewis Smith, of New York county. What better terms can characterise this paper than an exhaustive treatise, full of practical wisdom, and a model of direct statement? The subject is so well presented that extracts would only mar its coherence. Let the test be individual examination. "Diphtheritic Paralysis," by the same writer, said that no clear and unmistakable reference had been made to this sequence of diphtheria until near the close of the sixteenth century. He discoursed upon its clinical history, its time of commencement, and its different forms, such as loss of the tendon reflexes, palatal paralysis, multiple paralysis, cardiac paralysis, and rather favoured the view that this kind of paralysis was not due to central lesion. "Diphtheria," by Dr. E. F. Marsh, of Oswego county, is an encyclopedic article, valuable for its medico-historical references, its bibliography, epidemiology, aetiology, pathology, and treatment. Dr. Cronyn, in the course of a discussion upon this subject on another occasion, declared his belief that diphtheria was always a constitutional disease, and endorsed the monograph of Oertel as the best commentary so far printed.

Dr. J. M. Moore, of Albany county, furnishes in "The Therapeutics of Diphtheria" a masterly brochure. Dr. H. O. Jewett, of Cortland county, in the "Use and Neglect of Blood-Letting," indulges in a historical and controversial vein, while Dr. G. E. Fell, of Erie county, in several contributions on "Forced Respiration," with varying sub-titles, proves the superiority of forced over artificial respiration. This author, at different sessions, demonstrated the advantages of his method and appliances. "Specialists," by Dr. H. C. Van Zandt, of Schenectady county, brightens up the pages of the fourth volume with an arraignment of unsuccessful practitioners who have been lured into some special branch.

"Ergot: Its Uses and Misuses." Dr. J. K. Leaning, of Otsego county, has faith in the efficacy of ergot in atony of the bladder, uncomplicated with prostatic enlargement or urethral stricture; also in some forms of leucorrhoea, in haemoptysis, and in the mitigation of profuse expectoration. He thinks that under certain conditions ergot may prove to be an anti-abortifacient, and that in post-partum haemor_rhage it is an essential drug. In Dr. Leaning's opinion the foetal head receives too much pressure when large continuous doses are given. "Bichloride of Mercury: Its Uses and Abuses," by Dr. Chas. S. Wood, of New York county. The writer, in inveighing against its indiscriminate use, claimed that "the expectation of arresting any disease of an acute infectious character, produced or increased by any of the micro-organisms, must, from the very nature of the case, prove fallacious." "Chlorate of Potash: Its Abuses," by Dr. H. O. Jewett, of Cortland county. In this paper the toxical effects upon the mucous surfaces are pointed out, and the popular use of the chemical is especially tabooed. "The Therapy of the Chlorides: Antisepsis a Prominent and Important Factor in Their Medicinal Action," by Dr. Nelson L. North, of Kings county. After reference to the matter of chlorides, the author concluded that "treatment is not so much an effort to sustain the patient till the crisis is past, as it is an effort to destroy the *materies morbi.*"

SURGERY.

Your reporter may encroach upon surgical grounds in mention of the following:

"The Use of the Aspirator in Hydrothorax," by Dr. E. D. Ferguson, of Rensselaer county. The claim made is that pyo-thorax may be produced by the aspirator itself, and a rule is proposed not to remove more than a pint of fluid at one aspiration, either to relieve dyspnoea or to induce absorption. Otherwise the friable walls of the recently formed blood-vessels beneath the fibrinous material may give way, particularly if by continuous withdrawal of the fluid the pressure be relieved. "Pneumotomy for Relief of Tubercular Abscess and Gangrene of the Lung Twice on the Same Patient," by Dr. J. Blake White, of New York county. Drs. Truax and Ferguson expressed their thanks for the contribution, and supplemented the writer's experience with their own. They endorsed the views expressed of the feasibility and success of the procedure, especially with the strict antiseptic precautions in vogue.

"Report of a Case of Biliary Calculi, Diffused Hepatitis, and Hydrothorax," by Dr. Chas. S. Allen, of Rensselaer county. A unique case, illustrating a remarkable tolerance of diseased conditions during life. "Fatty Stools Due to Organic Disease of the Pancreas," by the same writer. Dr. Allen in his rare case was unable to obtain an autopsy, but suspected carcinoma, or some organic disease of the pancreas. "Intestinal Obstructions, with Reports of Cases," by Dr. B. L. Hovey, of Monroe county, who gives a résumé of the causes, and relates several cases which ended in recovery.

"Removal of an Enterolith: Presentation of the Specimen," by Dr. W. B. Sabin, of Albany county. The description is of a mass weighing four and a half ounces, of which more than · half an ounce has been lost by crumbling. The analysis gave phosphate of lime as the main constituent. "A Case of Intra-Rectal Larvae with Gastritis in an Infant," by Dr. C. S. Allen, of Rensselaer county. The doctor concludes that these larvae, which the microscope declared to be those of the blow-fly, developed from eggs that may have been deposited on the nipple of the nursing-bottle, or perhaps on the surface of the milk, and that they must have passed along with the food into the alimentary canal. Dr. R. H. Sabin, of Albany county, after his paper on "Gall Stones," presented a certain quantity of sand-like elements found in some alvine dejections, which on microscopic examination proved to be seeds, subsequently discovered to be those of the raspberry.

"Ataxic Paraplegia," Dr. Darwin Colvin, of Wayne county, maintains, is not to be confounded with locomotor ataxia, for in ataxic paraplegia the lateral columns are alone involved. Squibb's solution of the arsenite of potash in gradually increasing doses, beginning with five-drop doses, until symptoms of saturation show the limit of toleration, is recommended as a remedy, rather than Charcot's method of extension by suspension for the relief of sclerosis of the posterior columns, which is the pathology of locomotor ataxia. "A Case of Acute Mania Following Articular Rheumatism," by Dr. J. C. Hannan, of Rensselaer county. The learned doctor, even after an autopsy which precluded the existence of meningitis, could not classify the nervous phenomena, for his patient, being an exemplary youth, could not be suspected of any depraved habit or perturbed emotion as an excitant of the mania, nor, again, was the writer prepared to subscribe to the doctrine of metastasis. The negative conditions piqued him with vague guesses only.

"Report of Two Cases of Morphia and Cocaine Habit," by Dr. Judson B. Andrews, of Erie county. After a brief allusion to the still insufficient knowledge regarding the toxic effects of cocaine, especially when associated with morphine, the author embodied the written experience of an ex-patient, whose sensations were vividly described. Hyperaemia of the brain, gradually merging into incurable insanity, seems to be the penalty of the misuse of these drugs, especially when combined one with the other.

"Chronic Catarrhal Gastritis, Fatal from Complication of

Sudden Enlargement of Thyroid Body," by Dr. Wm. H. Thayer, of Kings county. The bronchocele in this case was responsible for the death by pressure on the larynx of a suddenly enlarged thyroid, recovery independently of the exciting condition being quite possible. "A Case of Cancer of the Kidney," by Dr. John Shrady, of New York county, in a three-year-old child, in whom the diagnostic points were contrasted in a differential way. Roberts' explanation of the absence of haematuria, explicable either by the pressure of the tumor or the extension of the disease into it, was accepted in the present instance. "A Peculiar Foreign Body in the Stomach, Concretions of Hair, Thread," etc., by Dr. W. Finder, of Rensselaer county. An interesting paper, giving the literature of the subject admirably collated; the conclusion of the author was that early surgery is preferable to expectant methods.

Still further additions to our literature may be mentioned in passing, such as "Intestinal Obstruction," by Dr. Avery Segur, of Kings county, in which the writer somewhat vigourously opposes the exhibition of cathartics, and instead enjoins rest in the horizontal position, with *per orem nihil*, morphia and atropia hypodermatically and nutrient enemata. Among the advantages of the enemata he claims the suppression of vomiting and increased flow of urine. "On the Duration of Contagiousness after Acute Infectious Diseases," by Dr. A. L. Carroll, of New York county. Dr. Carroll, as known to all, has done yeoman service as editor, contributor, and debater.

Another gift to the common stock is a paper by Dr. G. E Fell, of Erie county, entitled "The Death Penalty: Does the Garrote or Hanging Ever Produce Instantaneous Unconsciousness?" The author states that, in his opinion, the probable law is that a paralysed brain and an instant heart-stoppage give us the only assurance that death occurs without an intervening period of consciousness. The heart acting along with the continuing function of the cerebrum, consciousness may exist for a time, even when hanging or garroting has been successfully performed.

MEDICO-HISTORICAL MATTERS.

" Medical New York in 1800," by Dr. John Shrady, of New York county. This is a medico-historical sketch of the opening of the present century, designed to show the many rapid advances of the polyglot city. It contains also many sketches of old-time physicians, their habits, opinions, and modes of practice.

"A Short Review of the Fever Epidemic in Kingston, Ulster County, During the Winter of 1884–'85," by Dr. H. Van Hoevenberg, of Ulster county. The cause of this epidemic, according to the doctor's opinion, was the stirring up of a large quantity of decomposed and decomposing material in the cleaning of cesspools, water-closets, etc., at the behest of a new and zealous health board.

"Winter Cholera in Poughkeepsie," by Dr. J. G. Porteous, of Dutchess county. The writer ascribes the cause to the river water, despite the absence of proof and the negative results of analysis. He thinks that the danger must increase with the increase of sewage incident to a larger population, and further, that the Hudson river towns must find some other supply than the river water.

The papers on the "Kingston Epidemic" and the "Winter Cholera in Poughkeepsie" may be read with profit along with the one on the "Bacteriological Test of Drinking-Water," by Dr. E. K. Dunham, of New York county. The direct verdict of the sanitary value of water depends, according to the writer, on the relations between the water and the natural, uniform distribution of the various species of bacteria. The significance of these relations must be determined by our knowledge of the causation of disease.

" A Case of Anaesthesia by Nitrous Oxide, Supposed to be the First on Record," by Dr. G. P. Hubbard, of New York county, gives the details of a case, with corroborations, as called for by the title of his paper, which fixes the date of the incident November 5, 1821. The subject was a young man who had stealthily taken his fill of the gas by turning on the

5

stop-cock of the gasometer in a room adjoining the one in which the exhibition was given.

"Small-pox in Brooklyn; Defective Isolation and Defective Vaccination," by Dr. N. L. North, of Kings county. The writer pointed out many lapses on the part of the laity; particularly did he denounce the tendency on their part to conceal cases, and the "business lies " told by some vaccine purveyors as regards the freshness of their virus.

"A Cursory Review of the Epidemic and Endemic Diseases of Sullivan County during the Last Thirty-Four Years," by Dr. Isaac Purdy, of Sullivan county. The author, now deceased, gave a reflex view of old-style treatment when the sthenic idea of disease prevailed, during the autumn of 1861, after diphtheria travelled from Philadelphia in 1859–'60 to Mongaup valley. He stated that a single home would furnish as many as six patients at a time. During the winter of 1861–'62 the epidemic again prevailed in a virulent form on the high grounds, and the winter succeeding gave place to a petechial fever, which yielded to milder and more supporting measures. A spirited debate, chiefly of a reminiscent and comparative character, arose out of this paper.

"Medicine and Pharmacy Abroad," by Dr. Edward R. Squibb, of Kings county. Our esteemed Fellow awards to Denmark and Sweden the palm of best conserving the interests of these kindred vocations. As regards his observations of the proportionate number of physicians' offices in the large European cities, Boston, New York, Philadelphia, and Baltimore are far in the van. Our European confrères also make less display, visit by public conveyance or on foot, and in spite of their modest bearing have more influence with the masses. As regards pharmacy, our writer tersely concludes that "here there is probably better pharmacy and more of it than there, but here there is an enormous amount of bad pharmacy to contrast with a very little there."

CASES OF INTEREST.

A certain degree of attention was likewise given to cases from "the rich stores of experience." These were voluntary in character, and in the main excited discussions, which sometimes were desultory although instructive, and at other times reflected the individual views of the debaters. The general tenor of these challenges to investigation may be inferred from the somewhat incongruous grouping to follow. Here may be detected therapeutic hints and side-lights on obscure diagnosis, divergent procedures, etc. "Some Aetiological Factors in the Acne-Form of Diseases," by Dr. Geo. E. Fell, of Erie county. A paper imparting information of much interest regarding the *Demodex folliculorum*, a mite infesting the sebaceous glands, usually harmless but in large colonies capable of producing pathological changes of no mean intensity. The experimenter gives a happy experience with an ointment of sulphur and the hydrargyrum oleatum. "Paraplegia," by Dr. C. W. Brown, of Washington, D. C. This was a case with remarks upon difficulties of diagnosis, as to whether or not the paraplegia was due to exposure, a gonorrhoea, or to a mild myelitis. Dr. H. S. Williams, of New York county, remarked that myelitis was often not so pronounced as supposed, and referred to a case of his own which ended fatally within a week, and where the lumbar cord was chiefly affected, as shown by the microscope, and yet there was no sign of paraplegia. "A Case of Supposed Partial Twist of the Intestine," by Dr. G. E. McDonald, of Schenectady county. This, fortunately, passed from a surgical problem to a medical enigma, and having ended in a sudden recovery, left only the differential diagnosis to be discussed, which was ably done by several members. "A Remarkable Case of Obscure Toxaemia," by Dr. J. C. Hannan, of Rensselaer county. Dr. Hannan submitted his well described case to the Association, when Dr. E. M. Moore discussed it from the standpoint of malaria. Dr. J. Cronyn gave his personal experience in diphtheria, which originated some curious facts of coördination. Dr. E. H. Hamill believed that malaria simply brought the periodic tendencies of animal life into prominence, and that it was not the cause of periodicity. Drs. S. T. Clark, Caleb Green, H. D. Didama, and the author of the paper continued the discussion, with views more or less divergent. " Report of a Case Sudden in Attack, History Uncommon, Symptoms Severe and Alarming, with Doubtful Diagnosis," by Dr. B. L. Hovey, of Monroe county, sphinx-like, utters without expectation of response. He · merely gave reasons for the doubts within him.

"Abscess of the Liver." In this contribution Dr. Janeway, in his lucid style, gave the history of several cases, with comments upon the difficulties of diagnosis. Among his many valuable conclusions, the following, as regards treatment, appear important: "All accessible abscesses due to adherent liver are best dealt with by free incision, washing out with an antiseptic liquid, the introduction of a drainage tube, and antiseptic dressing." "An early and safe exit for the pus " is another of the doctor's golden maxims.

MISCELLANEOUS TOPICS.

Some of the minor topics considered were " Dermic and Hypodermic Therapeutics," by Dr. S. F. Rogers, of Rensselaer county ; " The Microscope in Diagnosis," by Dr. G. E. Fell, of Erie county ; " The Functions of the Auricles," by Dr. U. A. Lynde, of Erie county ; " Psoitis and Peri-Psoitis," by Dr. S. T. Clark, of Niagara county ; " The Relations of Physicians to their Medical Supplies," by Dr. E. R. Squibb, of Kings county, who says, " Perfunctory routine in the observation of cases soon leads to a routine practice of treatment." " The art and skill of the physicians," said Dr. Squibb, " will be worth still less than they receive for them if they allow the control of the quality of the supplies, as an essential element of their success, to slip away from them. This is their reasonable demand, and as such, should be met." " Chronic Intestinal Catarrh," by Dr. John S. Jamison, of Steuben county. " Seaside Hospitals for Sick Children," by

Dr. C. A. Leale, of New York county, illustrates the practical side of Dr. Leale's character, showing the benefits to be derived from a charity managed on the basis of business and economy. Dr. Leale, in "An Easy Method of Feeding Patients After Tracheotomy," resorts to a well oiled No. 8, velvet-eyed, soft rubber catheter (American), passed through the nostril directly backward into the stomach. A two-ounce solid syringe, worked by one hand and attached to the free end of the catheter, is made to conduct in all eight ounces for each meal. Water and medicines may be administered in the same way. This the writer claims to be superior to the ordinary oesophageal tube introduced by way of the mouth.

Dr. E. J. Chapin Minard, of Kings county, settled the question in the affirmative, " Does the Menstrual Flow Originate in the Tube ?—Act of Menstruation Viewed from an Inverted Uterus." Dr. C. G. Stockton, of Erie county, in his "Aetiology of Gastric Ulcer," intimates that some distinct and persistent nerve perturbation may constitute a cause. -

"Suggestions Relating to Improvement of Quarantine," by Dr. Stephen Smith, of New York county, is not disappointing in its title. Dr. G. R. Martine, of Warren county, in "A New Plan of Treatment for Pneumonia," embodies a claim that death does not result from high temperature, but from high arterial action and consequent heart failure. His method is to hold the pulse at eighty, his means veratrum viride.

Dr. W. H. Robb demonstrated an office battery, a contrivance of his own,—portable, reliable, and occupying the minimum of space. Dr. Joseph C. Greene, of Erie county, read a paper on " Leprosy," and exhibited a map showing its course of travel and most pronounced habitats.

Thus, Mr. President, Fellows, and Friends, has your reporter, reviewer, or critic—call him what you may—given you but an imperfect résumé to date of the proceedings of your body, in all honesty avoiding excuses and apologies. Thus has he endeavoured to descant on your work without extravagant eulogy, to do justice to every collaborator, and to omit no deed or contribution of earnest effort.

He is sensible of having fallen short of his intentions, as he can never know all the struggles for the common good, nor appreciate the perseverance of the many who, amid the exigencies of their professional lives, are forced to rebuild the temple with the trowel in one hand and the sword in the other.

He is well aware that theories may have been broached which have been merely half-truths or cloud-forms of medicine's future, but, in common with yourselves, he has his convictions that they were better uttered than suppressed. At all events, as your spokesman, he consoles himself with the assurance that the voice of this Association has been heard only when work for improvement was to be done, or courage for patient research was required.

Let us hope, therefore, that if our toil has been unfruitful, our motives may not be impugned. Still more was it your writer's wish, amid the whirl of busy interruptions, to spare a tribute to those who, once our colleagues, have gone to the hush of death. Let us emulate their example and deserve their reward.

PREVENTION OF DISEASE.

By J. G. Porteous, M. D., of Dutchess County.

October 10, 1893.

The often reiterated injunction in regard to the treatment of disease, "remove the cause," naturally brings the suggestion, Why not remove the cause first, and thus prevent the disease ?.

From the earliest times the use of the charm and amulet shows the desire to prevent disease and death, and perhaps the case of Achilles shows how small an oversight may admit them; and, even now, it is often easier to secure the use of an infinitesimal dose of belladonna to prevent scarlet-fever, or the wearing of a camphor-bag charm for any contagious disease, than to secure the use of common sense and intelligent precaution.

How many of you have ever convinced a woman, or, for that matter, a man, that their wearing narrow shoes had anything to do with producing corns, or that they were not more comfortable than broad ones? They may admit that their neighbour suffers from a tight shoe or dress, but not they; and it is the same with almost every community in regard to their water-supply or their filthy streets.

The study of the cause of disease is one of the most fascinating, and naturally precedes the consideration of measures of prevention; but so much has been said and written on the subject, especially since the discoveries of Pasteur, Koch, Shakespeare, and a host of other investigators in bacteriology, and while much more is to be achieved in the same line, I will confine this brief paper to the every-day application, instead of the theory or history of the matter.

It is only by the persistent, constant, and intelligent application of these great truths by the mass of the medical profession, that the greatest good can accrue to mankind.   Very
few deny the immense benefit derived from, and shown by,
the practical stamping out of small-pox, the intelligent control of cholera and typhoid fever, the prevention of that
dreaded group of diseases, septicaemia, hospital gangrene,
and traumatic erysipelas, which formerly followed the knife
of even the most brilliant surgeon, and are now so seldom
heard of—yet it must be admitted that in some ways they
have been indirectly responsible for a certain amount of
harm.   The feeling of immunity from immediate death has
led to many an unnecessary operation, and, I believe, the
needless unsexing of many a poor woman.   The after-results
have not always been so carefully studied.

The discoveries and experiments of Pasteur and Koch have
been drawn on, the shadow of their methods added to the
glamour of mystery, and used to impose on a credulous public such institutions as the " Keeley Cure," the " Silver Ash
Cure," and the "Auric Cure," and given a certain class of
physicians and self-styled philanthropists a chance to cloak
their greed for dollars under the pretence of benefiting suffering humanity.

The celebrated Dr. Hart says of this class of practitioners,—"As to the rule which prohibits the medical man possessing or profiting by any secret remedy, not only is this an
offence against professional morality, but it is a source of
great public danger as well.   From traditional law, and in
virtue of the mission of the physician or priest, both are alike
the. common birthright of humanity, and any man who, for
profit, keeps as a secret a new treatment, or a new doctrine,
is a traitor, not only to his profession, but to all humanity.
Moreover, no respectable physician should advertise : that is
a method of a quack."

And " there is no distinction between the quacks who have
medical degrees and the quacks who have not."   There are,
perhaps, a few men in the profession, even in this country,

who would do well to ponder the words of the great English
editor, when they see their names flaunted in the daily
press, or posted on fences and telegraph poles in connection
with the wonderful cures, or as medical directors of these
quackish institutions, sanitariums, and patent treatments.
But all this makes it more an obligation on the legitimate,
honest profession—of which we are all proud—to carry out to
practical conclusions the discoveries of our great leaders in a
way which shall afford the greatest good to mankind, and in
a way to show the world that we have higher aims and interests than the mere gathering of shekels.

The extensive prevalence of typhoid fever—properly considered a preventable disease—is due more to the indiffer-
ence and parsimony of municipalities and local boards of
health than to a lack of effort among physicians. When a
community, either town or city, will persist in drinking their
own or others' sewage, especially that containing human
excrement, and tolerating filthy streets and premises, they
must expect diarrhoea and this form of fever, and these diseases will not be done away with while dollars and cents are
valued above life and health. To aid in preventing the
spread of diphtheria, scarlet-fever, typhoid fever, and tuberculosis, the milk-supply should be supervised by the state, so
that the dairies, stables, and cows may be regularly inspected
as to the health of the cattle and cleanliness of stables,
utensils, and methods of handling the milk; and this cannot
be properly done by local boards of health. The state in-
spectors now have power to examine and condemn cattle
and milk, and, in certain cases, impose or collect fines; but
it is done so seldom that it loses half its force, and there is
little doubt that disease is at times conveyed through this
important article of food. The amount of filth in milk, as
delivered by farmers to condensed milk factories, is disgust-
ing; but the process of manufacturing, and the admirable
and scrupulous cleanliness in every department of these factories, make it much less dangerous than milk containing
similar filth and not subjected to cleansing and heating. I

have seen men, while milking, deliberately dip their fingers
in the milk, and then continue the milking, practically washing both their hands and the cows' teats in the milk which
some one was expected to drink.

Little can be done by the state to prevent syphilitic diseases in the face of present public opinion and a large portion of the daily press. Many wish this matter ignored, and
raise their hands and voices in holy horror when state control is mentioned, though the same paper may have columns
of advertisements for cures—which do not cure—couched in
the seductive terms of "renewing manly vigor," etc.; but
they bring dollars, while the disease drags along its weary
way, and leaves its trail of ruined men and women and their
tainted offspring.

The prevention the physician can offer is slight, as the
harm is generally done before it comes under his observation,
and his advice for prevention, given without authority, has
little weight.

Perhaps in no single disease is there at present so broad a
field for prevention, and which calls so decidedly for constant care and untiring vigilance among physicians, as tuberculosis, which is credited with destroying the most lives of
any single disease. It is undoubtedly infectious, and, like
cholera, only communicated by the introduction of a specific
germ, the bacillus tuberculosis (discovered by Koch, and the
discovery publicly announced, March 24, 1882), into the system of a healthy person, principally in three ways: First,
through the stomach; second, through the lungs; or third,
through an open wound. I quote from a tract issued by the
Pennsylvania Society for the Prevention of Tuberculosis:

Through the Stomach.—"When people eat imperfectly
cooked tuberculous meat, drink milk from badly diseased
tubercular cows, eat food out of the same dishes or with the
same eating utensils as consumptives, eat food with unwashed
hands after having been in contact with tubercular patients,
eat food that has been handled by persons suffering from
tuberculosis, put coins, articles of toilet, or other small

objects that have been handled by persons suffering from tuberculosis into the mouth, use musical instruments or implements which when in use are placed to the lips or in the mouth, and which have been used by consumptives, kiss upon the lips persons suffering from consumption, swallow tubercular pus in the form of dust, which has accumulated in the throat or fauces during the act of respiration."

Through the Lungs.—" When people inhale dried-up tubercular pus in the form of dust."

Through Wounds.—" When people get tubercular pus into an open cut, or an abrasion of the skin."

There is a chance that the exposing of dressed meat on the sidewalks may be a source of danger, as it could easily be infected by the filthy dust from the street, and possibly by the industrious fly, who divides his time impartially between the gutter and the meat.

Thousands of dollars have been spent, and very properly, in the last two years to prevent cholera in this country, and with most gratifying results; while practically nothing has been done to prevent tuberculosis, which is credited with more than one hundred thousand deaths each year in the United States, and according to Dr. Farr, for every death there are, on an average, three years of sickness.

Dr. De Lancey Rochester, of Buffalo, distributes a very practical paper of instructions to his patients, entitled "Directions to Prevent the Spread of Consumption," and the Pennsylvania Society for the Prevention of Tuberculosis issues a couple of tracts, with quite full directions to the patients and those who come in contact with them.

For some time I have been distributing the following card among my patients :

TO PREVENT CONSUMPTION.

Remember that it is an infectious disease, communicated principally by the matter coughed up and spit out.

THE PATIENT

should spit in a cup or wide-mouthed bottle, containing a little carbolic acid and water, and frequently washed with hot water. Use carbolic acid and water in commode.

Never spit on the street, or floor of house or cars.

Sleep alone, and if possible in an airy and sunny room. Have separate bed and table linen; these should be boiled before washing.

Use individual table utensils, washed separately.

Wash the mouth twice daily with soda and water.

Do not kiss anyone.

THOSE WHO ARE WELL

should remember that it is an infectious disease, communicated principally by swallowing the germs, by inhaling them, or by having them introduced through a wound.

Therefore, do not buy or use food that has been handled by a consumptive.

Do not share the food or drink of a consumptive.

Do not sleep with a consumptive.

Do not put coins or small articles in your mouth that may have been handled by a consumptive.

Do not use clothing until it is thoroughly disinfected if it has been used by a consumptive.

Do not kiss anyone on the lips if they have a cough.

Do not take food without first washing your hands.

It is brief, and more easily kept in view than verbal instructions; it is not as good or full in description or instructions as either of the others, but answers for a beginning, and now that I know of the tracts, I give them in addition, especially where there is a consumptive in the house. The injunction to burn all the sputa of a consumptive is good, but was not put in this card because it was found impossible to have it followed to any extent, especially among the poor, and in the summer when there is not much fire used. In most cases the sputum finds its way to the closet, and into the sewers—where there are sewers,—and probably adds somewhat to the danger in cases where the sewage enters the water-supply; but it is only one more abomination added to the sufficiently dangerous mixture, and should be another reason for not using it.

Dr. A. Gihon, medical director of the United States navy, in his opening address to the section of hygiene in the recent Pan-American Medical Congress, gave a graphic description of his experience on cars and steamer while travelling with consumptives, and the dangers of ordinary travellers from this cause; yet it should be remembered that most of these consumptives, crossing and re-crossing the continent by thousands, are usually doing so by direction of their medical attendants, and generally without the slightest instruction as to protecting their fellow-travellers.

The Society for the Prevention of Tuberculosis says,— "While science does not yet offer a certain cure, it has demonstrated that the disease can be avoided and prevented. It is now believed that tuberculosis can be exterminated among civilised people."

This, however, to be fulfilled, will require a vast amount of constant, faithful, and pecuniarily unrewarded work by the entire brotherhood of the great profession to which we belong.

AN ADDITIONAL NOTE ON NEPHROTOMY AND NEPHRECTOMY.

By E. D. Ferguson, M. D., of Rensselaer County.

October 10, 1893.

Since my report of cases of renal surgery at our last meeting, I have operated four times upon three patients, and the methods pursued and the results obtained have sufficiently differed from my former experience to induce me to report them.

In nine operations of nephrotomy or nephrectomy, no instance has occurred in which I have been able to certainly recognise tuberculosis as a cause, though in only a part of the cases was the evidence distinctly negative, while, on the other hand, pulmonary tuberculosis was present in one case. Renal calculi existed in but one case. The absence of these common causes of renal disease was notable. The origin of the pyelitis in each instance was by the propagation of simple inflammation from the bladder through the ureter to the pelvis or substance of the kidney. The origin of the cystitis was not clear in all of the cases, but in the main was due to urethral disease. In one case it was apparently due to an injudicious, and probably non-aseptic, sounding of the bladder. In this case it was evident that lithuria had been the sole pathological condition present, and that it had existed for some time without producing cystitis, or any turbidity of the urine, until shortly after the instrumentation referred to above. The symptoms of lithuria had recurred from time to time, but had failed of recognition by the physician who introduced the sound.

In my former cases of nephrotomy I had depended, for the purpose of drainage, upon the use of rubber tubes, allowing the wound through the superimposed tissues to close around the tube as rapidly as it would, or even hastening its closure by means of sutures. The trouble and discomfort connected with the use of these tubes, and the probability of injury being done to the renal pelvis by them, and thereby inducing suppurative nephritis where pyelitis alone existed, seemed to obtain in certain of my cases, and led me to adopt the open method. This procedure consists in making a *free* incision through the renal substance, so as to communicate thoroughly with the distended pelvis, and then packing with gauze, simply from time to time reducing the size of this packing so as to allow only a gradual reduction of the wound to a sinus. The effort has been rather to keep the wound free than to hasten its reduction in size. In this way the changes in the renal pelvis are kept under observation, and the formation of pockets rendered less probable.

The first case was that of a man between thirty and forty years of age, who had contracted a cystitis from non-venereal causes, and after about two years developed a pyelitis of the right kidney. His protracted illness had produced serious inroads upon his general health, and the continued presence of the cystic trouble rendered the outlook, even with operation, very grave. Still, the septic condition due to the pyelitis was so profound that I offered a nephrotomy, which was accepted and performed in September, 1892. The renal structure seemed to be so sound, and his weakened condition precluding the idea of nephrectomy, the operation was limited to that of simple nephrotomy; even this procedure was followed by grave symptoms.

After the operation he improved for a time, gained sufficiently to be able to be about his room, and was, in fact, quite comfortable, when he began to have a series of septic attacks, which I was inclined to ascribe to the imperfection of the drainage, but which I now consider were due to the effect of the drainage tubes producing injury to the lining of the renal pelvis, thus inducing a series of renal abscesses. All that had been gained was now lost, and it became manifest that a fatal issue was near at hand. In June of this

year, in spite of the immediate risk associated with any operation, because of the extremely feeble condition of the patient,
and in disregard of the small probability of a complete cure,
on account of the persistencè, in a modified degree, of the
original cystitis, it was decided to remove the offending
organ. The separation of the kidney from its surrounding
tissues was readily accomplished, but the unlocking of a pair
of forceps and the slipping of one of the primary ligatures,
subsequent to the excision of the kidney, was a serious accident, for although promptly controlled, the loss of blood was
necessarily considerable. His condition for some time was
critical, and at times a moderate degree of albuminuria without casts existed ; still, after a time, he began to improve,
and, though unable to use the right leg comfortably and
freely in walking, on account of the flexure of the thigh on
the body during his confinement to the bed, at last accounts,
two or three weeks before the date of this communication,
he had gained in flesh and strength, and had so far recovered
as to be able to go down stairs and about the house.

One curious circumstance connected with the events subsequent to the operation, misled and puzzled me. As he resided at quite a distance, I could only see him occasionally.
The wound, as already stated, was dressed with gauze, it
being purposed to keep it open until the bunch of ligatures
rendered necessary by the accident mentioned above should
separate and be removed. When I saw him, about two weeks
after the operation, I found a sinus of a tortuous character,
leading to the lowest portion of the wound, and which I was
unable to explain. The ligatures failing to come away, I
again saw him in about three weeks, and on separating the
ligature loops from the pedicle I found that one long end of a
ligature had been pushed by the gauze deeply into the wound,
and had become buried, by the process of healing, into a tortuous and looped position, in such a way that it was quite
troublesome to effect its removal. After the removal of this
ligature the sinus promptly healed, and at last accounts the
patient was comfortable and hopeful.

You will see in the specimen which I present, a cavity in the substance of the kidney, which cavity was completely closed at the time of the removal of the organ, and which contained about one half ounce of thick pus, similar to that found in an ordinary boil.

The next case occurred in a woman, about thirty years of age, and who was about three months advanced in pregnancy when I saw her. She had been having several epileptoid attacks daily for some days, had a moderate pyrexia, and gave a history of cystitis of uncertain origin and of some weeks' duration. Examination showed in the right renal region a movable cystic tumor of a size sufficient to contain nearly a quart of fluid. This was diagnosticated as a movable kidney, with torsion of the ureter and retention of urine, as it was found to increase in size, and again diminish with an increased vesical discharge. To confirm the diagnosis some of the fluid was removed, and was found to contain urea and a moderate amount of pus. The gestation being terminated soon after by a miscarriage, a nephrotomy was done. The incision into the dilated kidney was made as free as the anatomical limits would possibly permit; the borders of the wound in that organ were then secured to the wound in the loin by a row of interrupted stitches, these being placed so deeply as to give a good anchorage for the movable organ. The cavity of the kidney and the wound in the loin were kept open by being packed with gauze, and the patient began promptly to improve.

The epileptoid seizures became very infrequent, and she was able in a few weeks to resume her household duties, which required considerable strength and implied considerable fatigue. I saw her but once subsequently, some three weeks after the operation, and the impression of the kidney then gained was that it had rapidly contracted to about its normal proportions. At last accounts she was comfortable, the vesical urine was normal, and the large packing had been omitted for some weeks; still a sinus continued to discharge a goodly amount of healthy appearing urine. It seems to me

6

desirable that the sinus should continue, but no special
efforts have been made to maintain it, aside from small strips
of gauze inserted for a short distance.

The remaining case was also in a woman, about thirty
years of age, married, but never pregnant. She had suffered
for a long time from cystitis, which had eventually impaired
her general health. After having been confined to her bed
for a long time, I was requested to see her, with a view to
relief of the vesical symptoms. I found her so enfeebled
that a formidable operative procedure would imply a serious
immediate risk. The bladder had become very much contracted, and there was a tumor in the left renal region, which
was regarded as undoubtedly the kidney distended with pus.
There were also signs of incipient phthisis in both apices of
the lungs. A careful review of the history of the case, the
details of which are not necessary for our present purpose,
led to the conclusion that the first link in the chain of the
morbid processes had been a vulvo-urethral inflammation,
then a cystitis, then ureteritis, next a pyelitis, and finally,
though probably an independent trouble, incipient pulmonary
changes. As the patient resided two hundred miles from my
home, and as I was about to leave home for an absence of
three weeks, I could not undertake to determine the simple
or tubercular character of the inflammatory process in the
bladder, the kidney, or the lungs.

The vesical symptoms were so troublesome that I decided
to establish a vesico-vaginal fistula, thereby draining the
bladder and placing it at rest. This is a procedure which in
many cases is of great value, particularly when we seek to
protect a remaining kidney from consecutive pyelitis. The
cystotomy was done, and no evidence of tubercular ulceration was found.

On opening the pelvis of the kidney and evacuating eight
or ten ounces of pus, a careful exploration of the kidney was
made, with negative results aside from the pyelitis.

Since the operation I have not seen the patient, and
though my last account, received about three months after

the operation, was very gratifying so far as the fact that the patient had been relieved and had gained in strength and flesh was concerned, yet certain of the details of the report led me to fear that my instructions as to maintaining a free drainage by gauze packing had been neglected on account of her comfortable condition, and I presume, if the pulmonary trouble does not furnish a contra-indication, that she will need an operation to reëstablish drainage or to remove the kidney.

One of the most important reflections connected with these cases relates to the problem of drainage. I am now satisfied that when we are dealing with a pyelitis of considerable duration and not due to renal calculus, we should maintain the drainage by means of gauze, and that the incision through the kidney structure should be sufficient to give thorough drainage to not only the pelvis of the kidney but also to any diverticula which may exist; and this should be maintained until it is probable that good drainage through the ureter has again recurred, or that a small external sinus has become established which will serve that purpose.

DISCUSSION.

Dr. JOHN CRONYN, of Erie county, said that having seen a number of instances in the hospital with which he was connected, in which nephrotomy and nephrectomy had been performed with greater or less success, he had been led to a consideration of that most important feature—the diagnosis of the condition of *both* kidneys. It is not so difficult to determine that one kidney is diseased, as the patient is usually very accurate in his description of the symptoms. Some years ago a lady came to the hospital who had suffered for many years with all the evidences of stone in one of the kidneys. A pyelo-nephritis was present. She complained chiefly of the right side, but post-mortem examination revealed the fact that not only was the kidney on that side entirely diseased, and its place occupied by three large spiculated stones, but one half of the other kidney, which had given no symptom of disease, was filled with a single large stone. This showed that the removal of the right kidney in this case would have been of no material benefit. If those who were specially engaged in this department of surgery could only tell us how to determine that one kidney is without doubt healthy, then he would advise nephrectomy in all cases, so as to remove all of the disease at the first operation. He thought an examination with the cystoscope might eventually accomplish this desirable end.

Dr. THOMAS D. STRONG, of Chautauqua county, said he felt more than a usual interest in this subject, from the fact that he then had under his care a patient with cystic disease. She is a girl of fifteen years, whom he first saw in a severe attack of renal colic. After convalescence from this, it was suggested that investigation be made into the cause of this colic. There was at this time a urethritis and cystitis, and probably also an inflammation of the kidney, and it was suspected that there was a calculus of the bladder or kidney, or both. She was brought to the Presbyterian hospital in New York city, and was under the care of Drs. McCosh and Brown at that hospital. They examined the bladder and found no stone, but on cutting down on the left kidney they found a renal abscess, from which about two ounces of pus were evacuated. There were multiple abscesses in the substance of the kidney.

Regarding the matter of diagnosis in this case, he would say that all those who had seen the patient believed that it was a case of tuberculosis, but after hearing this paper he was of the opinion that the trouble was originally due to a urethritis and a consecutive cystitis. There had been some pus and blood in the urine from the bladder for the past two years. One observer thought he found tubercle bacilli in some of the secretion from the kidney, but in all the tests made in New York city by a number of gentlemen no tubercle bacilli were discovered. There was no history of tuberculosis on either side of the family, and the patient herself was finely developed and presented a healthy appearance. At present there is an open wound in the loin which discharges blood and urine, but during the four weeks since her return from the hospital her strength has been steadily increasing.

He was especially pleased to learn from the author that such cases may originate from other causes than tuberculosis.

Dr. FERGUSON said it seemed to him that the majority of these cases are not tubercular in the beginning. At first, the inflammation is an ordinary one, usually beginning at the lower portion of the genito-urinary tract, and then ascending and involving the kidney, where it may become a tuberculous inflammation by furnishing favourable conditions and the entrance of the tubercle bacillus into the body.

Two or three points had occurred to him in connection with the remarks made in the discussion. The recognition of the presence or absence of disease in the other kidney is a very important subject, but one hedged around by many difficulties. Many plans had been suggested for effecting this differentiation, but some were inefficient, and others involved too much violence or too much risk. In these cases of renal surgery the symptoms are sometimes entirely misleading, as for instance, when the discomfort is referred to one kidney, while the disease is really located in the other. Such facts are not explicable by our knowledge of physiology or pathology. In ordinary cases there will be the physical signs to aid the surgeon. When we have a tumor to deal with, it certainly furnishes an indication for an exploratory operation, and this, in his judgment, is not as serious as some of the methods recently advised for excluding disease in the other kidney. Of course, if the other kidney be diseased, we are dealing with a very serious, although not necessarily fatal, case. In any, even the most favourable, case, there is a risk of anuria following operations on a kidney.

Last year he presented a specimen of horseshoe kidney, in which there was a pyelitis and suppurative nephritis in one portion. The patient died on the table from the chloroform, but in any event she could not have survived the operation long, for the band of union was so broad that any line of suturing through the isthmus of the horseshoe would probably have so interfered with the function of the organ that a fatal issue would have occurred.

In his opinion, in the great majority of cases of renal disease with which we have to deal, the process begins at the lower portion of the genito-urinary tract, and extends by continuity of tissue to the pelvis of the kidney. There are of course exceptions to this statement, but in the series of cases presented in the paper he had excluded those originating in renal calculus. The flow of urine is of course from above downward, and the washing tendency is to prevent the ascent of the disease, otherwise it would occur more frequently than it does, for cystitis is very common, while pyelitis is relatively infrequent.

Anything which is going to increase the cystitis is going to add to the hazard of propagating the disease upward through the ureters. The use of the cystoscope in the hands of the ordinary operator must be looked upon as a surgical procedure. The evidence secured from such a very limited view of the bladder is, moreover, generally very unsatisfactory: it is like hunting over a microscopic field with a high power objective, a large cover-glass and much material under the cover-glass, and very little time in which to make the examination. In many cases he would rather perform an exploratory operation than subject the patient to the additional risk of a cystoscopic examination.

He thought also that ureteral catheterisation should be looked upon as an operation involving some hazard. In expert hands it is possible to perform it in the male, and he might be willing to trust Dr. Gouley, for example, to make the effort, if he would do it; but even in the female, where it is more easily performed, it is still somewhat a matter of chance to enter the ureter, as it is very difficult in many cases to find those folds and anatomical points which are given as the landmarks. Moreover, even though the bladder may have been washed out previously, it is quite probable that disease germs may be carried on the catheter up into the ureter, and so favour the development of the very disease which we wish to cure. Dr. Kelly, of Baltimore, has written several articles, in which he very warmly endorses this mode of examination, but the speaker felt sure the reverse side of the picture would prove far different than the first impression. If he were the patient, he would much prefer an exploratory operation to ureteral catheterisation.

Dr. STRONG suggested that supra-pubic cystotomy would admit of treating the bladder, and at the same time directly observing the ureters and the urine discharged from each of them.

Dr. CRONYN asked if when the disease spreads by continuity from the urethra, bladder, and ureters to the kidneys, it was not specific in character.

Dr. FERGUSON replied that it is often impossible to exclude specific disease, but in the cases reported in his paper, the evidence had been conclusive to his mind that it was not specific. In the first case the trouble was dysuria, evidently due to lithuria. The urine was normal, and there was no evidence of any trouble in the urethra antedating the lithuria.

About one year ago he was requested to operate upon a patient with an abdominal tumor, which he had diagnosticated as a renal sarcoma. He was not inclined to operate, and he told the patient she would probably die on the table, or very shortly afterwards, from shock or haemorrhage. The patient, however, insisted upon at least an exploratory operation. An incision was made, but after a prolonged search he could find no point of attack which furnished a possibility of controlling the haemorrhage, so further operation was abandoned. Although during this operation the kidney was handled with much violence, she recovered, and since then has been in much better health.

Dr. GOULEY said he fully concurred with the author in his deductions concerning the exploration with the cystoscope. Such meddling with an inflamed bladder must be even more harmful than an exploratory operation. Such an operation in cases of pyelo-nephritis is not dangerous, and it possesses the great advantage, that if the diagnosis be confirmed nephrotomy may be at once performed. In such a case nephrotomy would be the only proper method to employ. If it become necessary to make a nephrectomy subsequently, the chances of a favourable result are much better.

THE TREATMENT OF EPITHELIOMA AND THE CANCROID ULCERS BY TOPICAL APPLICATIONS—PRINCIPALLY OF LACTIC ACID.

By N. L. NORTH, M. D., of Kings County.

October 10, 1893.

At a meeting of the Fifth District Branch of this Association, held at Port Jervis, August 27, 1889, the late Dr. W. B. Eager read a paper on "Some Observations on the Use of Concentrated Lactic Acid."

The short paper I have now to offer will be the report of cases, with observations thereon, growing out of treatment adopted in consequence of the suggestions of Dr. Eager's paper.

1889.—Mrs. B., the widow of a young physician, who had early succumbed to phthisis pulmonalis, and, like many another in the profession, who for the sake of appearances had lived up to, and a little beyond, his income, and left his wife but a small life insurance with a pretty large family, which she was trying to support by "going out nursing." Her difficulty was dated from the birth of her last child. She complained principally of excessive leucorrhoeal discharge of a muco-purulent, sometimes bloody, character. Examination showed a large, somewhat indurated os uteri, with a notch or fissure upon one side containing a growth of a spongy, irregular mass of abnormal tissue of a suspicious, although possibly not as yet of a malignant, character. The cervix was contracted upon that side through inflammatory induration, causing a tilting of the neck of the uterus to the side affected. Of course, the proper treatment for the case would have been to remove the fissure and its contained abnormal growth, bringing the divided parts into coaptation and retaining them with sutures, etc. But as that would necessitate a certain time in a hospital and a certain amount of means to back it, which was deemed by the patient an impossibility with the aforesaid family to support, I thought it a good case to try the effects of the lactic acid, which was applied from time to time—as often, in fact, as she could catch opportunities between her nursing cases—with evident good result. The growth lessened with every application of the acid, and in the course of some months it was entirely removed. The muco-purulent discharge became less and less, and finally simply of an ordinary leucorrhoeal character, while the pains of the back, limbs, and loins have mostly ceased. She has continued her occupation, and is now, after four years, in comfortable health.

1890.—Mrs. M., a married woman of about forty-five years of age, expecting her menopause, was seized with a gradual attack of cystitis, which having become severe, I was called. A careful general examination showed, in addition to the cystitis, uterine disease of an undoubted cancerous character. The patient was very "nervous"—greatly frightened lest she should be told of something serious in relation to her disease. She feared a cancer, yet would not be told of the nature of her complaint. She was horrified at the thought of a hospital or of an operation. A plan was adopted temporarily of a non-committal palliative character, and the lactic acid was applied tentatively to the diseased organ as far as was practicable in the case. It was evident that the growth was more internal than upon the os uteri. The neck and mouth of the organ were drawn inward like the retraction of the nipple in mammary cancer. I applied the lactic acid on cotton, wound upon the uterine applicator, carrying it well up into the os and cervix, using it every day at first, then every second day, giving at the same time salol in large doses, in connection with the morphine, for the cystitis. After a few weeks of treatment, with a decided improvement in the symptoms, she expressed a desire for a change, and it was decided that she should try the country at a near-by place for a week or ten days, the family to notify me when she should return. Some weeks elapsed, when I called to inquire, and was informed that Mrs. M. was "dead and buried." Naturally expressing surprise, I was told that upon the advice of friends the patient, on her return from the country, was induced to try a "specialist," who, when called, expressed great indignation at the course of treatment I had pursued, and advised immediate operation, with the result stated. I was not informed as to the character of the operation, whether amputation of the cervix—an operation which could certainly do no good in a case of the kind,—or whether an attempt was made to remove the entire uterus. Certainly it was an improper case for hysterectomy, as there could be very little doubt of the involvement of the bladder, at least, in the diseased condition.

1891.—Mrs. B., a case of cancer of the os and cervix uteri. When called, and having made a diagnosis, I felt great desire to try the lactic acid; but the case seemed a proper one for removal of the uterus, with the hope of a complete recovery, so I recommended her to my friend and colleague, Dr. L. S. Pilcher, who, after a careful examination, advised that she be taken to the Methodist Episcopal hospital in Brooklyn, where, in due time, Professor Pilcher successfully performed the operation of vaginal hysterectomy. The patient made a fairly good recovery, and was for a few (six to eight) months in a comfortable state of health, when the disease reappeared in the surrounding parts, and rapidly proved fatal.

The next case, as regards the uterine disease, presented symptoms practically the counterpart of the last given.

1898.—Mrs. E. consulted me for a severe attack of sciatica. A general examination of the condition of the patient resulted in the discovery of the fact that she had cancer of the uterus, involving the os and cervix. Evidence was present of the disease having been in progress for several months, and it was rapidly advancing towards the fundus of the organ by way of the mucous membrane. The surrounding tissues and glands seemed not to be involved. I thought it a good case for operation, and advised a hospital with that end in view, when I was met with an emphatic refusal. She stated in the most positive terms that she would neither go to the hospital nor submit to a surgical operation, saying that she had known of several cases, and among them recently one of her own particular friends, who had been taken to a hospital, had been operated upon, and who had died. She said if she had a fatal disease, she would die at home. Under the circumstances, I commenced using the lactic acid, applying it to the more external portions of the growth freely, in the concentrated form, upon the cotton withe, and, after curretting thoroughly the internal os and cervix, carrying the applicator well up into the uterus as far as the abnormal growth appeared to extend. I made the application every day for a time, then twice a week, once a week, once in two weeks, once a month. Improvement commenced from the first. The growth shrank and appeared smaller and smaller with every repetition of the treatment, and when last seen, about a month ago,— now some eight months since the first application of the acid,—the uterus presented the appearance of absolute health, the discharges had all disappeared, the woman was gaining in flesh, improving in appearance, and was cheerful and happy.

The following is one of a class of non-malignant growths which, nevertheless, are prone to recur and give the patient and practitioner a great amount of "bother," to say the least :

Mrs. C.—Disease, caruncle of the urethra of many years' standing. The growth was continuous around the entire mouth of the urethra and extended well up into the canal. "Excision" repeated cauterisations, astringent powders and lotions had been repeatedly resorted to, and still the thing returned,—a not unusual history in these cases where the growth is anything more than a polypoid or subsessile tumor which can be easily tied or "snipped off." It occurred to me that the spongy, erectile character of the growth would perhaps *absorb* the lactic acid, which seems to have an "affinity" for abnormal tissues, and so become disintegrated under its use. The first application proved the supposition at least partially correct. The spongy mass gradually assumed a brownish colour, and shrank, under the use of the acid, to a small point.

Time enough has not yet elapsed to know whether the disease will again return.

Mrs. M.—A case of well developed cancerous disease of the uterus, involving the bladder, the rectum, and the parametrium generally. Vaginal *injections* of a solution of lactic acid corrected the foetid discharge to a great extent, and appeared to give relief to some of the more serious symptoms.

Mr. S., an old gentleman of generally good health, showed me, with some alarm, a curious abnormality upon his arm, of about a half inch in diameter, circular in shape, and raised above the surrounding healthy skin. It was a growth of pinkish, spongy tissue, was very sensitive, and bled easily when touched. It had a suspicious appearance, and the first question asked of me was, "Is it a cancer?" I produced my lactic acid bottle and made a free application—the acid does not in the least affect the healthy tissues, except slightly on the mucous membrane, so that in a situation like this it may be poured freely upon the part you desire to be rid of. The tumor soon assumed a brownish appearance, and gradually shrank in size as we looked at it. A few applications destroyed the growth entirely, and a normal covering of healthy skin soon took its place.

Miss J., a woman of advanced age in the Brooklyn Methodist Old People's home, showed me an ugly sore on the bridge of her nose, which she said was for many years only a wart, and gave her no trouble, but which had recently begun to ulcerate and was now giving her pain and troubling her greatly. She was the more anxious about it because those near her complained of a disagreeable smell. The sore gave all the indications, upon examination, of the *rodent ulcer*. In this case I again had recourse to the lactic acid, with the result of correcting the dysodia and arresting at least the process of ulceration. I make the application by wrapping cotton or lint about a wooden toothpick, and with that well saturated in the acid, I rub it into the ulcer with force enough to break up the crusts, and when the acid has thus been in contact with the morbid mass for a little time, a considerable discharge will set up of a brownish, bloody liquid, which will gradually cease, and a kind of scab forms, which appears to check the ulcerative process for several days. On some occasions I hasten the scabbing process by covering the whole surface of the ulcer with powdered nitrate of lead, which appears to add force, at least, to the deodorising effect of the dressing. This case is still under treatment.

I have used the lactic acid in a number of cases of uterine and skin diseases, of both the malignant and non-malignant type, with considerable satisfaction—notably upon a severe case of lupus which has been coming to me off and on for a number of years. But I need not further trespass upon your time with the report of cases; enough has been outlined to indicate the class of diseases which may be treated with lactic acid with probable benefit. Suffice it to say, that it would seem to me that the remedy *ought* to be put to a further test of its merits, particularly in cases of malignant disease in which operative proceedings cannot be had, as also in those cases—and, unfortunately, they are numerous—in which operations must of necessity prove unsuccessful.

Surgical operations which are successful *only* in the operating-room, are not wise. They do not, I am sure, advance the interests of true surgery, nor yet give permanent popularity to, nor advance the welfare or usefulness of, the individual surgeon.

One word more. The action of lactic acid when applied to abnormal growths is peculiar. As has been said, it appears at first to be *absorbed* by the *diseased* growth, while it has very little effect upon the *normal* tissue. There would seem to be a kind of endosmosis and exosmosis going on.

The remedy is applied, and if watched for a moment, it seems partially to disappear. After a little more time, a liquid of a different colour—somewhat brownish—will appear, and in a larger quantity than that which was applied.

I wish also to emphasise the fact that lactic acid is *not* a caustic or escharotic; it does not produce an eschar which covers up the malignant process while the diseased action goes on beneath, but seems to penetrate the abnormal cell and change its character, and so holds out to us the hope that it, or something like it, may soon be discovered and used which shall penetrate the malignant mass deeper than the mere caustic,—deeper even than the surgeon's knife,— and so, reaching the germ of the abnormality, prove at once destructive to it—the germ—and to the malignant outgrowth of which it is the origin, the cause.

VIA, WITH REMARK ON TREATMENT.

By Z. J. Lusk, M. D., of Wyoming County.

Read by title October 10, 1893.

There is probably no complication of pregnancy where more satisfactory results follow the strict application of *every* detail, on all matters pertaining to the present or new mode of treatment, than placenta praevia, and none which is attended with such disastrous results under the old method of treatment.

By present mode of treatment, I refer to the induction of premature labour, to the strict application of antiseptics, and I am going to add the disuse of the tampon in controlling haemorrhage. The old method is understood to apply to those who oppose the induction of premature labour, who disregard the use of antiseptics, and who place great emphasis on *vis medicatrix naturae*.

It is a melancholy fact that in the light of present knowledge many physicians maintain that antiseptics is a new fad, born to live only a season, who ignore facts and statistics, and asseverate that the mortality of obstetric operations remains unchanged. The fallacy of such statements can be shown by the following statistics:

The late Dr. Simpson, of Edinburgh, compiled a table of 399 cases in which he said that the "result was fatal to the mother in 115 cases; one in every three of the mothers perished in connection with the complication.[1]" He likewise collected into a table [2] "140 cases of expulsion of the placenta, of which 10 mothers died, an average mortality of 1 to 14." It has been estimated by Müller [3] that the death-rate by older

[1] London and Edinburgh Journal, March, 1845.
[2] Ibid.
[3] Transactions New York State Medical Association, 1887, page 392.

methods, to mothers, was from 36 to 40 per cent., which is probably not an exaggerated statement. By prompt induction of labour, "Thomas[1] had two deaths in eleven cases, Hecker had three in forty cases, Hoffman two in thirty cases, and Murphy fifteen cases without a single death."

I have had seven cases in my own practice, and seen one case in consultation. Six of my cases I saw in time to be of service, and saved the life of both mother and child. One, a case of central implantation, several miles in the country, was beyond assistance when I first saw her; and the one I saw in consultation was rapidly sinking from septicaemia. Both of these cases were victims of the tampon, an account of which I will give later in detail.

The advent of haemorrhage, severe or slight, is the first announcement of disturbed gestation. The placenta outgrows its limits; the barren soil to which it is attached fails to supply adequate means for its growth and development, when a portion becomes detached and haemorrhage follows. The physician is now summoned, and on examination finds the os soft and dilated, usually admitting easily the index finger (the contrary is the exception); the diagnosis is placenta praevia; there is now only one course to pursue, and that is the induction of premature labour: hesitation and procrastination can yield only disastrous results.

In corroboration of this opinion, I will quote the language of two of our most eminent obstetricians. Dr. Thomas, at a meeting of the New York State Medical Association in 1887, said,[2] "A timid practitioner is apt to be misled by two fallacies, which should here be exposed,—First, that as 'meddlesome midwifery is bad,' the interests of the mother are probably, and those of the child certainly, furthered by delay; and second, that even should the patient die by nature's efforts, at full term, less responsibility would fall upon his shoulders. Both these postulates are false; the safety of the child is furthered by premature delivery. Its chances of

---

[1] Transactions New York State Medical Association, 1887, page 392.
[2] Ibid. 390.

life would be better with premature lungs than placental respiration with the placenta partially detached."

Dr. W. T. Lusk,[1] on the same subject, said, "If the diagnosis of placenta praevia is confirmed, the time for folded hands is past; only cowardice pleads for delay."

Physicians are occasionally met who advocate delay on the ground stated by Dr. Thomas, that "less responsibility would attend delay." Like the criminal who prefers life imprisonment with the faint hope of escape, they allow the case to continue, thinking there may be a possibility of favourable results. The two elements of danger in placenta praevia are haemorrhage and septic poisoning. The effort to control haemorrhage with the tampon is preëminently the greatest source of infection, and under no circumstances would I think of using it. The danger of infection through the open sinuses is so great, and the result so fatal, that I would not consider it for a moment.

In a discussion on this subject, Dr. George Tucker Harrison said,[2] "By superseding the necessity of the use of the vaginal tampon we eliminate a potent cause of sepsis." At a meeting of the British Medical Association in September, 1892, Dr. Herman[3] reported the death of a case following the use of a tampon of iodoform gauze and carbolised cotton; death was thought to be due to "entrance of air into the veins."

Dr. Joseph S. Healey,[4] in an article on the "Value of Thorough Vaginal Tamponing in Placenta Praevia," writes, "The treatment par excellence in placenta praevia is 'thorough vaginal tamponing;'" after lauding this treatment of a case, he adds, "notwithstanding all antiseptic measures, on the third day symptoms of septicaemia set in; on the fifth day the temperature was 103° with extreme tenderness of the uterus, accompanied by an extremely foetid discharge." Comment is unnecessary.

[1] Transactions New York State Medical Association, 1887, page 391.
[2] Ibid., page 857.
[3] Society Reports Medical Record. British Med. Association July, 1892, page 285.
[4] Ibid., page 705.

We may, in post-partum haemorrhage at full term, as a last resort, introduce sublimated gauze into the uterus, but the conditions are not parallel. The large muscular body of the uterus contracts, closing the mouths of bleeding vessels, thus preventing the introduction of septic matter; but not so with the lower segment, which is much thinner, its muscular structure less marked, being largely composed of circular muscular fibres with only a few longitudinal ones.

The safest and best tampon, one we always have with us, and can easily be made aseptic, is the hand. After clearing the vagina of blood clots, I introduce the whole hand into the vagina, then pass index finger through cervix and separate placental attachments as far as possible by sweeping the finger around inside of the cervix. Following this manoeuvre the haemorrhage has never failed to cease, giving time to make subsequent arrangements. The hand is also the safest and most rapid dilator. The technique is simple, and consists in introducing the hand into the vagina and the index finger through the cervix, then gradually the middle finger, and finally the whole hand. During this time bipolar version can be performed. I have never seen a case of placenta praevia where the os would not readily admit the index finger. Dr. Harris, in a paper read at the late Pan-American Medical Congress, claims that in most cases manual dilatation of the os uteri from the introduction of the index finger to the full hand can, under ether anaesthesia, be accomplished in about twenty minutes. In the seven successful cases of placenta praevia treated in this manner by him, all the mothers recovered. The dilatation of the cervix from the first finger to the full hand was accomplished in an average time of nineteen and a fraction minutes. The average time for completion of labour was twenty-five and one eighth minutes. Five of the seven cases had not a single pain prior to the introduction of the hand into the uterus.

My first case of placenta praevia occurred in the fall of 1876, before antiseptic tablets occupied a place in the obstetric bag; strict cleanliness, however, was always observed.

The case was,—

A multipara, thirty-two years old; eight months advanced on the fourth pregnancy; profuse haemorrhage occurred about 1 a. m. I was at once summoned; found the patient in deep faint; under examination found the vagina filled with clots; after removing which, I introduced my index finger through cervix; found the margin of the placenta loose, and separated the attachments as far as possible. Haemorrhage ceased at once. I then gave her stimulants, and after she had rallied sufficiently I began dilating the cervix by introducing the index and middle fingers. The cervix offered very little resistance, and I was soon able to introduce all the fingers and finally the whole hand. There was vertex presentation. The uterine contractions came on regularly, but were feeble; I located the feet by external palpation; ruptured membranes during a pain; seized both feet, and brought them down through the cervix. Good pains from this time followed, and the child and placenta were delivered within half of an hour. Gave 30 drops Squibb's fld. ex. ergot, with 15 drops deod. tr. opium. Good contractions followed, and the mother and child did well.

Cases II and III were repetitions of Case I, excepting that Case III had had two previous slight haemorrhages. These three cases were placenta praevia partialis, and the mother and child recovered in each case.

CASE IV.—Mrs. H., twenty-four years of age, second pregnancy, eight and a half months advanced, was taken about 2 p. m. with a slight discharge of blood. The husband called at my office and said his wife had been having slight discharges of blood during the past five weeks, without any pain; she was now having considerable pain, and wanted me to be on hand in case labour came on. I explained to him what such attacks meant, and that I had better see her at once, which I did. I found her in bed, and she said she was feeling better, and thought she was benefited by the loss of blood. On examination I found the os rigid and not dilated; I advised her to keep quiet, to remain in bed, and send for me should haemorrhage recur. I saw her again in the evening, and found the discharge had been slight but continuous; I made no examination at that time—a mistake on my part, for three hours later I was hurriedly called. She was in a profound syncope, with no pulse at wrist. I was at her side twenty minutes after this attack, yet she was almost exsanguinated; I at once freed the vagina of clots; found os dilated, easily admitting two fingers; the placenta completely covered the internal os. I separated the placenta as far as possible, and sent for Dr. Young, who administered chloroform. The cervix dilated readily, but in trying to work the hand up the side of the uterus the placenta became completely separated; I at once ruptured the membranes, seized the feet, turned, and delivered. The placenta came first, the waters and baby following.

A few spanks brought the welcome squall from the child, which, as well as the mother, did well, and both are living to-day. This was a case of central implantation.

CASE V was a repetition of the first three cases, except that the first haemorrhage occurred at the seventh month and continued slightly till I was called three weeks later, when it became profuse. The mother and child did well.

CASE VI.—Placenta praevia centralis. I was called about 8 p. m., and found Mrs. B. (German), mother of three children, about thirty years of age, pulseless and apparently moribund. On inquiry I learned that the haemorrhage began about 4 a. m. The midwife who had previously attended her had used part of an old skirt for tampon. This she had forced into the vagina without a speculum. The blood continuing to escape, she placed both hands over the vagina and pressed on the protruding portion of the tampon; but this failing to arrest the flow of blood, and becoming exhausted from applying continuous pressure, they sent for me. On examination I found the cervix almost fully dilated, the placenta centrally implanted, and no motion had been felt since morning. I separated the placenta, ruptured the membranes, and brought down the breech. The child being dead, I did not hasten the delivery, but looked after the weakened powers of the mother. She rallied slightly, and labour was soon terminated. No post-partum haemorrhage occurred, and the patient did well until the following day, when she had a violent chill, death following from septicaemia in a few hours.

CASE VII.—Placenta praevia lateralis. This case was seven months advanced in her second pregnancy. I saw her the following morning, after an attack of haemorrhage the night before, and on examination found the os slightly dilated, admitting the index finger. Arrangements were at once made for the induction of premature labour. The cervix dilated readily under chloroform anaesthesia; the pains came on promptly, there was a vertex presentation, and when the cervix was fully dilated I pushed up the loose margin of the placenta, ruptured the membranes, and labour proceeded as in a normal case. The placenta immediately followed the delivery of the child, and the mother and child did well.

In all these cases, with the exception of Case I, thorough antiseptic precaution was observed.

During last July, in answer to a telegram, I saw a case in consultation with a physician who had several times resorted to the tampon to control haemorrhage. The case was,—

A multipara, thirty-six years of age, the mother of six children. She was taken three weeks before, when seven and a half months advanced in pregnancy. The first haemorrhage occurred about 6 p. m., after a short ride. The physician called the following morning, when it had stopped. The second haemorrhage was ten days later, and not severe. The third haemorrhage was quite profuse and occurred one

7

week from the preceding attack. The doctor called and tamponed about
8 p. m., and removed the tampon the following morning. There was a
slight dribbling continued through the day, when about the same time
as the evening before the flowing became profuse, and she was seen
again by the family physician, who gave anodynes, made cold applications, and repeated tampon, which he did not remove until the next
morning. Her condition continued about the same as the day before,
until 5 p. m., when she had a chill which was followed by fever and
headache. Her bowels, being constipated, were moved with enemata,
following which she appeared better and had less headache. Clots of
blood occasionally came away; otherwise her condition continued unchanged until 2 a. m., when she had another chill followed with fever
and pains in the back, simulating those of labour; flowing became more
profuse, when the doctor in charge used the tampon again and sent for
me. At the time I saw her, pulse was 140; temperature, 104½; respiration, 26. I removed the tampon and gave a vaginal injection of hot
sublimated water, 1-8000. Upon examination per vaginam I found the os
dilated, admitting three fingers, the margin of the placenta loose and
nearly covering the internal os, and a vertex presentation. Chloroform
was given by the attending physician; the cervix yielded readily, and
when fully dilated I ruptured the membranes, brought down the feet,
and in a very short time she was delivered. Less than one half hour
was consumed, scarcely any blood was lost, and there was no post
partum haemorrhage. She rallied slightly, and appeared better for an
hour or two, when, at 10 a. m., she had a violent chill, following which
she sank rapidly, and died at 2 p. m. Who can doubt that if at the
advent of the first haemorrhage, or even at the second, gestation had
been terminated by inducing labour under strict antisepsis, her life and
probably that of her child would have been saved ?

In the introduction of the tampon, *however aseptic* it may
be made, the cervix with its bleeding vessels is exposed to
the air. What makes compound fractures so serious as compared with simple fractures? *Exposure to the air.* These
wounds can be made aseptic; *not so*, however, with the torn
and bleeding vessels of the cervix.

In conclusion, then, I contend that in the treatment of
placenta praevia,—

1. The only rule to follow in the treatment of this anom-
aly is to terminate gestation as soon as possible. I can conceive of no condition whereby this rule permits of an exception;

2. Haemorrhage should be controlled by the introduction
of the hand into the vagina and the index finger through the

cervix, and then separate placental attachments as far as possible ;

3. The tampon, being an admitted source of infection, ought not to be used ;

4. In dilating the cervix, the hand should be used after the manner described in this paper, it being more readily accomplished and with less danger of infection ;

5. Every detail of antiseptic treatment should be observed.

DISCUSSION ON LESIONS OF THE PLEURA.

QUESTION I.

WHAT ARE THE FACTORS OF PLEURISY? ITS
FORMS AND CONTRIBUTIVE CONDITIONS?
WHAT ARE THE PATHOLOGICAL
CHANGES IN A CASE OF
PROGRESSIVE PLEURISY
ENDING IN RECOVERY?

QUESTION II.

WHAT ARE THE POINTS OF DIFFERENTIAL DIAG-
NOSIS IN PLEURISY AND OTHER AFFEC-
TIONS OF THE CHEST?

QUESTION III.

WHAT IS THE TREATMENT OF EMPYEMA, WITH
RELATIVE VALUE OF ASPIRATION, RIB-
RESECTION, AND FREE OPENING
WITH TUBE DRAINAGE?

REMARKS INTRODUCTORY TO THE DISCUSSION.

By JOHN SHRADY, M. D., of New York County.

October 10, 1893.

In introducing the present subject for discussion, there
need be no expectation of any novelty in its presentation.
Possibly there might be some re-arrangement of accumulated
knowledge regarding modes of treatment, for much thought
in recent years has been given to the subject, as well as

much analysation of cases. Pleurisy, none need be informed, as being the most obvious of maladies, was well studied by the ancients, and not badly treated upon the sudorific plan, which, independently perpetuated by the aborigines of our own soil, constituted a rude therapy for the general riddance of noxious agents from the body. The genesis of every varied treatment necessarily began in the belief that a principle of, evil, having taken refuge in the body, must be expelled, either by exorcism or by incantation. The body, too, being regarded as sacred, and surgery as a murderous art, much pathological knowledge could not well be gained, except in a comparative way by the inspection of the sacrificial offerings to a Supreme Power. Hence, to this day, the hands of the Hebrew butcher must freely sweep around the walls of the chest and abdomen as a safeguard against adhesions. It is fair to presume that this inspection of the lower animals, as the basis of anatomical research, gave the first inkling of the cause of that lancinating pain and sudden sense of suffocation which usher in an attack of pleurisy. As cold was interpreted as being the cause, heat must be applied; and if fluid were present, what more obvious than its expulsion through the pores of the skin? The same methods are essentially in vogue to-day, though the explanation of the wherefore somewhat differs.

Hippocrates, as well as his predecessors, had a somewhat hazy idea of the precise seat of this disease, evidently differentiating it from pneumonia by the " stitch in the side." It was not until Pinel, philanthropist and alienist, by substituting the analytic for the synthetic method in general medicine, as late as the eighteenth century described pleurisy as an independent disease, classing it among the inflammations of serous membranes.

What wonder this delayed progress, since pathological anatomy was neither a requirement nor a pursuit. The relics of ancestor worship had sanctified the human corpse and made dissection a crime. The occasional inspection of slaughtered animals furnished the only enigmas, which some may have solved and explained to a few, who soon forgot the lesson. To us, however, in our allotment to this era of exceptional achievement, the disease in question presents but few mysteries.

Aside from the traumatic, the forms of pleurisy are easily comprehended under the divisions of the dry, circumscribed, pleurisy with serous effusion,[1] and suppurative pleurisy. There may be some objections to the nomenclature on possibly transcendental grounds, but this classification about suits our present purpose.

Of course it is expected, in the inflammation of the enclosing sac of the lungs, whose function is to facilitate the movements of respiration, that mechanical embarrassments must arise, but they may be of such slight degree as to escape detection during life. Autopsies, running into high numbers, prove, by the observed adhesions, the existence of many a pleurisy literally without a symptomatology.

Many problems arise in the consideration of this subject, none more curious than the greater proclivity to attack of the left side, and mayhap, as claimed by some, a greater mortality. The converse of this in infantile cases is held by some to be an irrefutable fact. But let us quit at once the realm of speculation, with a saving credence in the futility of statistics, since the object of our discussion is to bring out the practical points.

The key of the diagnostic situation is in the shifting line of dulness at the upper margin, as indicating the presence of a fluid in a sac of some dimensions and capacity. As will be observed, the serous form is taken as the type, and the rule must not be made applicable to the circumscribed form of traumatic origin, or the interlobar deposits of pus, which formerly passed muster as pulmonic abscesses. Conceding this line of dulness as a basis, very little difficulty in coming to a correct opinion of the disease need be experienced. On the other hand, much aid need not be expected from the

---

[1] M. Gabriel Andral, of Paris (1797-1876), first called attention to this condition as a rapid sequel of inflammation.

auscultatory signs, pure and simple, owing to the failure of procuring fremitus, or corroborating the pleural râles of Leaming.

Aside from cold, wet, and traumatism, there are not many factors of pleurisy—that is, when complications like cancer of the stomach, chronic renal disease, gout, pulmonary phthisis, pneumonia, scarlet-fever, and whooping-cough are unconsidered. As a cause of pericarditis, or the fact of its association with cancer of the liver, it may also be overlooked.

A progressive pleurisy ending in recovery shows the following changes, as verified upon the lower animals, killed at different stages of the experiment, and given upon the authority of Dr. Prudden: 1, congestion; 2, production of serum and fibrin; 3, growth of new connective-tissue cells, and their extension in the superficial layers of the pleura, the layer being of fibrin; 4, cells in the fibrin still increasing, with the appearance of blood-vessels; 5, serum gradually absorbed, fibrin decreasing, cells increasing; 6, fibrin at last disappears, and a basement substance takes its place.

Without ceasing to be elementary, it may be conceded that the following classification of the forms of pleurisy answers all the purposes of description: 1, dry, circumscribed pleurisy; 2, pleurisy with sero-effusion; 3, sero-fibrinous; 4, acute fibrinous (plastic); 5, suppurative pleurisy.

The points of differential diagnosis in pleurisy and other affections of the chest are not as easily detected as at first sight supposed. The late Dr. Leaming *always* diagnosticated pleurisy, since it was his pet thoracic malady. He knew it by the intrapleural râles, conducted to his ear through thick layers of lung-tissue, notwithstanding that breath-sounds were transmitted much better through a collapsed lung than through a mass of fluid.

The hollow needle can usually settle the diagnosis. If the pleurisy be traumatic, there may be blood in the aspirated fluid; in the tubercular form, there are the same signs as in the serous and purulent. Family tendencies and personal history have their weight. Remember, that pericardial and peritonaeal symptoms point to tubercle, and that the secondary forms often foreshadow a pyopneumothorax.

In carcinoma there is blood in the exudate and carcinomatous matter in the microscopic field. Blood in aspirated fluid, according to Osler, may be found in,—1, asthenic state, carcinoma, morbus Brightii, and cirrhosis of the liver; 2, tubercular pleurisy; 8, cancerous pleurisy, primary and secondary; 4, blood from wounding the lung by the aspirating needle or trochar.

Malignant growths affect the pleura secondarily by extension from the mamma, the bronchial glands, the mediastinum, or other neighboring tissues. They stud the surface as growths, with a proneness to isolation. The usual forms of these adventitious products are the medullary and melanotic, which also readily explain the sanguinolent character of the effusion.[1]

A few words regarding the medical treatment of pleurisy may be in order. The indications are two-fold,—1. To limit the exudate, if in the early stages to allay the pain with opium, relax the bowels, and reduce the fever by sponging. 2. Promote the absorption, which is not so easy, as the fluid cannot get out, owing to the blocking of the lymph-paths. These are substantially Osler's recommendations. Still, he does not long hesitate before passing over to the surgical view. He believes in dry diet and brisk saline cathartics, and if at the end of ten days the exudate persists, and is at the level of the fourth rib in the erect posture, he says aspirate, and repeat again in a few days if the fluid re-accumulates. "So far as I know," says Osler, "there are no greater risks in the tuberculous than in the simple sero-fibrinous cases, and it is very important to relieve the lung early of the compression to which it is subjected by any large quantity of fluid."

Many have been the laws propounded for the operation of aspiration. 1. Begin early, says one. "Being a serious matter," says Dr. R. C. M. Page, "it should not be performed

[1] Pathological Anatomy—Jones & Sieveking, London, 1854, p. 472.

during the acute stage." 2. Should be done to relieve the
dyspnoea, which is often very urgent. 8. Imperative when
great amount of fluid threatens syncope from pressure,
and where there is improbability of its absorption. 4. Fluid
sufficient to produce intermittent orthopnoea. 5. Fluid filling half a pleural cavity and showing no signs of being
absorbed after a month. 6. Double pleurisies, where sum of
fluid would fill one pleural cavity. 7. All cases of pus.
These are mainly the rules of Dr. R. C. M. Page, and they
appear to be in accordance with reason.

Dr. Matas gives as a rule, " when fluid can be detected on
a level with the second rib, operation is indicated."

Dr. Jos. Ransohoff, of Cincinnati, who has recently written on the subject, gives the following: "1. Aspiration limited to one or two trials for empyemas of the meta-pneumonic
type, as seen in adolescents and children. 2. For all other
cases, free incision and drainage. 8. Never let an empyema
grow old."

There are a few "kinks" about the instruments, aside from
the aseptic lavatures. Here is one: Dr. F. O. Marsh (Cincinnati *Lancet and Inquirer*, Vol. XXXI, new series, p. 154)
advises a sharp three-cornered trochar in lieu of the specially
thick needles for exploration, as being not so apt to cause
pain, and to push the membrane in advance of the instrument. He also claims an advantage by picking up a fold of
skin with the haemostatic forceps at the intended point of
puncture and spraying with ether.

Another hint of value is that given by Dr. Carl Beck, of
this city, who, when the pus cannot be made to flow, resorts
to the wire of the needle, which, when on withdrawal, if
coated with pus, settles the diagnosis.

In preparing for the operation of aspiration, if we may
dignify the simple procedure of puncture by that name, we
may calm the perturbations of the patient, particularly if an
adult, by a little suggestive ceremony, such as pinching up
the skin with a small forceps and spraying with ether, or
dispensing with these procedures and hypodermatic injections

of cocaine, the operator may use menthol and chloroform, 1
to 15. Or, again, the operator, after Janeway's method, may
simply inject a syringe-full of water beneath the skin in the
region selected, perhaps with or without aseptic precautions.
One writer recommends boiling the trochar and canular separately for twenty minutes in a solution of sodium bicarbonate, one drachm to a pint of water. After this, dry and im-
merse them in a sterilised bottle of absolute alcohol.

In a child, however, these procedures need not strike with
awe, as though Moses were about to smite the rock. He
may simply enfold his arms around his parent's neck, and
the nervous attendant may control the struggles behind the
paternal back, since there is no classical point for operation
beyond selecting a point near the fluid. Avoid the point of
the shoulder blade, and so the discomfort of moving in bed;
also the ninth rib, as being perilously near the diaphragm.
And yet, as the books say, there is a " place of election ;" it
is the *sixth interspace, close above the upper border of the
seventh rib and in a line with the middle of the axilla.* Be
not too eager or hasty, as a sudden evacuation might produce
syncope ; a sanious discharge might indicate the wounding
of some vessel, perhaps a lung, a cough might warn to desist
for a moment. Also bear in mind that a cough may aid in
emptying the sac. When fluid ceases to flow desist, barring
the needle be not plugged by a flake of lymph. Through
with the operation, use the antiseptic pad.

Empyema, or intra-pleural accumulation of pus, much
oftener double in character than supposed, is a secondary
malady, ascribable to the final lesion of a surface. It is the
sequel of such diseases as typhoid fever, scarlatina, osteo-
myelitis, influenza, perhaps croupous pneumonia, and of the
complications of the tubercular process. In passing, we may
call attention to the term " meta-pneumonic empyema," a
very happy coinage of Gebhardt. The centres of infection
may be outside of the pleurae, as in such instances as pyaemia and puerperal septicaemia.

The empyemas of adults are, in about one fourth of the

cases, due to pulmonary tuberculosis, or to state the law more distinctly, the simple serous effusions of tubercular origin may become purulent, or they may start as such. Even the dry variety of pleurisy is held to be in effect tubercular, with a purulent focus elsewhere. At all events the explanation is to be hunted for in the lymphatic system rather than by a refuge in any doctrine as applicable to deteriorated blood changes. In a bacteriological sense, the microbe must have found a suitable soil, even without the history of a traumatism. Here the pneumococcus also is found, and Thire, of Christiana, who obtained cultures of this micro-organism, found blockades of the lymphatics leading to the pleural cavity. Criticism may question the office of these microbes, but their line of march is certainly indicated.

Fraenkel enunciates the doctrine that these pneumococci showing the previous existence of lobar pneumonia, also explain the cases of spontaneous recovery by perforation into the bronchi, although there are greater difficulties in the way when the rarer form of perforation of the diaphragm is concerned, for here their course cannot be made so clear. Since then we must, in some form, or by some minor reservations, accept the rôle of the tubercle bacilli as causing a primary effusion, destined to be serous if the bacilli be encapsulated, but purulent if they gain access to the pleural cavity, we are certainly armed with better therapeutic measures. The germicidal action of the blood itself may count for something, but not much, as a reliance; certainly nothing as a forlorn hope. Evacuation is therefore to be the only resource, unless precluded by a hectic condition, which can only divide the responsibility between death and the procedure.

Now how is this to be effected? We answer—as in the simple serous variety—by aspiration, for which many instruments more or less simple in principle have been devised. These range from the simple canula and trochar, to those on the suction principle, with pump and measuring receiver complete. The shops afford a wide range of choice, although as regards modes no essentially new features have been developed.   Continuous siphonage has been substituted by immersing the outer end of a tube in an antiseptic fluid in a receptacle at the bedside during the night and about the person during the day.   But as the books say there is no great tendency to re-accumulation, why all this annoyance?

As in the absence of absorption the presence of pus does not make itself manifest, our suspicions are not readily excited; we may explain away the fluctuations of temperature as being dependent upon tubercular conditions or upon insignificant pockets of pus unevenly distributed.   Perhaps the dyspnoea is overlooked, much less the bulging intercostal spaces, for when the latter by palpable appeals to the eye compels the timid thrust of the hypodermic needle, the merest tyro has made the diagnosis, and knows at once that neither can the exudate be limited nor its absorption promoted.   Our tyro has also learned from his cliniques that in children a single aspiration may cure in less than a month, from the fact that the lung tissue is still elastic and the chest wall yielding.   He has already mentally adopted "the sooner the better policy."   Bowditch, of Boston, after all did not leave us very much to learn: he was first rational, then bold, and therefore lucky.   Even he did not expect chills for even the vast accumulations of pus; he merely looked for a means of exit.

Rib-resection has its advocates, although not among our hospital surgeons.   The statistics are unfavorable, but only because, say these advocates, that desperate chances are taken.

Dr. Carl Beck, in a paper—"Empyema and its Proper Surgical Treatment," read before the "Pan-American Medical Congress" at its recent session in Washington, D.C.,[1]—advocates resection as the best of all methods, safe, clean, and easy to perform.   He maintains that you have room to sweep the finger around inside and clear away the adhering lumps upon the surface of the pleura, which no amount of washing can remove.   He lays stress upon the preservation

[1] Medical Record, Vol. 44, p. 877.

of the periosteum for rib-reproduction, and condemns aspiration as delaying the cure and as relegating to surgery the opprobium of having received its cases just late enough to spoil the statistics.

Perhaps the reasoning may be valid, more especially if active depletion of blood serum by hydrogogue cathartics has been tried along with the limited ingestion of fluids—after cups and blisters—after blood-letting and other makeshifts. Perhaps, too, its insidious approach, the suspicion of an incomplete resolution of pneumonia, have waived off the operator; and last of all, the days before bacteriological research may have produced less accurate observers. In section for removal of portion of rib or for drainage, keep the incision in the axillary line, not lower than the fifth or sixth intercostal space. Nearer the spine, the inter-space is held to be too small and the danger, if any, from the lower branch of the intercostal artery greater, while pus-burrowing in the outer-muscular septa is more likely. An incision made below these points may occlude the opening, and so make it valvular by the ascent of the diaphragm. Some of the rules, collated without credit and condensed for space-saving purpose, the writer subjoins.

If there is not sufficient room for thorough drainage, excise a portion of the lower rib,—a semi-circular cut by saw or bone forceps, not necessarily the entire width of the rib, may answer every purpose.

If the *entire width of the rib* must be removed, incise over the middle of the rib, detach periosteum, and remove about an inch. Secure *intercostal artery before opening* the pleura. Freely lay open the pleura, insert finger, and break apart any bands of lymph that may form separate pockets of pus. Insert drainage tube without side holes with one-fourth inch calibre, and stitch to the skin by wire or silk sutures.

It may be mentioned here, as showing the perfection of prophylaxis, that Sir William Stokes turned the flap of the periosteum over the end of the rib to obviate absorption of the discharge by the cancellated bony tissue.

The after-treatment in rib-resection consists in washing out the pleural cavity with a carbolic acid solution (1:40), beta-naphthol (1:4000), salicylic or boric acid, once in twenty-four hours by the hydrostatic pressure method. One or two pints of fluid may be introduced at once, and repeated until very little, if any, pus traces remain. This to be continued for several weeks. The time for removing the tube depends upon the amount and character of the discharge.

Among the sequelae, contractions of the chest and curvatures of the spine are the rule. These are, of course, traceable to the long-continued effusion and the subsequent discharge with contraction. Unfortunately, recommendations for relief are numerous, and range all the way from carefully devised gymnastics to costotomy, or the removal of ribs in a triangular form near the spine. One fact is claimed to be overlooked by some observers, and that is, the great anatomical law that the soft parts modify the hard and that the elasticity of the lung is gone.

There are many points yet to be mentioned, enough, in fact, to use up the time of a long congressional session; but as none of us are expected to speak in folios, or to use up the opportunities of others who have more established opinions to promulgate with more fervour and more tenacity, the writer therefore yields the floor to those who are able to entertain this learned body with much greater edification.

QUESTION I.

WHAT ARE THE FACTORS OF PLEURISY? ITS FORMS AND CONTRIBUTIVE CONDITIONS? WHAT ARE THE PATHOLOGICAL CHANGES IN A CASE OF PROGRESSIVE PLEURISY ENDING IN RECOVERY?

By Wm. McCollom, M. D., of Kings County.

It will not be wise, in the brief consideration of the questions propounded, to specifically note the long established and fully recorded facts of the pathological changes occurring during the course of serous and sero-fibrinous exudative pleurisies.

Pleurisy is an exudative, adhesive inflammation of the serous membrane lining the thoracic cavity.

The producing causes are several, and the specific cause, in a given case, not always easily determined.

The varied combination of symptoms in the several types of the disease, associated as it is so frequently with other diseases, allows it to pass without being diagnosticated.

That pleuritis, in some form, is exceedingly common, is evident from autopsies made for pathological study. I think it is not an exaggeration to say, that in about one half of the bodies examined pleuritic adhesions or exudates, or both, can be found. If it be so common, and often so insidious in its onset that it passes unrecognised, it is well to critically study and frequently discuss the subject, inasmuch as it is so far reaching in its baneful effects. The importance of the subject is being recognised of late in all countries, more, perhaps, than ever before; or at least the pathogenesis of inflammations of the serous membranes, and of the pleura in particular, is being more scientifically studied.

The principal primary division is dry pleurisy and pleurisy with effusion. In dry pleurisy, exudative, adhesive action is present, with resulting plastic matter and organised membrane, but not appreciable serous effusion at first, though serous or sero-fibrinous effusion may follow a dry pleurisy.

It is common to divide pleurisy with effusion into two classes, serous or sero-fibrinous and purulent, but these conditions constantly run into each other, sero-fibrinous, sero-purulent, or pus mixed with blood. In dry pleurisy, most common in the apex of the chest, where but little plastic exudate occurs, adhesion of pleural surfaces results, the plastic matter is removed by absorption, and the damage completely repaired, save an adhesion of the pleural surface.

In cases of sero-fibrinous pleurisy, layer upon layer of plastic matter is thrown out, which becomes organised into dense, heavy membrane, of a thickness at times of a quarter or half an inch. This mass, or organised exudate, may remain, with little change after a few months, during life, with little trouble to the individual other than what results from lessened volume of the lung and diminished respiratory power. This favourable result does not occur when the disease is caused from tubercle bacilli, which some investigators believe to be the most common cause of sero-fibrinous and suppurative pleurisy. Goldschrider claims that from forty to eighty per cent. of such cases have their true origin in tubercle. Dr. Wm. Osler, in a Shattuck lecture delivered in Boston the present year, gives the results of a careful study of the tubercular origin of pleurisy, and concludes that such origin is more common than previous teaching had established. This is somewhat a matter of opinion, and requires further study.

When the lung is crippled, its volume lessened, and respiratory power much impaired, pulmonary tuberculosis will often result, the pleurisy preceding the pulmonary tuberculosis. Only a bacteriological examination of the effused fluid after aspiration can determine the matter, in the absence of other evidence of tubercular infection, and this method is unsatisfactory, for tests, when a small quantity of fluid has been withdrawn, often fail to show the presence of tubercle bacilli in true tubercular cases; in fact, studies seem to show that in only a small per cent. of cases have such bacilli been found. It is difficult to demonstrate the presence of tubercular germs in plastic exudates; a failure to find the germs after aspiration is not conclusive evidence, however, that the disease is not tubercular.

The recent French writers teach that a majority of pleurisies are of tubercular origin, and there is a growing belief among those making a special study of the subject that a large per cent. of cases of sero-fibrinous and suppurative pleurisies have their origin in tubercle bacilli.

Fluid remaining in the chest a long time, by interfering with the nutrition of the body in general as well as the lungs in particular, will predispose to the development of phthisis pulmonalis. When pulmonary tuberculosis immediately follows pleurisy, in a person in good health up to the particular seizure, it is fair to presume that the pleurisy is of tubercular origin.

Suppurating pleurisies rarely terminate in recovery when left to nature's efforts. When a pyogenic membrane has formed, absorption of pus rarely takes place, and the cavity must be opened up and kept free for the discharge of purulent matter until such time as the pathological condition has changed and suppuration has ceased. A large per cent. of such cases recover under good treatment.

The more recent studies of the aetiology of exudative pleurisy, by the microscope and biological methods, have thrown a flood of light upon the causes and pathological conditions present in the different forms and conditions of the disease.

The progress made in the study of microphytic diseases in the last decade has shown that pathogenic micro-organisms are prolific causes of well defined forms of inflammatory lesions of the serous membranes, the pleura, the peritoneum, the pericardium, and the cerebral meninges. Pleurisy and

8

peritonitis from tubercular infection, from the specific germs
of puerperal and typhoid fevers, are examples.

More recent bacteriological study, by men eminent in this
department of scientific work, seems to have established the
fact that micro-organisms, and especially the tubercle bacillus, the pneumococcus, the streptococcus, and the staphylococcus play the most important part in the production of
exudative pleurisy.

The work and writings of Netter are of especial interest,
his studies being more extended. In his analysis of one
hundred and fifty-six cases of empyema, he found in twenty-
one cases the staphylococcus pyogenes, not alone, but associated with other pyogenic germs in a less number of cases.
Other than the ordinary pyogenic germs are found in purulent cavities.

In his analysis of one hundred and nine cases, he states
that the streptococcus pyogenes was present in about forty
per cent., the pneumococcus in about twenty-six per cent.,
and the staphylococcus pyogenes in about two per cent.; he
teaches that in empyema the streptococcus is often present
in adults, and in children the pneumococcus predominates.

Fraenkel studied twelve cases of empyema. In three cases
no cause could be traced; the pus only contained streptococci pyogenes, three only pneumococci. The presence
of streptococci in suppurating pleurisy is not proof that
these micro-organisms are causative agents because they are
present when the disease is secondary to pneumonia and
pulmonary tuberculosis. The pneumococcus has more diagnostic significance, and would indicate that—when found in
suppurating pleurisy—pneumonia had preceded the pleurisy,
though recent study appears to show that the pneumococcus
produces lesions of the serous membrane without the co-
existence of pneumonia.

In four of Fraenkel's cases, the origin was tuberculous.

In Ehrlich's nineteen cases of empyema, in seven, tubercle bacilli were found.

E. Levy, in a communication republished in the London

Lancet, November 29, 1890, reports his bacteriological examination of fifty-four cases. Thirty-seven of these were
serous, and seventeen purulent. Six were associated with
typhoid fever, "five were serous, and one purulent;" "nineteen with pneumonia and influenza, ten serous and nine
purulent;" fourteen cases tubercular, thirteen serous, and
one purulent. Levy concludes that in the great majority of
sero-fibrinous pleuritic effusions no pathogenic micro-organism is present, and that the absence of micro-organisms in
purulent effusion indicates the cause to be a tubercular one.

Koplic states that in twelve cases of empyema in children,
the pneumococcus was present in seven, the streptococcus
pyogenes in three, the bacillus tuberculosis with streptococcus in one, and the staphylococcus in one.

Dr. T. Mitchell Prudden, in a communication to the New
York *Medical Journal* of June 24, 1893, reviews the more
important bacteriological study of the aetiology of exudative
pleurisy, as it relates to pathogenic micro-organisms as causative agents, and records his morphologic and biologic examination of forty-five cases. Of these, there were twenty-one
cases of sero-fibrinous, twelve of which were uncomplicated,
and no bacteria were found in the exudate. Among six
metapneumonic cases, the pneumococcus was present in two.
There were twenty-four cases of empyema, eight cases not
associated with other diseases; in seven of these cases the
streptococcus pyogenes existed, and the staphylococcus
pyogenes aureus in one. In nine of the eleven cases associated with pneumonia, the pneumococcus was present. In
the twenty-four cases of empyema, bacteria were found in all.

In this brief imperfect revision of the more important bacteriological studies of the aetiology of pleurisy, it will be seen
that while different investigators differ somewhat in detail
and in minor results, there is sufficient unanimity of teaching
to establish a belief that pathogenic micro-organisms are
potent factors in causing pleurisy. That different observers
should not always be in harmony in matters of detail could
be expected, for simple serous exudates gradually change to

the purulent, as all have observed who frequently aspirate the pleural cavity. The first aspiration of clear serum is followed in later aspirations by a change in the character of the fluid withdrawn, it becoming sero-purulent, and purulent after a few aspirations.

The examination of the aspirated fluid made at different stages of the disease would account in part for the resulting differences.

Some of the pathogenic germs, like the pneumococcus, have a brief life, and the changing character of the fluid favours the death of some and the growth of others.

We do not forget the effect of cold and dampness, and that taking cold is a potent factor and the most common predisposing cause of pleurisy and pneumonia, in this, our brief review of the germ theory of the origin of the disease.

QUESTION II.

WHAT ARE THE POINTS OF DIFFERENTIAL DIAGNOSIS IN PLEURISY AND OTHER AFFECTIONS OF THE CHEST?

By J. BLAKE WHITE, M. D., of New York County.

At the last session of this Association an interesting paper upon the subject of "Acute Pleurisy" was presented by Dr. Frank S. Parsons, of Northampton, Mass., in which he described, with admirable clearness, the usual symptoms accompanying pleuritic invasion, but in our present discussion we have to deal with the unusual manifestations of this malady and its differentiation from lesions about adjacent organs or structures which closely simulate, and when co-existing with pleurisy are likely to obscure, the evidences of the existence of pleurisy itself, and often render a diagnosis an extremely difficult undertaking.

When such complications are present, it is my experience that little reliance can be placed upon the ordinary symptoms, individual idiosyncrasy having much to do with the character and intensity of the symptoms as they are developed.

Hence it is that the highest diagnostic acumen is required of the physician to correctly interpret, in a vast majority of instances, the signs which are presented to his attention in this class of cases.

We should not lose sight of the fact that chill, which authorities lay so much stress upon as an early and most constant symptom of pleurisy, is not only equally indicative of other affections of the chest, but may prove the primary cause of pleurisy, and suggests the importance of always being on the alert for such attacks following a chill.

The liability of a rheumatic or gouty diathesis to pleuritic invasion should receive due consideration, and may afford useful assistance in making a diagnosis. Furthermore, the debility of any illness, or malarial poison, predisposes to pleurisy, but one of the most potent factors in its causation, though receiving far less notice than its relative importance in this regard would seem to merit, is the depression superinduced by overwork, business harasses, and mental anxieties. The very near relation which some forms of pleurisy bear to the physical depression attending mental perplexities, has received support from the pen of the late Dr. Leaming.

Anaemia, with leucorrhoea, in the female, mal-nutrition, with dyspepsia and constipation, more or less aggravated and persistent, deserve mention among other general conditions predisposing to pleurisy.

The significance of local pain, referred to by all authors, cannot be looked upon as characteristic of pleuritis, because it is present in so many affections of contiguous organs or structures, though certain modifications of pain, to be hereinafter described, may afford some help in diagnosis, if otherwise sufficiently corroborated. Pain in pleurisy is not infrequently referred to parts remote from the seat of lesion, as the loin or abdomen, thus inviting attention to the possibility of mischief elsewhere, and leading the investigator who places too much reliance upon it as a symptom into serious error.

Dyspnoea is another ordinary symptom of pleurisy upon which it is not safe to rely, though when associated with pain and cough its significance is enhanced.

Osler,[1] after a careful investigation of a number of cases, places the relative importance of these three symptoms in the following order: cough, dyspnoea, and pain in the side. But his investigations were chiefly with reference to tuberculous pleurisies, in which class of cases I have found the same order of frequency of these symptoms maintained. In simple acute pleurisy, however, these symptoms are present in

[1] Boston Medical and Surgical Journal, July, 1898.

exactly the reverse order, the first and most frequent symptom being pain in the side, then dyspnoea, and cough. The tuberculous type of pleurisy usually attacks in an insidious manner, and without the warning that generally characterises the frank onset of a simple acute attack.

The pain in the side, which all authors refer to, is of a sharp, incisive character—the "stitch" of the old authors—more or less lasting, but aggravated by every attempt at inspiration.

The dyspnoea is difficult to describe, but, to a certain extent, is characteristic. It appears to be of a double nature, of an inability to breathe from a mechanical hindrance to lung action, with a dread to make the attempt for fear of the pain that will result. Hence patients will preserve invariably an apprehensive expression, considered by experts as quite diagnostic.

Cough in the early stages is not always prominent, and in the passive types of pleurisy it is seldom present until the affection has considerably advanced.

In the diaphragmatic form, symptoms of disturbance of the digestive system are manifested, accompanied by aggravated hiccough. This phenomenon will sometimes prove the earliest indication of pleural invasion at or near this site, and has, on some occasions, first excited my suspicion of inflammation involving the pleura, which subsequent auscultation verified.

The cough in pleurisy, when present, is dry, harsh, and ineffective, but in this respect is not always as significant of pleurisy as the two other symptoms to which I have referred; but the constant desire which some have to clear the throat without throat lesion, is eminently characteristic of pleurisy with adhesion. The character of the effort of clearing the throat affords an indication of the locality of the adhesion. A quick cough, or equally quick attempt at clearing the throat, usually is a sign of adhesion high in the chest, whereas a prolonged effort at clearing the throat points to adhesion low down in the chest, generally at the base.

These are interesting occurrences in pleurisy to which I have never seen any allusion. The symptom is purely reflex, and transmitted to the throat, giving rise to a disposition to clear the throat. It calls attention to the fact that some lesion is to be found in the chest, and I venture to assert that any one affected with this constant tendency to clear the throat without local causes manifests a symptom which substantiates a pleurisy with adhesion.

In the later stages of pleurisy the diagnosis is comparatively easy through the aid of auscultation and percussion, but it is in the more obscure and early stages that these aids to diagnosis are to be more fully understood and applied. If applied perfunctorily and unintelligently, they will prove of no value, since a correct understanding of the use of auscultation and percussion, with the results, depends solely upon a full comprehension of the principles of physical examination.

Pericardial friction may be mistaken for a pleuritic friction, and pleural adhesions may be mistaken for endocardial as well as extracardial lesions. The distinction of pericardial from neighbouring pleural friction mainly depends upon its difference of rhythm. Cardiac action sometimes produces friction in an inflamed pleura adjoining, without the pericardium being affected.

If, however, the pleural lymph has produced, by its contraction, a puckering of both the pleura on which it lies and an adjoining part of the pericardium adherent to itself, the occurrence of cardiac friction sound of this anomalous mechanism will be materially facilitated. This kind of 'friction, pleural in site and cardiac in rhythm, is not always an easy matter to differentiate; though commonly limited to the confines of the cardiac region in front, it may be audible in the back on the 'left side, and is sometimes limited to the time of expiration, when the pericardial friction sound is also most generally marked.[1]

The limitation of the sound to either edge, generally the

---

[1] Walshe and Wilkinson.

left, of the cardiac region; fixity in one or more particular spots; cessation complete or, what is more common, occasional, with certain beats of the heart when the breath is held after expiration, and marked unsteadiness in the intensity and quality of the friction which is heard to one side and not in front of the heart, are all circumstances which argue in favor of friction of cardiac rhythm being of pleural and not pericardial origin.[2] It is well to bear in mind, furthermore, that change of friction into creaking is far more common in the pleura than in the pericardium.

As the properties of sounds vary greatly with the conditions of the fundamental cause producing them, so the force, loudness, or intensity of a sound depends on the relation which its seat of origin bears to the surface, and also to the quality of the conducting medium afforded by the organ or tissue intermediate between the surface and the seat of a sound.

Auscultation should not be considered complete until the entire area of the chest has been carefully examined, for diseased conditions are often found in situations where the ordinary symptoms would least have led us to look for them. I have placed much value upon quick, forced expiration, as in the act of blowing out a candle, when auscultating the chest for the purpose of facilitating differentiation of pleural and cardial or pericardial lesions. The expulsion of air from the lungs in the manner described, renders them better conductors of sound than when inflated or partially so; and the ear thus brought nearer to the seat of the sound, auscultation is materially facilitated.

I recall, over a year ago, an interesting case where this practical test greatly assisted me to determine the true character of an obscure lesion of the pleura, supposed to be due to valvular disease, that disappeared, with all the distressing accompanying symptoms, under appropriate treatment.

A fibrinous adhesion, as a result of pleuritis, had united the lung to the posterior pericardial surface, and occasioned

[2] Walshe.

not only praecordial pain but distressing dyspnoea. On auscultation, a peculiar creaking sound was detected over the
left posterior thorax, heard most distinctly under the lower
angle of the scapula. In the ordinary act of respiration the
sound was very much like the loud murmur of a mitral insufficiency, but when a quick expiration was effected, as if
blowing out a candle, the grating, vibratory, and creaking
sound, so characteristic of adhesion external to the heart,
could be distinctly perceived, and the diagnosis was easily
established. It was subsequently a satisfaction to me to
have the presence of this lesion verified by the late Dr.
Leaming.

Pleurodynia may readily be confounded with the acute
and subacute forms of pleurisy in what is called the "dry
period." The pain in the side in this affection, however, is
more of a nature of a catch to the respiration than the sharp,
darting, and more durable pain of pleurisy. There is no
better means of differentiating these two affections with pos-
itiveness than to administer a hypodermic of morphia and
atropia, which very promptly relieves the acute pain and
permits free and full use of the lung, when the slightest deviation from normal respiration may be discerned by the
experienced auscultator. The hypodermic method is mani-
festly preferable to the internal administration of morphia,
because the relief is so nearly immediate and the indications
are usually very urgent.

An impression exists, that in the late stages of pleurisy,
after effusion, the diagnosis is always easily made, but experience will controvert this notion in not a few instances.
Complete and extensive dulness, absence of elasticity of the
chest wall, of respiratory murmur and of vocal thrill, under
ordinary circumstances, will make clear the diagnosis, and
we have ample authority for stating, that if resonance below
the clavicle is detected, the high-pitched character of its
sound points very conclusively to the presence of fluid below.
We do, however, meet with cases where neither this resonance nor the vocal thrill is present, and as their absence may

be also due to the presence of intra-thoracic tumors, it will be seen that these symptoms will often prove *per se* of little service in substantiating a diagnosis of pleurisy.

To differentiate between exudations and pulmonary consolidations is equally difficult. In acute pneumonia we have the initial chill more or less pronounced, fever, and the characteristic expectoration, which does not, however, appear for several days when the congestion of the lung is deep-seated. It is much safer to rely on the evidences revealed by auscultation. With pleurisy, the conditions about the seat of lesion so often vary through respiratory effort, position, etc., that the diagnosis is necessarily more obscure, and our sole reliance is to be placed upon keen and neat auscultation.

The relations of dulness and absence of respiration to other parts of the chest demand notice, for, gravitation of fluid taking place, the lung is forced to float upon its surface, and breath sounds become audible in localities where they were previously absent, affording strong confirmation of pleuritic effusion. But even this circumstance would not always prove a reliable guide, since adhesions sufficiently strong might take place and limit the quantity as well as the locality of the fluid, the lung being bound in a manner to prevent its changing position upon alteration of the patient's posture.

Extensive adhesions produce deficiency of resonance, which is especially perplexing in children, where the parietes are thin and there are consequently very great changes of resonance.

Phthisis ranks as the most important affection which may readily be confounded with pleurisy, though perhaps not so likely to mislead an expert as might at first be readily supposed. The two conditions are often associated; it is even generally thought that pleurisy results from a tubercular diathesis, but I think it not so much the direct result of this particular diathesis as the general somatic dyscrasia superinduced by its debilitating effects; pleurisy exists in not a few instances as a primary affection, and through its depressing influences determines tubercular complication.

It is impossible to settle this matter in all cases, either by
ante-mortem examination or post-mortem investigation, but
the simple discernment of tubercular invasion can be determined, I am convinced, in all cases by careful auscultation,
together with other indications always to be found in these
cases. Cachexia and progressive emaciation are symptoms
common to both tuberculosis and passive exudative pleuritis,
and are therefore not indications of diagnostic value in either
affection without corroboration.

We have it on the authoritative statement of Vosburg,
that pulmono-pleural congestions result sometimes from a
diseased state of the vessels and parenchyma of the lungs.
Such effects do undoubtedly arise from morbid conditions
about the heart, and though hypertrophy of the left heart
may be a cause, by far the larger number of cases can be
attributed to unsoundness about the mitral orifice. It is,
then, in these secondary pleurisies that the pleural involvement and complication—without the most assiduous physical
exploration—is most likely to escape notice and result in a
fatal issue, which, if early detected and appropriately treated,
could be averted.

The relation of bacteria to the symptomatology of pleurisy may be considered in a few words. At the risk of being
thought behind the times by some who may think themselves
advanced, I venture to assert that no investigation yet made
gives conclusive proof of pleuritis having been originated by
microbic influences. I admit the great difficulty that exists
in substantiating the facts, but this need not lessen the
eagerness to know more upon the subject, or lessen the caution with which every true student will naturally view theories in relation to this subject.

The fact of discovering pathogenic micro-organisms in
pleuritic exudations does not establish their previous presence as a causative agent by any means. It is just as reasonable and probable, in the light of such knowledge as we at
present possess, to conclude that these micro-organisms are
the result of pathological processes, as that they originate

these processes. It is very certain that no way has yet been devised whereby micro-organisms of destructive character can be discovered outside of morbid tissue, therefore the influence of bacteria in the symptomatology of pleuritis must of necessity receive secondary consideration.

In the case of tuberculosis, which offers the strongest arguments of its bacterial origin, the bitterest partisans of this theory will acknowledge that to defer a diagnosis until the bacillus is recognised is too uncertain and hazardous. He is an unskilled diagnostician who, failing to appreciate all other evidences of disease, patiently waits only for such evidences as the powerful lens of a microscope may reveal to his dull senses.

In a most admirable paper on the aetiology of exudative pleuritis, Prudden[1] sums up his careful and authoritative examination of a number of cases in the following manner: "These studies would seem to justify, more than most of those already published on the same subject, a belief in the comparatively frequent occurrence of a simple exudative pleuritis, with sero-fibrinous exudate which is not tubercular and not demonstrably associated with bacteria of any kind, and bearing more favourable prognosis than any other form of exudative pleural inflammation."

I cannot omit in this discussion a brief allusion to differentiation of pneumothorax, which might ordinarily be recognised by the merest tyro in examination of the chest; but air may be generated in the pleura through decomposition of effused fluid, or admitted by thoracentesis, in which case the existence of previous pleurisy must be acknowledged. A local tympanitic resonance and modification of the respiratory sound are caused by the air rising to the upper part of the pleura, and could be mistaken for a pulmonary cavity by a too hasty examiner.

In the language of Barclay,—"Such a diagnosis is always hazardous, for what are supposed to be the most common signs of phthisis may be exactly simulated by those of pleu-

risy with accompanying bronchitis, while there is no tubercular deposit whatever in the lung." It will not be a very
difficult matter to make sure, after careful examination, that
the resonance in pneumothorax is too high-pitched for any
other state than the presence of air in the pleural cavity,
and the auscultatory sounds must necessarily be deficient in
distinctness, while the tympanitic resonance, through change
of the patient's posture, could be made to alter its seat.

QUESTION II.

WHAT ARE THE POINTS OF DIFFERENTIAL DIAGNOSIS IN PLEURISY AND OTHER AFFECTIONS OF THE CHEST?

By J. G. Truax, M. D., of New York County.

Perhaps it would be better first to name the kinds of pleurisy, and the physiological signs and symptoms which characterise them. Thorough familiarity with these varieties will enable the diagnostician almost invariably to distinguish between pleurisy and other diseases of the chest.

The history of the origin of a disease is often very valuable, and must not be forgotten or overlooked by us when at the bedside; but its consideration does not belong to this question. Simply to call your attention to its importance is all that is required on this occasion.

Dry Pleurisy.—There is one sound which, when it can be heard, is almost complete evidence of the presence of lymph. It is the "friction sound," or "pleuritic rub." The name indicates plainly enough its aetiology. It may be profitable to recall a few of the peculiarities of this rub. It is not generally heard over a large part of the chest wall at any one time. Seldom is it present for a long time in any one spot. It changes as new areas of the pleura become involved in the inflammatory process. The "pleuritic rub" can be felt as well as heard by placing the flat hand on the chest wall. It needs sometimes a deep inspiration to produce the sound. The effusion of liquid will destroy it. The part of the chest at which it is most likely to be heard is in the region of the axilla, or below the nipple. This may be accounted for from the frequency of the inflamed pleura of the lower lobe of the lung, and on anatomical grounds. In dry pleurisy it may be heard a few hours after the disease commences, and it may persist for weeks. The last, but by no means the least, important fact connected with this rub to which I would call your attention is, that one must learn to recognise the sound, or it will often be overlooked or mistaken for bronchial crepitation.

Pain is the first symptom of which the patient will complain. So severe may it become that all chest movement is apparently lost. The respirations are short, jerky, or superficial, the object being to lessen as much as possible the friction between the two pleuritic surfaces.

Dulness on percussion is not generally as complete in the dry as in pleurisy with effusion. In most cases of pleurisy liquid is effused in great quantity and very rapidly. This is called wet pleurisy. At first the fluid is non-purulent, but later may become thicker, more opaque, with an increase of leucocytes. This is called empyema.

When there is a large quantity of liquid in the pleural cavity, percussion and auscultation show a complete absence of resonance and respiratory murmur. In other words, liquid and lung cannot occupy the same space at the same instant.

If the lung has been bound down by previous pleuritic adhesions, a bronchial breathing may be heard when fluid is present in a large degree. This condition may also prevent the line of dulness from changing when the patient is placed in a sitting position. Generally speaking, this is the only disease of the chest in which the area of dulness changes with the change of position. Old pleuritic adhesions may prevent the liquid from gravitating to the most dependent part of the chest cavity. The question may be asked, and very properly, Does not the fluid always gravitate to the lowest part of the serous cavity? My answer will be, To the lowest part of the cavity in which it is confined. The pleural cavity may be divided into several spaces, and each space must of necessity have a bottom, or one part lower than another.

Touch and sight will frequently show an increase in width or a fulness of the intercostal spaces when only a moderate amount of liquid has been effused. Naturally this sign will be more pronounced as the fluid increases, and associated with it will be the displacement of the chest organs, as evidenced by the change of the position of the apex beat and heart sounds. The writer has seen the fluid present to such a degree that many of the abdominal viscera were crowded from their proper places.

When the effusion is limited to one side, as is usually the case, a careful measurement will show the affected side to be larger than the other. The pressure of the effused liquid upon the heart and vessels will sometimes cause murmurs, which may lead one to suspect complications which do not exist. It is sufficient to call your attention to this fact; I will not consume your time by naming them.

The voice sounds are changed, either by being entirely lost or modified. These changes are called bronchophony or aegophony. Dyspnoea is a striking symptom of pleurisy. Cough is seldom absent. The pyrexia is generally moderate. The disease rarely begins with a high fever, but after the effusion becomes purulent the temperature may run up to 106°. It may be higher on the affected side than on the other. This peculiarity was first noticed by the writer in the year 1881 (in March). He called the attention of the then Dr. Austin Flint to the fact. Some authors have claimed that under some conditions there may be a pleurisy with great effusion and no elevation of temperature. Namely, when there is disease of the kidneys, etc., oedema of the subcutaneous tissue and hectic flush are signs that empyema is present. A metallic sound is said to be another sign. The writer is of the opinion that it is a sign of something more, namely, that there is an opening from the lung into the diseased cavity, If such an event were to occur, the fluid contained in the cavity would quickly become purulent.

What are the other diseases of the chest for which the list of symptoms I have just enumerated could be mistaken?

9

One is inclined to answer, upon first thought, There is none. Experience has taught us that such a reply would be far from the truth. Pneumonia, phthisis, pulmonary collapse, pericarditis, abscess of the lung, and abscess of the liver have all, to the knowledge of the writer, been diagnosticated as pleurisy with effusion. Fibrinous or plastic bronchitis might with greater ease be mistaken for pleurisy than some of those I have named. Cancer and aneurism must not be forgotten.

Pain is a symptom common to almost all diseases of the chest. The history we are not to take into consideration. The signs revealed by percussion and auscultation are the ones which should mainly command our attention. Percussion will show a greater dulness in pleurisy with effusion than in any other disease of the chest; it will also be more uniform. We must always keep in mind the exceptions mentioned in my signs of pleurisy. In no other disease will the line of dulness change with the change of position of patient. In dry pleurisy, percussion as a diagnostic sign is not so valuable. In this variety of the disease auscultation comes to our aid. If there be the friction murmur or rub, or if the normal respiratory murmur is not lost, one may naturally conclude that the dulness was caused by the effused lymph. Cough is almost always present in pleurisy, and is common to the diseases with which it is most likely to be confounded. We should find in pneumonia the dulness on percussion to be less pronounced. There would be the fine, crepitant râle, bronchial breathing, increased vocal fremitus, and sometimes amphoric breathing. The history would show that the disease commenced with a severe chill, which was followed by great prostration and a high temperature. Pain is usually less pronounced than in pleurisy.

The slow development of phthisis pulmonalis, the increased expectoration, moist râles, haemorrhage, cavity, loss of flesh, night sweats, and the discovery of the bacillus tuberculosis in the matter expectorated, are signs which would enable one to decide between it and pleurisy.

Abscess of the lung is not always easily diagnosticated, and may be mistaken for empyema, even after the lung has been aspirated. However, it can be done by excluding pleurisy, through absence of many of the signs which have been named as always belonging to the latter disease.

Pericarditis can be recognised by the muffled heart sound, the normal position of the organ, the area of dulness remaining unchanged when the patient is placed in an upright position; and if there be a friction sound present, it will correspond with the heart and not the lung movement. It has been the object of the writer to avoid details. In this short paper only suggestions have been made which will aid in making the differential diagnosis between pleurisy and such other diseases of the chest as would be most likely to give rise to error.

QUESTION III.

WHAT IS THE TREATMENT OF EMPYEMA, WITH RELATIVE VALUE OF ASPIRATION, RIB-RESECTION, AND FREE OPENING WITH TUBE DRAINAGE?

By Charles A. Leale, M. D., of New York County.

The great variety of pathological changes that are seen after death, when the lungs and pleurae are examined, plainly demonstrate the impossibility of formulating abstract rules to govern operations for the relief or cure of intra-thoracic diseases.

A study of the anatomy of the thorax and its contents teaches us that its conical frame-work, formed partly of bones and partly of soft tissues by which the bones are connected, requires special consideration, as it contains the heart and lungs, without which the continuance of life is impossible, and that these organs require protection to a sufficient degree to maintain the integrity of the heart for blood circulation, and an adequate useful portion of the parenchymatous lung-tissue for the necessary respiratory function.

Many of my observations prove that an entire lung may be destroyed or rendered useless, and that fully one half of the remaining lung may be diseased beyond utility; yet if the body be kept in moderate repose, sufficient oxygenation of the blood may ensue to continue the life of the individual.

We must, therefore, bear in mind that a useful portion of the lung is as necessary as the heart itself, and that we cannot, as I have seen suggested, with impunity simultaneously open both cavities of the thorax. Consequently, we can understand why calcareous or otherwise pathologically changed pleurae cannot be removed as offending parts, but must be tolerated so long as life endures. So it is with certain portions of the diseased lung, as—after the cure of pulmonary tuberculosis by adhesive consolidations—cheesy or chalky deposits, shutting off one lobe or more, thus causing a reliance on the remaining portion of the lung, and no one experienced in surgery would hazard the trial of well recognised impossibilities, for the opening of the thoracic cavity is far different from that of the abdomen, where an incision extending from the ensiform cartilage to the pubes may be followed by complete recovery in a few days.

It is true that we may have a circumscribed lung abscess, or a generally or locally defined empyema. These may be once emptied by the most simple method and the parts immediately closed, or the thorax thoroughly irrigated with a non-irritating antiseptic liquid, resulting in a perfect cure without any subsequent treatment.

In such cases we simply remove the offending material and nature continues the beneficial course until complete recovery ensues ;—or, as I also have often seen, spontaneous opening may take place and the abscess of the lung or the empyema be cured by an opening into the bronchus, and from thence the pus is ejected by the mouth. I have, on a number of occasions, observed and reported instances of perfect recovery after such events.

Again, in regard to the results of an inflammation of the pleurae, leaving either a serous or a purulent effusion, we may, under auspicious surroundings, have complete recovery by absorption.

In an article of mine, published in the Transactions of the New York Academy of Medicine, I cite an instance of complete restoration of the function of the lung and pleura in a boy, whose parents did all that was requested. Here, after about two years' attention to diet, clothing, and different climatic advantages, all the pus was removed by absorption, and the lung and pleura left in a normal condition at the end of five years. But experience has taught, that without such advantages, a good result could not usually be obtained, as the following illustrates :

A boy, the son of a New York physician, had complained of shortness of breath and a palpitating heart whenever attempting any unusual exertion. His father brought him to me, and on physical examination I discovered left empyema. I removed a pint of pus, hermetically closed the wound, with an immediate result of improved breathing and unrestrained heart action. His convalescence was complete after a stay of three months in the Catskill mountains.

In this instance, a simple aspiration between the ninth and tenth ribs, below the angle of the scapula, while the boy was held in the erect sitting posture, was all that was necessary.

But I can recall a number of instances where such results could not be attained by a single aspiration, or even a free opening. Here we had pathological conditions which were continuing, and which must be eliminated, or else we would have the never ceasing, hacking cough, the hectic fever, and great exhaustion.

In my last instance of such, there was tuberculous disease, which apparently was checked whenever a free opening permitted the discharge of the offensive pus; while, if the opening were permitted to close for more than two days, alarming symptoms quickly supervened.

Here pathology steps in to our aid, and shows us that it would have been impossible to have removed the diseased or useless part of the lung, as the disease was diffused in places throughout both lungs; and although the pleurae of both sides were at all places somewhat diseased, yet even in their pathological conditions they were of sufficient utility to perform all absolutely necessary work, and that a large cavernous opening in the thorax would have been a cause of more agony.

During the War of the Rebellion, as surgeon in charge of the ward at the U. S. A. general hospital, Armory square, Washington, containing all the patients with wounds of the thorax, I had one young officer, whose chest wall had been extensively torn away by a large gun-shot wound, where portions of the ribs had been removed from the side and below the angle of the scapula, somewhat as recommended by the advocates of rib-exsection. Every time the suffering captain sneezed or coughed, large volumes of the before confined air would be forcibly expelled, with frightful noise and acutely painful gasps for breath.

He never was free from agonising pain, and could not sleep except while under the influence of an anodyne—and here permit me to state, that nothing in the materia medica produces soothing results better than opium or its alkaloids. The large opening in his thorax was a source of great annoyance to him, and any one who had heard his appeal to " close that opening " would never, without due deliberation, repeat, under the name of surgery, the frightful act of war.

In another instance, I had a colonel in my ward whose anterior portion of the left thorax had been entirely shot away, including a portion of his pericardium. He had extensive pyothorax, suppurative pericarditis, and a progressively extending necrosis of several ends of his broken ribs. The large opening into his thorax represented a similar condition to that left after some of the operations for exsection of the ribs.

The results of my personal experience have been that where we have a thick laudable pus in the thorax of an otherwise healthy individual, one removal, as a rule, will suffice for a permanent cure ; but where the pus is putrid, we must have antiseptic irrigations and free drainage.

GENERAL DISCUSSION.

Dr. THOMAS H. MANLEY, of New York county, said that last year Dr. F. Parsons read a paper on pleurisy which, in a general way, reflected the opinions of modern French authorities as to the aetiology of pleurisy and the value of plastic operations on the thorax. He had hoped to hear more in the preceding discussion about aspirating in simple serous effusions of the pleura. One year ago last winter, when the subject of the treatment of pleuritic effusions was the theme for a protracted discussion in the Parisian academy, Verneuil stated that pleurisy is not as well treated now as formerly. His experience had led him to think that this is partly due to the excessive and injudicious use of the aspirator, for he was free to confess that he had never aspirated a patient for serous effusion who recovered. By this he meant that his patients subsequently acquired a suppurative pleurisy. The speaker said that this remarkable statement from Verneuil led him to look back over his own cases, and he found that not one of them had lived more than three years.

With reference to simple serous effusion in the pleural cavity, in the absence of extreme cyanosis and imminent suffocation, he believed the aspirating needle to be a deadly instrument: the opening of the pleural cavity is always a serious affair. With reference to empyema, there is no way that pus can be as safely drained as that way which nature provides, *i. e.*, through a bronchus to the mouth. His experience confirmed the statement made by Dr. Leale, that the pleural cavity possesses the property of safely confining a suppurative accumulation, and that the pyogenic germs will die, and ultimate absorption will take place, with complete recovery.

He cited a case of an old man who came to him with suppurative pleurisy on the right side, and a discharging fistulous opening in the fifth intercostal space on the axillary line. On cutting down on the fistula, it was found that the pleural cavity contained numerous plaques of bone of all conceivable shapes. Several ribs were resected in order to allow of proper falling of the chest walls. The interesting feature in this case was, that there was not the slightest evidence of septic poisoning.

Regarding the surgical treatment of pulmonary cavities treated of by Dr. Dandridge, he would say that a careful examination of the structure of the thorax showed that the pleural cavity has no analogue in the human body: it is a continuous tubular cavity. In cases where the pulmonary cavities are superficial, the question of the future will not be, How shall we treat them? for it is conceded that it must be by surgical means; but, rather, How shall we perfect our methods of diagnosis?

Dr. CRONYN said he was sorry to hear the preceding speaker say that aspiration of serous cavities, especially of the pleura, is attended by such serious consequences. He had done the operation frequently, and he believed in doing it as soon as the inflammatory action showed there was effusion into the pleural cavity, and percussion indicated that this amounted to about a half pint. Of course some care is essential in introducing the needle, to prevent the introduction of air. He held that pus, as such, can remain in the pleural cavity to the end of the patient's life without doing harm, if there be no change in its composition. Physiology teaches that the pus corpuscle is larger than the blood corpuscle, and hence it cannot reach the circulation and do mischief. If absorbed as pus, it would do no harm: it must become poisonous or septic pus.

He was not in favor of Estlander's operation of resection of the ribs: there is no necessity for it. The old valvular operation for removing pus in Pott's disease of the spine will answer just as well in relieving empyema. Such an opening allows the pus to run out by gravity, and there will be no danger of air entering, and very little of relapse. He thought if pleurisy in its earliest stages were seen by the skilful physicians composing this Association, they would scarcely allow the pleurisy to become suppurative.

"Dry pleurisy" is an old expression, but not one which he considered quite correct. Dryness of the sides of the pleura is the first step in an inflammatory action; this is true of all serous surfaces. Effusion is the second stage of the inflammatory action.

If active measures, and not placebos, be adopted at the very onset, there should be very little danger from pleurisy. As had been already said here to-day, pleurisy is not as well treated as it was years ago. The same observation may be made about pneumonia.

He would advocate, in the treatment of pleurisy, the application of either the dry or wet cups, and then the administration of a brisk purgative, followed by opium for the relief of pain.

Dr. Leale's remarks regarding the infectiousness of tuberculosis recalled to his mind a striking case. A lady, supposed to be dying of tuberculosis of the lungs, was married to a hearty farmer. She was thought to be on her death-bed. Although there was no doubt at the time about her having tuberculosis, she unexpectedly recovered, and subsequently went to live with her husband. She had a large family, and lived to be seventy-eight years old. After thirty years her husband died of consumption, and all except two of her children have died of the same disease. The speaker said he had not the slightest doubt about this man having contracted tuberculosis from his wife.

He believed he had mentioned here once before the curious fact that metastasis is very frequently the cause of curing one disease while producing another. He remembered a young man in the hospital who had all the usual evidences of tubercle in the lungs—haemorrhages, cavities, etc. One night he was taken with a violent maniacal attack. The speaker gave him chloroform, had his head shaved, put a large blister upon it, and administered three drops of croton oil. After a few days he became quiet, and his cough disappeared. This was twenty-two years ago; he is now alive and well, and weighs two hundred and sixty pounds. He had seen the same cure by metastasis occur in other cases. Why may not this account for many other extraordinary cures? The guiding rule in our treatment should be, to rectify nature only when she makes mistakes, which she never does if she can help it. It is therefore impossible to lay down more than the most general rules, which require to be intelligently applied to each individual case.

Dr. FERGUSON said, regarding Question III, which had been thus far less considered in the discussion, that it is now a matter of common observation, particularly in young patients—and these furnish the larger percentage of cases of pyothorax,—that opening and drainage result, as a rule, in a cure. We do find cases of this kind, however, in which the purulent effusion is very limited, and if we are fortunate enough to make the diagnosis, we can remove the pus with the aspirator very successfully. This had happened under his own observation in a case where only one or two ounces of pus were removed from an intra-pleural effusion. In several cases of this kind a cure had followed a single aspiration. This fact shows that the greater operation of resection is not, as a rule, called for. In a small number, however, where the lung is bound down and there is much adventitious matter which cannot be absorbed, and the rigid parts fail to become adapted to the necessary process of contraction, more severe surgical procedures are indicated. In a certain proportion of cases, resection of ribs will prove favourable, but these cases are more serious at the outset, and essentially a somewhat distinct class.

Dr. McLEAN, of Detroit, said he hesitated to offer any remarks at the present time, owing to his not being present at the beginning of the discussion. However, he would like to speak about the relative value of aspiration as compared with rib resection and free opening with tube drainage. It might be that he was extreme in his views on this subject, yet the fact remained that for a long time he had almost entirely laid aside the aspirator as a curative agent, whether the fluid were in the pleural, abdominal, or pelvic cavities. He looked upon this instrument as a broken reed, for it seldom happens that one can completely evacuate a cavity with the aspirator, on account of the almost constant presence of shreds or flocculi which block up the needle. As a means of diagnosis in a doubtful case, the aspirator is sometimes helpful, yet his own conviction was that this was as far as the aspirator could be trusted. He had had very little satisfaction with this instrument in his own practice.

He had always looked upon resection of the ribs as fulfilling one of the most important rules of surgery—the establishment and maintenance of free drainage. He had operated frequently on cases of empyema in this way, yet he had had no disasters to record. Two years ago he was able to exhibit to the Michigan State Association a little boy on whom he had performed this operation. Very soon after the operation, the boy was transformed from a puny little invalid to a healthy, strong boy. Yet the aspirator had been used before this, and without success. He was greatly in favour of free and generous incision in cases where there is pus to be evacuated.

Dr. DANDRIDGE said he was entirely in accord with the preceding speaker in regard to the value of resection of the rib in these cases. In his own experience, it was very exceptional for him to treat empyema without resection of the rib, for he did not think the intercostal space sufficient for proper drainage; even though it be sufficient at the time of the operation, it soon falls in and renders drainage defective. The aspirator is, however, useful in the treatment of recent pleurisy, to assist the expansion of the lung. As soon as the chest wall is freely opened, the atmospheric pressure on the outside is equal to that on the inside; if, on the other hand, the chest wall is not opened, there is a certain negative pressure, which certainly assists very materially in the expansion of the lung. Here there is a real scope for the aspirator—not that you will not have to make an opening subsequently in that chest, because you probably will, but simply in order to get the benefit resulting from this negative pressure.

Dr. LEALE related an instance recalled to his mind by the remarks on metastatic cure of tuberculosis. A young lady having a family history of phthisis married a strong farmer. He suddenly developed mania, and died in this condition. Two prominent pathologists in the city examined his brain, and they found increased secretion in the arachnoid, and the arachnoid membrane dotted over with miliary tubercles.

He also wished to speak of the great utility of removing a portion of the serum from a recent accumulation. If we examine this serum chemically and microscopically after removing it from the thorax, we shall find it contains a large amount of fibrinous substance, which soon becomes a solid mass. He had removed a pint of serum from the thorax, and had seen it become a mass of jelly within a half hour. By removing this mass we take away a large amount of foreign substance, which would, he thought, in itself increase that plastic exudate which has a tendency to bind down the lung, and which Dr. Leaming so persistently urged was one of the most frequent causes of pulmonary tuberculosis.

THE SURGICAL TREATMENT OF PULMONARY CAVITIES.

By N. P. DANDRIDGE, M. D., Cincinnati, Ohio.

October 10, 1893.

The surgical treatment of pulmonary cavities, with its proper limits and restrictions, is well worth serious discussion and careful consideration at this time, for on the one hand there is an undoubted tendency on the part of some to boldly push its application beyond the just limits of reason and safety, and on the other hand there is a hesitancy to admit its application to those cases where it has already been shown that it may be properly applied, and where experience has demonstrated that we possess no other adequate means of combatting conditions which tend to a necessarily fatal termination.

A large number of experiments upon animals has unquestionably shown that considerable portions of the lung may be removed without serious impairment of health, and that the lung may be punctured with comparative safety, and that for this purpose local obliteration of the pleural sac may be induced by artificial means. These experiments have undoubtedly been of great service in establishing the possible extent of operative interference in man, and have determined many important steps in the methods and technique of these operations. Their comparative safety in animals, and the possibility of avoiding fatal consequences by proper care and experience, have, however, often led to conclusions beyond the limits of just deduction, and have justified operative interference beyond the proper bounds of prudence. Simply because a patient's survives some operative interference, by no means proves that he is ultimately the better for it, or that the same end might not be better and more safely, even if more slowly, attained by other less hazardous means. The experimental work on animals, which has done so much for this department of surgery, has so often been fully described that it is not necessary to recall it in detail, except to offer the suggestion that here as elsewhere the work of the laboratory has proved a very insufficient basis for the actual work of the surgeon.

Peyrot, in his recent work on surgery, divides pulmonary lesions, in their relation to surgical interference, into two classes,—1st, Limited or localised lesions, in which he includes gangrene of the lung, most abscesses, and hydatid cyst; 2d, Diffused lesions, pulmonary cavities, and bronchiectasis. This division is of practical importance for the purpose of this paper, for the complete removal of a limited lesion, if possible, relieves the patient of his trouble, and if he does not succumb to the operative attack restores him more or less fully to health ; on the other hand, the removal of a local lesion in a generalised or diffused disease must of necessity be incomplete and leave the general pathological state unchanged. Evident as this is, and of great importance to bear in mind concerning the subject we are considering, too much stress must not be laid upon it, for we are constantly confronted with cases where the influence of a local pathological lesion dominates the general state and becomes the controlling factor in the dangerous conditions present. This is notably true in regard to tubercular cavities in the lung. The presence of foul, decomposing secretions in these cavities gives rise to a series of profound septic conditions, which materially aid in developing the general disease, while, by causing frequently recurring attacks of distressing cough, they weaken the patient by loss of sleep and strength, and so materially diminish his resistance to the influence of the general tubercular trouble. Furthermore, the discharge of the foul-smelling secretions by the mouth often nauseates, and so diminishes the little capacity there is for taking the necessary food. This unfortunate circle of influences is due to the

fact that there exists a focus of pent-up secretions, under
conditions most favourable for putrefaction, and where the
conditions are most unfavourable for disinfection or the
thorough removal of the materies morbi. If, now, surgical
interference can remove or modify this local trouble, which
is the direct cause of such serious consequences, and can so
modify for the better the general condition of the patient,
even if it does not control the other phases of the disease, it
is not only justifiable but strongly indicated. This course,
indeed, is constantly pursued in other portions of the body,
where operations are performed simply for the relief of suppurative processes which are sapping the strength of the
patient. What surgeon would hesitate to drain or scrape
out a tuberculous abscess in other parts of the body which
were accessible to interference, because there happened to
be evidence of commencing disease in the lungs or tubercular foci elsewhere? The presence of such new and extending processes of disease calls with increasing force for the
removal of the source of septic infection. What applies to
tubercular cavities applies also, but possibly with less force,
to bronchiectatic cavities, for here we find much less frequently a single cavity so far in advance of the dilatation,
more or less diffused, as to be the evident cause of the septic
state from its retained secretions.

As to the efficiency of operative measures in these cases,
Powell, in the last edition of his work, bears strong testimony. In speaking of a case in which a bronchiectatic cavity had been opened and drained, he says,—"I was much
struck at the extraordinary effect draining of the cavity had
upon the cough and expectoration. The amount of expectoration was reduced from sixteen to twenty ounces a day to
almost nothing."

Because the conditions favourable to operation are not
present in the majority of cases of bronchiectasis, or because
they are rarely found, is no reason for withholding the operation when a favourable opportunity does occur. The
results which have thus far been attained by surgical interfer-

ence in pulmonary cavities have been to provide free drainage and disinfection of cavities and abscesses, and the removal of gangrenous masses and foreign bodies.

The propriety of operative interference depends, therefore, upon the possibility of accomplishing these aims and upon the danger of the operation; and further, upon the presence of a septic condition dependent upon the local cavity or lesion; and finally, as to whether other forms of treatment have been satisfactory and successful. This last element in the problem may, I think, be readily disposed of. "All attempts," says Shurley, "to modify or disinfect lung cavities by injection or disinfection have proved in the vast majority of cases ineffectual." That foul and decomposing secretions found in pulmonary cavities are in themselves most hurtful, and modify most unfavourably all forms of chronic lung disease, is so universally admitted that it is not necessary to prove it by specific authority.

In the following paper I shall confine myself to the opening and draining of pulmonary cavities, and pass without further consideration those daring attempts, based largely upon experiments in animals and false pathological analogies, in which portions of consolidated lung have been removed. Tuffier, indeed, has reported a case where a solid apex was successfully removed from a man of twenty-five, and Watson, more recently, another, where an infiltrated mass as large as a fist was taken away by an operation most ingeniously conceived. In spite of such isolated success, the time has certainly not yet come when the words of one of our most advanced surgeons—words spoken, indeed, before the state society of this very state, eight years ago—can be said to have become prophetic, when, in speaking of Bloch's case of pneumonectomy for tubercular disease, he said,— "While I would not say that we are just yet prepared for this sort of thing, I would not be surprised at its attempt by some venturesome spirit, nor condemn it; and I look forward to the time, perhaps just before the millennium, diagnosis and technique having in the mean time been perfected, when

excision of the tuberculous apex may be the recognised treatment." Peyrot, in his recent work, condemns these operations most strongly: "I would say, most willingly, with
Keonig, that to practise these operations one must ignore all
the acquired knowledge of pathology, and that we ought to
protest against such wholly unjustifiable attempts."

The various forms of pulmonary cavities which come
under the care of the surgeon for operative interference,
may be enumerated,—1st, abscess of the lung, pulmonary
gangrene, and hydatid cyst; and 2d, tuberculous cavities,
bronchiectatic cavities, and pyopneumothorax. The second
class presents much the largest number of cases in which the
question of operation will have to be considered, and here
also we find the greatest difference of opinion as to the propriety and efficiency of surgical interference.

Turning now to the treatment of tubercular cavities, it
will be of interest and profit to know what some of the
recent systematic writers, who view the matter from a medical stand-point, have to say upon this subject. Douglas
Powell says,—"Surgical treatment in phthisical cavities offers
little prospect of advantage, because, first, cavities are usually situated at the apex, and their drainage per vias natu-
rales, by the bronchia, is fairly maintained, so that interference is not often called for; secondly, cavities are not often
single with any activity of symptoms; and third, excavation
in phthisis is a conservative process, so far as it results in removal of morbid materials that are far more injurious than
vacuity. Half the history of phthisis is made up of this elimination process, with which the hectic phenomena are identi-
fied, and with the accomplishment of which they cease, if the
perfected elimination be not overlapped by activity of process
in other centres. Hence, pulmonary surgery, in regard to
phthisis, has not, I fear, a hopeful future. But," he continues, "cases now and again present themselves in which the
extent of the excavation, superficialness of cavity, restriction
of disease to one side, and a large amount of secretion strongly
suggest external drainage." This is a very concise statement

of the case, and one which fairly offers encouragement for the surgeon in properly selected cases.

Exaggerated claims for operative interference are to be most strongly deprecated, but in a certain number of cases, as practically admitted above, the conditions are such that operation for the purpose of external drainage is justified and demanded. Burney Yeo writes in much the same strain : "It is doubtful if ordinary phthisical cavities will ever admit of successful surgical interference, either by drainage, injection, or aspiration. It is exceedingly rare in phthisis to find a single cavity without adjacent lesion, and most commonly there is an extensive surrounding pulmonary disorganisation, so that whatever alleviation of particular symptoms (profuse or foetid exudation, for example) might occur, it could only be temporary." Shurley, who has such undoubted confidence in the form of treatment in phthisis introduced by himself and Gibbs, has recently reported two cases of advanced disease, in which pulmonary cavities were treated by incision, and the inflation of the cavity with chlorine gas ; and, while neither of these cases proved successful, he advocates further efforts in this direction to secure free drainage, and to bring into contact with the tubercular tissue of the walls this agent, in whose destructive action upon the bacillus tuberculosis he has so much confidence.

In this connection I desire to report the following personal experience :

B. S., aet. 29, well developed and fairly nourished, entered the Cincinnati hospital, September, 1892. His father died of phthisis, and most of his relatives have died of the same disease. He has had the ordinary diseases of childhood, and in addition gonorrhoea and pneumonia, but denies syphilis; he admits free drinking. Patient says he had rheumatism all of last year, and last March he was in the hospital with symptoms of chronic inflammation, extending along the entire ascending colon, and since then he has always been sick. Patient came to the house complaining of severe pain on the right side upon inspiration, with dyspnoea and a continued dry cough. Appetite good, bowels regular, and tongue normal, pulse 108, temperature 99.4°. Physical examination showed some diminution of expansion on the right side of chest. Palpation negative. On percussion there was dulness on the right side as high as the seventh

10

rib in front and to the angle of the scapula behind, and diminished resonance at the apex. Auscultation negative on the left side; there was a
roughened and prolonged expiration upon the right side at the apex,
and tubular breathing at the seventh rib, and weak, moist, faintly audible sounds below. Soon after admission, Dr. Oliver, then on duty in my
absence, introduced a hypodermic and drew off some bloody fluid, which,
on microscopic examination, failed to reveal any pus corpuscles, and on
this score he expressed a doubt as to the presence of empyema, which
had been asserted, and gave his opinion that a cavity of the lung existed.
The general condition of the patient was such as to keep him constantly
in bed for several weeks after his admission ; the local condition remained unchanged. He was then submitted .to operation, and three
inches of the eighth and ninth ribs were removed in the axillary line and
the underlying cavity freely opened, and about half a pint of blood-
stained, purulent fluid, mixed with the debris of broken lung tissue and
caseous material, evacuated. Over this cavity the pleural surfaces were
firmly adherent, and the cavity reached to the surface of the lung. The
walls of this cavity were rough and irregular as in ordinary phthisical
cavities, and a large portion of the lower lobe was excavated. The cavity was washed out with a sterilised boracic solution, the skin incision
partly closed, and a double drainage tube left in place. The discharge
at first was very free, but soon diminished, and the drainage tube was
abandoned after some days and the incision readily healed. The general condition at once improved, and the man was soon up and about the
house. The area of dulness diminished, but did not entirely disappear,
and the respiratory sounds could be heard at a much lower level than
before. The condition of the right apex remained unchanged. This
man left the hospital in about two months, and since then nothing has
been heard from him.

This case presents the type of lung cavities most accessible and most favourable for operation—obliteration of the
pleura over a superficial basic cavity of considerable size, in
a patient not too much debilitated, and whose general nourishment has not already suffered. In such cases the operation presents no difficulty and but little danger, and few, if
any, would hesitate to recommend it. It is unfortunate that
the case could not have been kept under observation sufficiently long to determine the course of the disease in the
right apex. In cavities at the apex of the lung, the operation is necessarily more difficult, from the relation of the
parts; but even here Poirier finds that it is easy of performance, and secures very efficient drainage. Their situation
offers the condition favourable for freer drainage by the

bronchi, so that there is less likelihood of secretion being retained and undergoing putrefaction. Still, this condition does occur, and where sufficiently prominent the operation should be undertaken, and there is good prospect of benefit, and even of cure. Poirier and Jomnesco, in their report to the congress for tuberculosis, Paris, 1891, report that 29 operations in cavities of the apex gave 4 cures, 15 were benefited, 9 without results, and 1 unknown. A study of the general statistics of the operations on lung cavities of both apex and base presents curious contrast.

Hofmokl reports 24 cases, with 5 cures, 5 unimproved, 9 deaths, and 3 unknown; Lopez, 13 cases, 13 deaths; Slawitz, 13 cases and 3 cures; Seitz, 11 cases and 5 cures.

Such results are certainly not without encouragement, when the benefits of diverting the foul discharges are remembered, even if a cure does not result, and contains in itself a refutation of the condemnation which has been expressed against surgical interference in tubercular cavities. The objection which has been urged against operation in bronchiectasis, that the dilatation is never confined to a single portion of the bronchial tube, is certainly true of the majority of cases; but it is also certainly true that at times we meet with single cavities from this cause, so much larger and so far in advance of all others that they can be readily located, and which undoubtedly furnish the great mass of the putrid expectoration from which the patient suffers. In such cases, Powell speaks in hopeful and approving manner of operative measures. I have quoted him above as to the benefit to be expected by marked diminution of the quantity of expectoration. He further adds, " When the area of disease is definable, and the patient's health is becoming undermined in spite of all the resources of medicinal and climatic treatment, operative measures may be devised, and I believe good may be effected, although the cavity or area of excavation be not thoroughly drained, by setting up contractile changes in the tract of the tube," and this favourable opinion he considers supported by actual statistics of the operations thus far reported. Findley reports 5 cures and 15 deaths in 20 cases; Lopez, 4 cures and 8 deaths in 12 cases; Hofmokl, no cures, 8 deaths, 1 unimproved, and 3 unknown in 12 cases. The average operation in bronchiectatic cavities is likely to be much more difficult and dangerous than a like number in tubercular cavities, for the latter are much more apt to be superficial with adherent pleura, so that the danger of cutting through lung tissue will be avoided. Still, both Burney Yeo and Powell speak with approval of surgical interference in appropriate cases. In cases of abscess, gangrene, and hydatid cyst of the lung, there seems to be a growing unanimity of both medical and surgical opinion that an attempt to drain and evacuate these cavities ought to be made.

Abscess of the lung may occur as the result of septic emboli, when they are likely to be small and scattered throughout the organ. These do not fall within the range of operation. "Abscess formation is frequent in the deglutition and aspiration forms of pneumonia. They vary in size from a walnut to an orange, and have ragged and irregular walls, and purulent, sometimes necrotic, contents."[1] Foreign bodies may cause abscess by penetrating the wall, or by being drawn in through the trachea. In most, if not all, the cases reported from the latter cause, the foreign body has been accidentally discovered when the abscess was opened; and finally, abscess may break into the lung from neighbouring organs. In individual cases, the question of operation would depend simply upon the possibility of diagnosis and the definite location of the abscess, for all admit the extreme gravity of this condition when left to nature. Huber has advised against the attempt during the existence of an acute pneumonia, and this has been the course in the majority of cases reported. Lopez has reported 14 cases of abscess of the lung submitted to operation, with 12 cures, 1 death, and 1 case the result unknown; Hofmokl, 42 cases—14 complete cures, 3 with fistula, 24 deaths, and 1 unknown. The question of how far

[1] Osler.

the operation was responsible for the fatal cases cannot be determined from these statistics. Spontaneous evacuation through the chest wall sometimes occurs, but the drainage in these cases is seldom sufficiently free to insure a perfect cure, and fistulous tracks often remain open, and finally determine a fatal result. The following case bears upon this point:

Case of pyopneumothorax with a bronchial fistula, relieved by resection of rib and opening and draining of cavity. In March, 1891, I was called to see the patient by a friend who was temporarily in charge during the absence of the regular physician. The condition I found was as follows: There was an opening between the seventh and eighth ribs on the left side, in the axillary line, from which a foul-smelling discharge escaped, and through which air was forced, with jets of putrid matter, during the fits of coughing, which occurred at short intervals. Large quantities of purulent matter were expectorated from time to time. A probe was found to pass readily through the fistula, upwards and inwards, and at the depth of three inches entered a cavity of apparently considerable size. The connection of this cavity with a bronchial tube of large calibre was unmistakably demonstrated by the manner in which air and pus were forced through the external opening during the spells of coughing. A carbolic solution which was used to wash out the cavity was immediately tasted after being introduced, and always provoked coughing with expectoration of a quantity of matter smelling of carbolic. The heart was somewhat displaced to the right, and the upper part of the left side anteriorly was depressed. The respiratory sounds could be heard over the upper part of the lung in front, and throughout the back. The right lung appeared normal. It was evident that the cavity on the left side contained a quantity of foul, decomposing pus, for which there was a very inadequate escape, either through the bronchus or by means of the external fistula. The symptoms all indicated a profound septic condition. Severe and distressing chills occurred at short intervals, with high temperature and exhausting coughing spells, and for some days, when first seen, the man had been growing rapidly and progressively worse. The early history of this case which it was possible to obtain is somewhat meagre.

In January, 1890, more than a year previous, the patient had suffered from an attack of pneumonia, from which there was consolidation of nearly the whole left side. In March an abscess pointed, and was opened on the anterior aspect of the chest, and proved to be connected with the interior of the thorax. His physician, at that time, was uncertain as to whether this was due to an abscess of the lung, or an empyema. There was no pneumothorax at this time, and the date when this occurred could not be definitely determined. The man's condition, when I saw him, was such that it was evident death must soon ensue unless he could be promptly relieved of the constant absorption from the putrid pus in the

badly drained cavity. It was determined, therefore, to freely expose and
empty this cavity, and attempt its thorough disinfection. A large section of the sixth, seventh, and eighth ribs was removed through the an-
tero-lateral aspect of the chest. The pleural cavity was obliterated, and
the pleura greatly thiçkened. The fistulous track was traced upwards
and inwards with a large grooved director, and with this as a guide, a
large cavity was laid open with the thermo-cautery. The cavity was of
large size, and contained an amount of decomposed pus. The tissues
covering it, which were cut through with the cautery knife, were of a
dense fibrous structure, and had lost all characteristics of lung tissue.
This was freely destroyed by the cautery, and the cavity was irrigated
and a large sized drainage tube left in place. The improvement began
at once; the septic condition disappeared, and in a few weeks the man
was able to be out, and was soon restored to comparative health. The
fistulous opening in the side has, however, never completely closed, but
all evidence of connection with the bronchial tube quickly disappeared,
and if the patient had permitted the proper means to be continued in
order to secure sufficient drainage, a definite cure might have resulted.
He was, however, irascible and unreasonable, and would not tolerate
the presence of a drainage tube. As it is, however, he has enjoyed
nearly two years of comparative health and comfort. He is now, I understand, beginning to show amyloid degeneration of some of the inner
organs. Whether or not in this case there was originally an abscess of
the lung, there may be, possibly, some doubt. Certainly, at the time of
the operation a considerable cavity was found within the limits of the
lung, from which there was free communication with a bronchus of large
size.

In these cases of bronchial fistula, free removal of ribs will
probably always be necessary, and the fistulous track should
then be freely laid open until the cavity is reached, and for this
purpose the thermo-cautery is certainly the best instrument.
In this way a cavity, if it exists, can be more certainly
drained, and if none exists, any irregularity in the fistulous
track itself, which may prevent the ready escape of the discharges, be removed. In local gangrene, operation affords
the only practical chance, and when the disease can be
located the cavity should be opened freely enough to permit
the removal of the gangrenous mass. The suggestion made
by Delageniere, that the entire section affected should be
exsected, is not to be approved of, although he claims that in
these cases " failure is due to the fact that gangrenous foci
have only been opened and drained, and thus all the gangrenous tissue has not been fully removed."

Of the result in gangrenous cases, Lopez reports 17 cases of gangrene treated by opening the cavity, followed by 11 cures, 6 deaths, and 1 case unknown ; Hofmokl, 24 cases, 5 cures, 1 unimproved, 13 deaths, 2 unknown. Hydatid cysts give the larger number of cures where pneumotomy has been done, and the greatest percentage of recoveries. It has become a recognised procedure among the English surgeons of Australia, both before and after suppuration has occurred. Hofmokl and Lopez give, respectively, 45 cases with 37 cures, and 36 cases and 31 cures—certainly a most gratifying result.

The operation of pneumotomy may be extremely simple, or may involve very great difficulty. The difficulties depend upon whether adhesions have closed the pleural cavity where the opening is to be made, and upon the depth in the lung at which the cavity is situated. If situated any distance beneath the surface it may be easily missed by the knife or trocar, and the necessity for cutting through normal lung tissue certainly exposes to the risk of haemorrhage, and increases the danger of infection. It is of importance, then, to determine in all cases whether adhesions of the pleural surface have taken place or not. The introduction of the sterilised needle through the chest wall is said to indicate this with certainty. If adhesions have not taken place, movement of the pleural surfaces upon one another will be indicated by free movement of the free end of the needle. The value of this method is accepted by a number of writers upon this subject.

It may be a question as to whether partial consolidation of the lung might not so limit the pleural movement as to render it inoperative. The size and depth of the cavity it is of importance to determine if possible. Godlee says that the amount of discharge by the mouth is no indication at all of the size of the cavity. He has known cases where a pint was daily expectorated in which the cavity would not contain an ounce. Shurley has emphasised the difficulty of determining with certainty the location of cavities, and the distinguishing of pulmonary excavations from locular col-

lections in the pleural cavity, or of distinguishing bronchiectatic cavities from others. "I believe," he says, "it well
nigh impossible, with certainty, to determine the perspective,
so to speak, of a pulmonary cavity—that is, whether it be
half an inch or two or three inches from the surface, with or
without much intervening pulmonary parenchyma." Before
any operation is undertaken, the existence of a cavity should
certainly be ascertained by the introduction of a large-sized
aspirator needle, and its depth determined, so far as the
uncertain thickness of the thoracic wall will allow. And, at
the time of the operation, puncture should again be made
after the costal pleura has been exposed. The lung may
thus be punctured safely, in various directions, a number of
times, until the cavity is reached and its depth accurately determined. The canula, held in place, is a ready guide for the
cautery or knife. It has, indeed, been suggested to have the
canula grooved in order to facilitate its use for this purpose.

The opening of cavities at the apex is more difficult, and,
from the relation of the parts, likely to be more dangerous
than in the base. Poirier and Jomnesco have minutely
described the steps of this operation, and their description is
worthy of being followed. The first intercostal space has
an average breadth of two centimetres. The incision commences in the middle of the sternum, 4 centimetres, the
thickness of two fingers, below the supra-sternum notch, and
follows the interspace 9 centimeters. This incision is made
with the thermo-cautery, and includes the skin and subcutaneous tissue. The fibres of the pectoralis major, which are
seen, are separated by a grooved director. At the outer
angle of this wound the anterior thoracic artery and vein
may be seen, and at the inner the internal mammary vessels,
a centimetre from the edge of the sternum. The space
between is six centimetres. The intercostal pleura is laid
bare by a careful incision of the intercostal muscle. The
presence of adhesions of the pleural surface can now be
readily determined. If they are not present, the transpar-
ency of the pleura allows the movement of the underlying

lung to be seen. If present, the pleura appears thickened, resistant, and of a dull white colour, and conceals the lung-surface underneath. Any uncertainty, however, can be removed by the introduction of a needle and observing whether movement occurs in the free end. If adhesions are present the cautery knife is used, and made to penetrate the tissues in a direction slightly upwards and backwards. The cavity should be freely opened; and it is often necessary, in order to reach it, to pass through some thickness of tissue which is studded with tubercle. If adhesions are not present, the perforation of the lung is postponed for several days. Resection of the rib is deemed generally unnecessary.

There is decided advantage in commencing the incision in the middle of the sternum, for this permits of free separation of the edges of the wound, and so gives greater space for the deeper manipulations. In order to approach the lung from behind, the incision commences from the seventh cervical spine and extends to the internal superior angle of the scapula, passing through the skin and trapezius. The fibres of the rhomboidus are separated, and the posterior third of the second rib is exposed. Four centimetres of this are removed, and the pleura laid bare. This latter operation is reserved for exceptional cases, and I have not been able to find any report where it has been done in actual practice. The operation thus described should be practised in cavities at the apex, except that the knife may be well used instead of the cautery in the superficial incision, and resection of the rib may be made, if found necessary to secure sufficient room. The scapular region must be for the present considered beyond the reach of surgical interference. Whether it will remain so, time alone will tell. For the rest of the lung, especial care should be exercised to see that the puncture falls at the point where the symptoms of cavity are the most pronounced and of the greatest intensity; otherwise, the cavity may be entirely missed. A preliminary puncture should always precede operative interference. The incision through the thoracic wall should be made with care, until the parietal pleura is reached and the question of adhesions determined. Resection of ribs is usually advisable, and a sufficient number should always be removed to permit of free opening and full exploration of the cavity with the finger.

Most writers object to the washing out of the cavities with any kind of fluid, and advise their being packed with dry gauze. In this, I think, they have gone too far. A gentle stream of water, if free escape is allowed, would seem to be the safest and readiest method of removing secretions, often tenacious, and the debris of dead tissue, with the caseous masses, which are not infrequently found. Distention of the cavity must be most carefully avoided. I must deprecate mopping or swabbing the walls with dry gauze, however gently it is done, as liable to produce bleeding and open the door to infection. Bleeding may occur from two sources,—first, the walls of the cavity, and second, the overlying tissue cut through by the knife. Spurting vessels should of course be seized, if possible, and tied. In the bottom of the cavity with friable walls this will not, however, often succeed. Packing with simple or iodoform gauze is usually successful. The best preventive for bleeding along the incision is the use of the cautery in puncturing the cavity. This track may be enlarged, if necessary, by the same agent, or by the use of forceps, which are introduced closed and subsequently opened. The knife should not be used to open the pleura, or penetrate the cavity, unless the latter is very superficial and the former most certainly obliterated. If the pleural surfaces are not united, the opening of the lung should be, if possible, delayed. Adhesions may be induced by simply packing the wound with gauze, or by sewing the lung to the thoracic wall. Godlee, as far back as 1888, showed that the latter was feasible but very difficult. It has been done, but how often successfully, it is impossible to say.

Cases have been reported in which an empyema has promptly resulted, after opening the lung, where the pleura had been stitched together. Immediate opening in these cases should be avoided if possible, as this method of attaching the surface is by no means a satisfactory and safe barrier against the escape of the contents of the cavity into the pleura. In cases of pyopneumothorax, if the track through the lung can be traced, this should be enlarged with the cautery, using a grooved director as a guide. In this way any cavity or dilatation may be exposed, and irregularities of the track destroyed. The depth to which it will be safe to follow up these tracks, time alone can tell. Treated in this manner, there is a reasonable expectation that any communication with a bronchus will be permanently closed. The method adopted in one case, with bronchial fistula, by Guermonprez, is not to be commended. The opening in the pulmonary pleura was found, after an excision of a number of ribs, and was then closed, and a slow convalescence ensued. Such a procedure would not be without danger, and would probably result in the retention of secretions and a probable subsequent opening of the fistulous track. We may quote here, with approval, the suggestion of Thompson, of Manchester. In cases of empyema he advises the removal of ribs, and after the escape of the pus he explores the surface of the lung, and if any irregular indurated spots are found on the surface, he lays them open with the thermo-cautery. In this way tubercular food or superficial abscesses may be dealt with.

The above study justifies the following conclusions:

1. A certain number of lung cavities can be successfully dealt with by incision and drainage.

2. Tubercular cavities in the lower portion of the lungs—if single and superficial, and the general condition of the patient permits—should always be opened. Cavities at the apex should only be opened where free and persistent foetid expectoration is present and has resisted treatment, and the rest of the lung is not involved.

3. Abscess, gangrene, and hydatid cyst should be opened and drained whenever they can be located.

4. Closure of the pleura should be present before evacuation of a cavity is attempted.

5. In cases of pyopneumothorax the fistulous track should be explored, and any cavity freely laid open by the cautery.

6. Cavities that have been opened are best treated by packing with gauze, preferably iodoform.

7. The further careful trial of such agents as iodoform, chlorine gas, and chloride of zinc is desirable to determine as to whether the tubercular infiltration may not be modified by them.

8. It.is very desirable, for the further extension of surgical interference in pulmonary cavities, that the means of locating such cavities, and of determining their size and the exact character of the tissue that overlies them, should be perfected by further study, and for the accomplishment of this the surgeon must look to the physician.

REMARKS ON FERMENTATIVE DYSPEPSIA.

By Austin Flint, M. D., of New York County.

October 10, 1893.

There are few diseases that present greater difficulties in the way of treatment and of permanent cure than what may be termed functional dyspepsia. In using the term functional dyspepsia, I wish to be understood as meaning difficulty in digestion unconnected with ascertainable lesions of the digestive organs or of the alimentary tract, and not complicated with serious organic disease of other parts. While certain alterations may exist in the digestive organs, they are temporary—at least when the disease is not of long standing,—and they must disappear in cases of permanent relief. Almost all cases of dyspepsia of long standing are accompanied with more or less mental and moral disturbance, even though the periods of pain or discomfort may not be very long. These nervous symptoms I do not propose to describe. They are Protean in their character and manifestations, often relieved or mitigated by moral influences—such as change of scene or occupation—without much actual improvement in digestion. They almost invariably disappear as the normal digestive processes are restored. The long-standing "peripatetic" cases, with which physicians are unhappily too familiar, have been prominent among the unsatisfactory and discouraging experiences in general practice. Such cases usually are treated with but little expectation of permanent relief, and the most satisfactory result to be anticipated has been temporary improvement by means of palliatives, and a life rendered more or less miserable by a real or fancied necessity of constant attention to diet and general hygiene. It is in precisely such cases as these—unconnected with

gross excesses or indiscretions in diet, and especially with
the abuse of alcoholic beverages or narcotics—that modern
medicinal therapeutics seem likely to produce such results
as will render the treatment of fermentative dyspepsia of a
purely functional character almost as certain and satisfactory
as that of any acute trivial disorder.

Flatulence is a very common attendant of functional dyspepsia. This condition may be more or less pronounced, and
there are great variations in the degree to which it is tolerated by different individuals. The discomfort and distress
which accompany flatulence may amount to actual pain,
which is sometimes, though rarely, intense; but when pain
is habitual, remedies directed to its prompt relief are merely
palliative and usually do actual harm in the end. This
remark is specially applicable to all forms of opiates, whether
administered by the mouth or by subcutaneous injection.
Contrary to the popular, and to a certain extent the professional, notion, I must apply this remark as well to the various pepsins, pancreatins, *et id genus omne*, so commonly prescribed. I have fairly full records and histories of a score or
more of what may be called peripatetic cases of dyspepsia of
several years' standing, which have been subjected to nearly
every variety of routine treatment; and these constitute but
a small proportion of the cases that have come under my
observation. I have yet to see, however, a case in which
any of the pepsins, pancreatins, or the physiologically absurd
combinations of pepsin and pancreatin, logically seem to have
produced any benefit, even of a temporary character. In
certain cases in which they have seemed to act favourably as
palliatives, careful inquiry has almost invariably shown an
attention to diet and hygiene during their administration, to
which their apparently favourable effects have been fairly
attributable. If this statement be even in a measure correct,
it is most important that the fact should be recognised and
appreciated, in view of the gratuitous instruction in the
physiology of digestion and the pathology and therapeutics
of dyspepsia offered so freely to physicians in the advertising

pages of medical journals and in circulars by pharmaceutical manufacturers and even meat packers, and indiscreetly indorsed by members of the profession. Of late years my opinions have not permitted me to extend my experience in pepsins, etc.; but the histories of previous treatment in cases that have come under my observation, as well as physiological considerations, have convinced me that agents intended to supply an assumed deficiency of digestive enzymes are absolutely inert. I do not wish, however, to be understood as including in this condemnation the use of foods partially digested or peptonised, undoubtedly valuable in many cases.

This subject, to my mind, is so important that it seems proper to give my reasons for the decided opinion just expressed.

Digestion is one of the most complex of the physiological processes, and even now it is but imperfectly understood. Concerning certain facts, however, there can be no doubt. It is well known to physiologists that a combined as well as a successive action of the digestive fluids is essential to normal digestion. If the food be imperfectly masticated and insalivated, especially the latter, digestion becomes difficult. It is essential, not only that the saliva should exert its own chemical and mechanical action, but that it should become gradually mixed with the secretions of the stomach, and that the gastric juice should as gradually be mixed with the food, the pepsinogen being transformed as it is discharged from the peptic cells into pepsin, by the action of the hydrochloric acid produced by its peculiar cells. Assuming, even, that a few grains of what is called pepsin, extracted from a pig's stomach and dried, will have the same action in the human stomach that it has on minced food in a test-tube, it is by no means certain that the discomfort and distress which are sometimes observed soon after taking food are due to deficiency of pepsin. As a rule, these symptoms are produced by the undue formation of gases, which artificial pepsin is not known to have any power to control. Normally, the gases of the stomach do not exist in large quantity, and

probably are derived mainly from the air which is incorporated with the food in mastication, an evidence of which is
the presence of a considerable proportion of oxygen, which
is not found in other portions of the alimentary tract. When
gas is formed in the stomach, it is probably due to the action
of micro-organisms, and these organised ferments take no
part in digestion.

It is almost inconceivable that artificially extracted digestive enzymes can find their way into the small intestine in
such a condition as to exert any action in digestion. The
so called pancreatin has no existence, the enzymes produced
by the pancreas being trypsin, amylopsin, and steapsin.
Intestinal digestion, also, is an alkaline process; and it has
been abundantly shown by experiment that it cannot go on,
with sufficient efficiency to support life, in the absence of
the action of the intestinal juice, the composition of which
is unknown, and of the bile, the action of which has never
been clearly understood and defined. Life, indeed, cannot
be maintained in the absence of either the bile or the intestinal juice alone.

Gases are much more abundant in the small intestine than
in the stomach, and a certain quantity of gas is essential to
the proper movements of the alimentary mass under intestinal peristaltic action. The composition of the gas in the
small intestine—consisting, as it does, of carbon dioxide,
pure hydrogen, and nitrogen in variable proportions—shows
that it is in greatest part derived from the food, even if it be
admitted that a certain proportion of the carbon dioxide may
be evolved from the blood. When gases are produced in
excessive quantity in the small intestine, the action of micro-
organisms is probably involved. It is not pretended that the
so called pancreatin has any influence in modifying or restraining this action.

In cases of functional dyspepsia it is by no means invari-
able that the body is badly nourished, unless the diet is
greatly restricted. Many dyspeptics have an appearance of
perfect health. While digestion may be slow, laboured, and

attended with great discomfort and even actual pain, the processes may be efficient and complete, and general nutrition may be perfect. Although such cases are exceptional, they are not uncommon. It is seldom observed, however, that a strict diet, called, perhaps, anti-dyspeptic, secures immunity against dyspepsia, although it is desirable and useful to avoid notoriously indigestible articles and those which, in individual cases, have been found to occasion distress.

In my opinion it is seldom the case that undue fermentation in the alimentary mass begins in the intestinal canal. It usually occurs first in the stomach, and is continued in the small intestine. In the exceptional cases in which its origin is intestinal there is usually a deficiency of bile, and more or less active diarrhoea is present. In the great majority of cases, however, constipation is fully as common as diarrhoea, and sometimes the bowels are regular. When there is no gastric flatulence, when the digestive discomfort begins two or three hours after the taking of food, and when diarrhoea with flatus is present, it is probable that the fermentation is purely intestinal, and that it continues to an abnormal degree after the residue of food has passed into the large intestine. In all cases it is important to regulate the action of the bowels, either by laxatives or by agents that have the opposite effect. I have been lately in the habit of using Villacabras water as a laxative when constipation is obstinate. By carefully regulating the dose of this water, according to the effects observed in individual cases, I have found it acts most satisfactorily. Using it for any considerable time, the dose, as well as the frequency of its administration, may be diminished rather than increased, and the dejections are usually easy and painless. I give before breakfast enough to produce two or three evacuations; and for two or three days after, a daily movement follows. It may then be repeated if necessary, and given as required. A very important point in the treatment of dyspepsia with constipation is to see that the patient acquires the habit of

11

soliciting, without great effort, a movement of the bowels every morning at a fixed hour, resisting a desire for defaecation at other times. Attention to this will sometimes regulate the bowels without the use of laxatives. In cases of undue looseness of the bowels, the remedies administered with the object of restricting fermentation will often suffice. Opium or its derivatives should never be used, unless imperatively demanded by intense pain.

My main object in writing this paper is to call attention to the value of certain modern additions to the materia medica, that act as anti-fermentatives. For many years the late Dr. Austin Flint was in the habit of using salicin in doses of about ten grains before each meal, often with remarkable success. I have used this remedy very largely, and have frequently found it of great benefit; but I have lately employed other agents which seem to be much more efficient.

In nearly every case of functional dyspepsia that has come under my observation within the last ten months, I have begun the treatment by giving five grains of bismuth subgallate, either before or after each meal. In some cases it seems to act more favourably when given before meals, and in others its action is better if taken after eating. In studying my records and memoranda of cases, I find that the treatment by salicin has often been unsatisfactory. The proportion of unsuccessful cases was about twenty-five per cent.; but in some cases the effects of this remedy given alone have been remarkable. I have full records of one case of severe dyspepsia, of ten years' standing, that was completely relieved in one week, without any return, now for more than a year. The bismuth subgallate, however, is almost a specific in cases of purely functional dyspepsia with flatulence. While I have full records of a few obstinate cases, the histories of most are merely short memoranda, and of many I have no records. Since December 8, 1892, when I began to use the bismuth subgallate, I have noted only two cases in which it gave no relief, there being no evidence of organic disease. Both of these were in hysterical women. In both I used salicin and salol; and in one, salol, salicin, naphthalin, and aristol. These were cases of long standing, which had resisted treatment of every kind, and they soon passed from under my observation.

I was led to use bismuth subgallate by seeing it recommended as a valuable remedy in the diarrhoea of children, acting as a disinfectant. I first employed it in a case of dyspepsia of eleven years' standing, which is so remarkable, in some of its characters, that I shall give farther on an account of it somewhat in detail. Its action in this case was so favourable that I began to prescribe it very largely, almost invariably with remarkably satisfactory results, and I continue to use it almost daily. I have no records of many of my cases, but have been careful to note the few instances in which I have been disappointed in its effects, with certain cases in which its favourable action has been truly remarkable. I have already mentioned the two cases in which it seemed to be of no benefit. The following are a few of the cases of remarkably prompt and favourable action : A case of alcoholism of twenty years' standing, with habitual dyspepsia for the last five or six years ; bismuth subgallate gave almost instant relief; the flatulence and distress disappeared in twenty-four hours, and did not return, except in a very mild degree, when they were usually relieved by a single dose. While under other treatment for alcoholism, this condition was relieved. The patient has taken no alcohol for several weeks and has no craving for it. A case of dyspepsia of four years' standing, with chronic diarrhoea, was entirely relieved in five days by the use of the bismuth subgallate alone. A case of dyspepsia, of more than thirty years' standing, was promptly relieved by bismuth subgallate alone. In this case, every few weeks the trouble returns, and is relieved by two or three doses. I am indeed no longer surprised at results from the use of this remedy, which first seemed to me remarkable; and now I confidently expect prompt and favourable action. I have been in the habit of prescribing it in capsules containing five grains each, but lately have had it prepared in the form of tablets. In this latter form it is more convenient, and seems to act more favourably.

The following case, which I give on account of certain remarkable and interesting features, is the first in which I used bismuth subgallate:

On November 16, 1892, a gentleman, about forty years of age, tall and robust, with the appearance of perfect health, consulted me in regard to a long-standing dyspepsia. He had suffered from indigestion, with considerable pain, for a long time, and about eleven years ago, under the advice of a physician, had adopted an exclusively milk diet. Since that time he had taken milk and nothing else, consuming about five quarts in the twenty-four hours. He has been in the habit of taking milk about every half hour during the day and at variable intervals at night. If he goes more than an hour during the day without milk, he has gastric and intestinal pain, which soon becomes almost unbearable, but is soon relieved by about a half pint. With the pain he has great flatulence and violent eructations. During the past eleven years he has engaged in literary work, and has travelled extensively in this country and abroad. While taking milk, however, he has felt well, slept well, taken considerable exercise, and his bowels have been regular. His personal and family history is good in every respect, and a careful physical examination failed to reveal structural disease of any organ. He wished to be treated for what he called the "milk habit."

I directed him to cut off milk promptly and absolutely, and to take three meals a day, without restriction as to quantity or kind of food, except that he was to avoid sweets and pastry and be moderate in the use of wine at dinner. I prescribed ten grains of salicin four or five times daily, and always to take a dose after eating. On the evening of the first day of treatment he went to a dinner party, eating and drinking of everything. He described his sensations at the dinner as most delightful, enjoying his unaccustomed food immensely; but his teeth were sore and his jaws tired after eating, as he had not masticated for eleven years.

On the following day he reported that he had suffered intensely with abdominal pain and eructations, but nevertheless had taken breakfast, lunch, and dinner, and had abstained from milk. I continued the treatment, and directed him, in addition, to take sodium bicarbonate five or six times daily to relieve the flatulence.

On the third day he reported that he was doing fairly well, but still suffered considerably an hour or two after eating.

On the fourth day he was about the same. I discontinued the salicin and prescribed napthalin, five grains every four hours. During the entire treatment he took sodium bicarbonate freely, and as often as he felt much discomfort from flatulence.

On the fifth day, having eaten like other persons from the beginning of treatment, taking no milk, he had slightly improved. He thought the napthalin gave him considerable relief.

On the sixth day he was doing very well, and the treatment was continued. He had become so much encouraged that on the fifth and sixth days he took supper late at night, with some excess in eating and drinking.

On the seventh day he was not so well. The indiscretions in diet of the fifth and sixth days, as he thought, gave rise to considerable pain, with flatulence and vomiting. At night on the sixth day he took about a half pint of milk, which gave great relief. I discontinued napthalin, substituting five grains of salol every two to four hours, and allowed a glass of milk at night.

On the tenth day he reported that he had done fairly well. The treatment was continued, with the addition of a glass of milk on rising in the morning.

On the twelfth day he had improved, the salol acting well. The treatment was continued.

On the fourteenth day he reported as not so well, having had a great deal of flatulence. I continued salol and prescribed ten grains of salicin before eating.

On the sixteenth day he was about the same. I prescribed a teaspoonful of Listerine after eating.

On the twentieth day he reported no progress. The Listerine seemed to have no effect. I discontinued Listerine and prescribed ten grains of menthol as required.

On the twenty-third day he reported that the menthol seemed to act unfavourably. I then discontinued other remedies, and prescribed ten grains of bismuth subgallate three times daily after eating. On the following day he went to Washington for six days.

On his return from Washington—the thirtieth day—he reported that his diet had been unrestricted, and that he had been perfectly well since first taking bismuth subgallate. From time to time he took, in addition to the bismuth subgallate, sodium bicarbonate to relieve slight flatulence with eructations. He then left the city for an extended journey abroad.

In May, 1898, six months after, I received a friendly letter from the patient, in which he made no mention of any digestive disturbance.

In August, 1898, the patient called upon me, and reported that he had travelled extensively, at times subjected to very unfavourable conditions of diet; that he had been perfectly well and strong; had lost some flesh, which he regarded with satisfaction; had taken very little sodium bicarbonate, and occasionally, though rarely, a few doses of bismuth subgallate. His diet was unrestricted, and he considered himself permanently cured.

I have given rather an extended account of this case, to illustrate the unsatisfactory results following the administration of a great variety of anti-fermentative remedies until the bismuth subgallate was prescribed. This remedy promptly produced marked improvement; and, in the light of my subsequent experience, it seems to me that if it had been used earlier, the recovery would have been much more speedy.

It was not my intention to discuss the question of diet in the causation and treatment of fermentative dyspepsia. Of course a cure is established only when a diet practically unrestricted may be used with impunity. During the treatment of these cases, patients are simply directed to avoid excesses in food and drink and to eat little or no pastry or sweets.

DISCUSSION.

Dr. CRONYN said he had been extremely interested in the paper, for very recently he had had an opportunity of observing in his own person the nature of the disease. First, there was gastric flatulence, then duodenitis and obstruction of the gall duct and jaundice, and for five weeks he was dangerously ill. He thought there was a lack of hydrochloric acid in the stomach, and that consequently by administering this acid the same purpose would be accomplished as was fulfilled by giving the subgallate of bismuth in the cases reported in the paper. His physicians, however, insisted that this was not the case. At first the treatment consisted in giving two grains of blue pill in hot water, along with hot water applications, poultices, and leeching, to relieve the pain. One morning, after an attack of nausea and vomiting, he noticed that the juices which came up were quite sweet. This led him to think that his own theory was correct, and he accordingly prescribed for himself five drops of dilute hydrochloric acid in water every two hours. The improvement was immediate and decided. He was unable to take anything but milk, or a preparation of it called "junket"—peptonised milk made into rennet custard. This is quite palatable when taken cold. He lived in this manner for four weeks, but on the Fourth of July he tested his stomach, and at the same time commemorated the day by taking a good meal, and since then he had been well.

Fermentative dyspepsia is unquestionably the most intractable of all the forms of dyspepsia. He recalled a patient of this kind whose business required him at one time to go into the country, where he could not follow his customary careful diet. He accordingly ate the same food as the men, and this was the beginning of his cure and the end of his dyspepsia.

The value of bismuth, he thought, was due to its containing a very small proportion of arsenic, and he had found, in cases where bismuth was effective, Fowler's solution in very small doses was equally beneficial.

Dr. HENRY F. RISCH, of Kings county, said that he believed two kinds of fermentation only were possible in the stomach—the fermentation of hydrocarbons, and the fermentation of nitrogenous substances. Therefore, when a patient comes to him with functional dyspepsia, he first determines the kind of gases eructated. If it be carbonic acid gas, it is from hydrocarbon fermentation, whereas the gas from nitrogenous fermentation is known by its foul odour. Germs are the cause of both kinds of fermentation. If there be a hydrocarbon fermentation, hydrocarbons are excluded from the patient's food, and if there be the fermentation of nitrogenous substances, the patient is fed on hydrocarbons instead of nitrogenous substances.

Before stomach washing came so much in vogue, he was accustomed to give a patient about one drachm of ipecac, and when he became nauseated, directed him to swallow about two quarts of warm water, containing salt and a little boracic acid. This is a very effective method of cleansing the stomach. After this, he administered antifermentative remedies along with acids and pepsin.

Dr. C. A. LEALE thought the author struck the key-note when he said the cause of all these troubles was micro-organisms in the alimentary canal. During the past summer they had had over forty-four thousand infants at the St. John's Guild hospital, and the resident physicians had employed lavage of the entire intestinal canal quite extensively in children suffering from acute gastro-enteritis. They found almost always masses of undigested food in the stomach and colon, which undoubtedly increased the temperature of the body. After a thorough washing of the stomach and colon, and the action of some purgative remedy, they were given an easily assimilable diet. After this treatment, the little ones would frequently fall asleep and not awaken during the whole of the homeward trip on the Floating hospital. The results had been very gratifying. In a large number of these cases, the trinitrate of bismuth —an old remedy—was used in doses of from one to five grains, three times a day; also the liquor arsenicalis, one to three minims three times a day. As an intestinal antiseptic they had found nothing better than a solution of boracic acid. They also refrained from using at the hospital any milk which was not sterilised, for it would be irrational to thoroughly cleanse the intestinal tract and then introduce milk filled with micro-organisms.

He could recall many instances where the lamented Professor Flint had recommended, in consultation, the use of salicin, and he had seen it followed by remarkably good results.

Dr. FLINT, in closing the discussion, said he wished to emphasise the fact that he intended to treat only of fermentative dyspepsia uncon-

nected with any ascertainable organic disease.   He also wished to repeat
the statement that he was most thoroughly convinced that fermentation
in the alimentary canal is produced by micro-organisms, and therefore
he believed the only logical treatment is to employ such substances as
will destroy these micro-organisms, for it is then, and then only, that we
can ascertain how far the digestion itself is impaired.

UPON THE TREATMENT OF TUBERCULOUS DISEASE OF THE JOINTS.

By Thomas M. Ludlow Chrystie, M. D., of New York County.

Read by title October 10, 1893.

Tuberculous disease of a joint implies necrosis and caries of the contiguous osseous tissue, associated with suppuration. Before, and more frequently since, the advent of bacteriology —with its theories as to aseptic and antiseptic conditions— it has been and is customary to excise the diseased structures, with a view of eradicating the mischievous tuberculous disease and closing the sinuses which discharge the pus. The ultimate results, however, are not always successful from the patient's point of view, and investigation by subsequent candidates inspires them with a preference to adopt more conservative methods. Besides, where there are several joints in different parts of the body simultaneously affected, or where the disease attacks the vertebral joints, an operation cannot be seriously entertained. Many such cases ultimately drift to the orthopedic surgeon, and some are with him from the beginning of the attack, for suppuration will occur in cases of joint disease having a cachexia tuberculous or scrofulous in character, no matter what line of treatment is adopted. An early and complete exit for the pus is desirable, and, if on account of its distance from the surface, an opening there cannot be maintained, subsequent operations should be performed when there appear symptoms indicating the reaccumulation of pus at or about the joint, rather than resort to drainage tubes.

. A child with hip-joint disease presented, early in its course, a swollen, oedematous thigh, with an afternoon rise of temperature. No fluctuation, or other indication, could be found to localise the pus. A trocar

was inserted at the outer and upper part of the thigh, and pushed inwards and slightly upwards across and in front of the femur towards the
hip-joint until its end was felt to lie freely; the stylet was then withdrawn and the canula screwed to its aspirator, which was operated until
pus ceased to flow. Twenty ounces (ζxx) of creamy pus were withdrawn.
The thigh was shrunken from the suction of the aspirator, but no evil
effects ensued; the patient at once went about as usual—the joint protected by the hip-splint,—and the temperature at once became normal.
At the end of a month a rise of temperature and a general swelling of
the thigh reappeared. There was a similar procedure and result. No
anaesthetic was used, and by incising the integument to admit of the
easy passage of the trocar through it, pain was not experienced, so that
the patient was not at any time under such nervous dread as attends a
deep incision. It was necessary to repeat this procedure a third and a
fourth time at intervals of four to six weeks. After this the pus flowed
freely through a sinus formed in the track of the trocar, and the parent
was instructed how to knead, or pump out by a kneading process, the
last drop of pus each day. The sinus ceased to discharge, and healed
from the bottom at the end of eight months. The patient has had no
suppuration or signs of it since then, and hip-joint with limited motion
in a fair position was the result at the end of two years. About eighteen
months subsequently she was brought to me again, and cured of Pott's
disease (angular curvature) of the first to third lumbar vertebrae. There
could not be learned any history of an injury in either of these attacks,
but there was pulmonary consumption on the mother's side of the family. The child is now fourteen years of age, and in good health for the
past four years.

An important point in the treatment of sinuses discharging pus, in this class of cases, is to keep their openings
through the integument entirely free from superabundant
granulations, and to maintain them patulous. This can be
accomplished by cleanliness in regard to the dressings, and
by the local application of tannin pulverised very finely.
The ordinary condition in which tannin is dispensed is not
suitable for this purpose : it must be reduced to an impalpable
powder. Its application turns the granulations a greenish
colour, finally forming a black scab, which can be removed by
a dressing-forceps, or left to detach itself by adhering to the
dressing. Care must be taken not to remove this scab unless
it can be readily detached, otherwise the bleeding and irritation following its too early removal will increase the granulations. The tannin should be continuously applied until

the opening becomes patulous. It is a much more thorough and more easily applied remedy than nitrate of silver or other caustic remedies. Drainage-tubes, or injections of anti-septic or other liquids, I find not beneficial, and in the main injurious.

The most convenient and best absorptive aseptic dressing is Hartmann's wood wool tissue, to be obtained from the Hygienic Wood Wool Company, at 56 Broadway. Its use has in many cases kept the sinuses clean without further treatment, and I have experienced but little trouble in this respect since prescribing it during the past three years. When the dressings are changed, I direct that they be at once placed on a newspaper spread out conveniently near the patient, and shall be rolled up in it and destroyed by fire in the same room with the patient. They should not be laid aside, placed in a waste-basket or slop-jar, to wait the con-venience of some one to carry away the next day or week. This is as important as any point of cleanliness, and it is sur-prising how much carelessness obtains in this respect, when the welfare of the patient and those about him is so depend-ent upon the observance of this rule.

It is hardly possible to tell how long these sinuses will dis-charge, but with efficient orthopedic treatment and attention to keeping the openings in the integument patulous, the patient is soon able to go about and keep in the open air, with a corresponding improvement in health. What becomes of the sequestra of bone I have had no opportunity to ascer-tain. But for eight or ten years past—and even a longer time—patients have remained well, and to all appearance have sound limbs and joints, though not always symmetrical in form, when their previous condition indicated without doubt the presence of extensive necrosis and caries. I have had some cases where perfect restoration of function and form has occurred, but there seems no treatment by which such a result can always be assured.

The internal administration of cod liver oil is beneficial, though occasionally it is not tolerated. I prefer a small

dose—not more than a teaspoonful for children, and a tablespoonful for adults—not oftener than once a day. But its
value depends on its being continued daily throughout the
year. If it occasions digestive disturbance, the dose should
be lessened; there is nothing gained by taking a large quantity at a time. The pure Norwegian oil is best—that prepared by Peter Möller in the original imported bottle, with
the year of its preparation punched in the label pasted on
the bottle. A point in taking the oil is cleanliness. The
mouth of the bottle, and likewise the spoon, should be wiped
dry with paper, which is then destroyed. If the oil of a previous dose adheres to the bottle or spoon, it becomes rancid
and dusty, and the oil for a fresh dose passing over it par-
takes of this character. It is impossible to cleanse off the oil
by washing with water. To obviate the taste at the time of
administration of the oil, as well as after, the spoon should
be immersed in *cold* water, and *cold* water be drank before
and after the dose. The *cold* moisture on the spoon and
fauces, preceding the contact of the oil, prevents its adhering
thereto. Many cases, however, have done well and recovered
without oleum morrhuae. But its value is undoubted in cases
of poor nutrition with a cachexia, and I always urge it as a
necessity where there is suppuration.

In caries of the vertebrae the pus often becomes enclosed
in a sac, which cannot of course be located with sufficient
accuracy to admit of any attempt to reach it with a trocar
or simple incision. This reservoir eventually discharges its
contents at the surface of the body, and does not do the
harm in the abdominal cavity which we are led to expect
from the accounts relative to abscesses arising in that location from other causes. They dry up after discharging their
contents, under treatment previously related about other
cases. In the thoracic region they are apt to give more
trouble, and may there lead to a fatal result, but the pus is
in most instances contained safely in its sac, and often
reaches the surface of the body without doing any injury.

A young woman presented herself twelve years ago with Pott's disease, which had destroyed the bodies of the fourth to seventh dorsal vertebrae and occasioned a corresponding kyphosis. She was helpless from a paraplegia of eighteen months' duration, and with reflex muscular spasms. A cavity in the left lung and clubbed finger-nails indicated a decided cachexia. A "spinal assistant" was applied with benefit. After a few months a swelling over the upper edge of the right trapezius appeared, at the level of the spine of the first dorsal vertebra, *above* the level of the kyphosis. It was incised and the pus given an exit. The paraplegia disappeared entirely, coincident with the escape of the pus, which continued to discharge from the opening by which it first had exit. Later it would occasionally cease to flow, though the opening through the integument was patulous, and then a cough appeared, persistent and threatening to wear out her life. After some weeks the cough would disappear as pus resumed its flow. Acting upon this, I introduced a rubber catheter through the opening. Passing it gently downwards and forwards, its end would become engaged in some obstruction, which, by aid of a movement of the patient's scapula, I could generally pass with ease and insert the catheter for six or seven inches from the surface. Attaching it to the tube of an aspirator, there were withdrawn twelve to eighteen ounces of pus, without any distress to the patient and with entire relief to the cough. This I did once or twice a year. She was seen by Dr. Loomis, who suggested that there was no means of telling whether a pulmonary cavity or the sac of a vertebral abscess was drawn upon. For the past five years the cough has not troubled her enough to resort to this procedure. Her health is fair. She goes about much as others do, wearing a "spinal assistant" without inconvenience, the sinus discharging pus slightly, which is caught in a pad of salicylated tow. An ordinary observer would not detect anything the matter with this patient. She is the only case among a large number in which the suppuration has not permanently ceased. However, she is not a candidate for exsection, and enjoys life as fully as others.

In giving exit to the pus, as well as to ascertain the character of the tumor before an incision, I find an exploring needle to be useful in some instances. The hollow needle of the hypodermic syringe appears to have driven it out of the ordinary pocket-case, but the hypodermic needle used for this purpose is apt to be injurious as well as painful, and its minute calibre often makes it useless. The exploring needle in my possession is flattened and grooved on one side and round on the opposite side. It is $\frac{1}{16}''$ wide. It presents a point sharpened at its edges and slightly turned towards the concave (round) side of the needle.

Two years since I was consulted in a case of extensive suppuration and numerous sinuses discharging pus, located at
the upper part of the left thigh, over the brim of the pelvis,
and over the sacrum and coccyx.   He had hip-joint disease
fifteen years previously, and these sinuses had been forming
ever since then.   There was a painful swelling of the left
crus penis.   The exploring needle gave exit to pus without
the necessity of incision into so frail a structure, and discharged for several months.   Under a more precise orthopedic treatment, which permitted, under a firmly limited extent, a better and fuller use of the limb, and a plan of treatment for the sinuses as previously outlined, this case is now
practically well, with all the sinuses healed and many cica-
trices of the integument loosened from their attachments to
the bone and tissue underneath.   He is still under treatment,
as I see him twice a year, though actively engaged in a large
manufacturing business.

BLOODLESS AMPUTATION AT THE HIP-JOINT: A REPORT OF FORTY CASES BY THE AUTHOR'S METHOD.

By John A. Wyeth, M. D., of New York County.

October 10, 1893.

As recently as 1881, Prof. John Ashhurst, Jr., one of the highest authorities in modern surgery, wrote,[1] "the removal of the lower limb at the coxo-femoral articulation may be properly regarded as the gravest operation which the surgeon is ever called upon to perform, and it is only within a comparatively recent period that it has been accepted as a justifiable procedure."

This author further voiced the accepted opinion of surgeons when he adds, "The most pressing risk in any operation at the hip-joint is that of haemorrhage."

Beginning with aortic compression by digital or mechanical means, as advised by Pancoast, Lister, Abernathy, and others, and later the intra-rectal lever of Davy for compressing the common iliac artery against the pelvis, the first really practical and valuable suggestion for controlling haemorrhage was the figure-8 elastic bandage of Jordan Lloyd,[2] which included the posterior aspect of the thigh in its grasp, and then passed over the rim of the pelvis, making compression of the external iliac by means of a roller bandage placed beneath the elastic bandage and over this artery. This was, in fact, a figure-8 bandage around the thigh and abdomen.

As far back as 1865[3] Dr. A. Hewson, an American surgeon, first employed acupressure in an amputation at the

---

[1] International Encyclopedia of Surgery, vol. 1, p. 669.

[2] Lancet, 1883, p. 897.

[3] Am. Jour. Med. Sciences, vol. 52, p. 82.

hip-joint. There was much loss of blood before the needles were placed, and the patient died without reaction.

In 1880 (July 28), Trendelenberg, at the suggestion of Newman,[1] first employed acupressure as a means of controlling haemorrhage in hip-joint amputation. "A steel needle 38 centimetres long, 6 millimetres broad, biconvex on cross section, and 2 millimetres thick in the thickest portion or centre, was inserted just below the anterior iliac spine and carried in the direction of the perinaeum, passing between the neck of the femur and the vessels and emerging on the inner aspect of the thigh near the perinaeo-femoral crease. A figure-8 ligature was then thrown over the ends of the needle and in front of the thigh, thus constricting the femoral artery and vein. The limb, having previously been emptied of blood, by the application of Esmarch's bandage as high as the middle of the thigh, a long knife was carried through the front of the thigh 2 centimetres beyond the needle and parallel with it (Lisfranc), and a flap formed by cutting by transfixion. The vessels were then tied, the needle and figure-8 loop removed, and the head of the femur disarticulated. The needle was again introduced behind the bone, the figure-8 carried posteriorly, and the posterior flap then formed."

In 1886 (Aug. 10), Dr. Muscroft, of Cincinnati, employed a similar method.[2] "A needle one eighth inch wide, slightly bent at the point, about the thickness of a dime, and four inches long, was introduced perpendicularly into the front of the thigh, about an inch and a half below Poupart's ligament. The exact point of entrance was one fourth of an inch internal to the combined sheaths of the vein, artery, and nerve. The point was pushed beyond the vessels and turned outward until the needle had passed beyond them ; the point was then pushed out through the integument. The needle was then behind the vessels and nerve. A piece of cord was passed under the heel and point of the needle, forming a figure-8 ligature."

[1] Archiv. fur Klinische Chirurgie B. 26, S. 861, 1881.
[2] Cincinnati Med. News, April, 1887.

Myles,[1] of England, advised a steel skewer to be passed through the thigh, the point entering an inch below Poupart's ligament, going external to the femoral artery and internal to the neck of the femur, emerging a little above the gluteal fold. An India-rubber cord, in figure-8 fashion, is then thrown over the ends of the skewer and the inner aspect of the thigh. Amputation by lateral flaps.

In theory and practice any method of constriction which only controlled a part of the blood-supply at the hip, when in the formation of flaps the other portion was exposed to haemorrhage, must prove less satisfactory than one which permits the operation to be completed with absolute compression of every vessel passing the level of the coxo-femoral joint.

In 1888 I removed the outer half of the clavicle, the glenoid, acromion, and coracoid processes, and part of the body of the scapula, together with the upper extremity, of a patient suffering from a large sarcoma of the upper end of the humerus. Not wishing to do a preliminary deligation of the subclavian in its third division, I transfixed the pectoralis major muscle about three inches from the shoulder with a stout mattress needle, and about the same distance from the joint on the dorsum scapulae I introduced a second needle in such a way that when I carried a strong rubber tube several times around the shoulder under strong traction, above these needles, the compression was so great that haemorrhage was well controlled during amputation. It occurred to me then that the same idea was equally feasible at the hip.

In 1890 I had the good fortune to apply it successfully, and as I now, in the light of subsequent experience, believe, to establish an operation in which haemorrhage at the hip-joint is as safely and easily controlled as at the middle of the thigh. In 1890 I demonstrated the method at the meeting of the American Medical Association at Nashville, at the International Congress in Berlin, and at Louisville before the Mississippi Valley Medical Association.

[1] British Med. Jr., Nov. 9, 1889.

12

Under strict antisepsis the operative technique is as follows: 1. With the patient in the usual position for a hip-joint amputation, the limb should be emptied of blood, either by elevation of the foot and lowering of the trunk, or by the Esmarch bandage applied from the toes to the trunk. Under certain conditions the bandage can be only partially, or may be not at all, applied. When a tumor exists, or when septic infiltration is present, pressure should only be exercised not quite to the diseased portion, for fear of driving septic matter into the vessels. After injuries with great destruction, crushing, or pulpification, of course the Esmarch bandage is not applicable, and one must trust to elevation to save as much blood as possible.

2. While the member is elevated, or before the Esmarch bandage is removed, the rubber-tubing constriction is applied. The object of this constriction—and it is the chief point in the method—is *the absolute occlusion of every vessel at the level of the hip-joint safely above the field of operation.*

To prevent any possibility of the tourniquet slipping, I employ two large mattress needles, or skewers, about three sixteenths of an inch in diameter and ten inches long, one of which is introduced one inch below the anterior superior spine of the ilium and slightly to the inner side of this prominence, and is made to traverse superficially the muscles and fasciae on the outer side of the hip, coming out on a level with, and about three inches from, the point of entrance.

The point of the second needle is entered one inch below the level of the crotch, internally to the saphenous opening, and passing squarely through the adductors, comes out an inch below the tuber ischii. The points are shielded at once by bits of cork, to prevent injury to the hands of the operator. No vessels are endangered by these skewers. A piece of strong white-rubber tube, half an inch in diameter and long enough when tightened in position to go five or six times around the thigh, is now wound very tight around and above the fixation needles and tied. If the Esmarch bandage has been employed, it is now removed.

Dr. Lanphear succeeded in holding the constrictor in place with only one (the outer) needle. Dr. Deaver dispensed with both needles, using a strip of bandage, passed under the tube in front and behind, which were held by assistants who made upward traction. The needles are absolutely safe, easy and cheap to obtain (a piece of telegraph wire will suffice), and entirely out of the way. I see no benefit to be derived by their disuse, and should be afraid to operate without them.

3. In the formation of flaps the surgeon must be guided by the condition of the parts within the field of operation. When permissible, the following-method seems ideal:[1] About six inches below the tourniquet a circular incision is made, and this is joined by a longitudinal incision, commencing at the tourniquet and passing over the trochanter major. A cuff, which includes the subcutaneous tissues down to the deep fasciae, is dissected off to near the level of the trochanter minor. At about the level of the trochanter minor the remaining soft parts, together with the vessels, are divided down to the bone by a circular cut, and in order to facilitate the search for the vessels the soft parts are rapidly removed from the femur for several inches below the line of the divided muscles. At this stage of the operation the larger vessels, *veins* as well as arteries, should be tied with good-sized catgut.[2]

As suggested by Dr. Murdoch, of Pittsburgh, I now leave the entire extremity intact, and use the full length of limb as a lever in dislodging the head of the bone. When the larger and easily recognised vessels have been secured, the

[1] At Bardstown, Kentucky, in August of 1806, Dr. Walter Brashear amputated at the hip, in a negro lad seventeen years old, on account of a severe fracture of the femur and laceration of the soft parts. A circular incision was made, the muscles divided well below the hip-joint, and the vessels secured as the operation progressed. Then a longitudinal incision along the outer side of the limb exposed the remainder of the bone, which, being freed from its muscular attachments, was disarticulated at the socket (Prof. D. W. Yandell in *American Practitioner and News*, 1890). Dieffenbach's name has been associated with this operation prominently among other surgeons, but Dieffenbach did not take his degree in medicine until 1822, sixteen years after the pioneer Kentuckian had performed his operation, the first hip-joint amputation done in the United States.

[2] I employ catgut in all cases, and have never had a secondary haemorrhage.

muscular attachments to the upper extremity of the bone are
lifted off with scissors or knife, keeping along very close to
the bone.   Holding the soft parts away with retractors, the
capsular ligament is exposed and divided in its circumfer-
ence.   Forcible elevation, abduction, and adduction of the
thigh permit the entrance of air into the socket, and at the
same time ruptures the ligamentum teres, and the disarticulation is thus easily and rapidly effected.   Properly con--
ducted up to this point, not a drop of blood has escaped,
except that which was in the limb below the constrictor when
this was applied.   If now the tourniquet be carefully and
gradually loosened, each bleeding point may be determined,
and the forceps applied as required until the tube is entirely
removed.   Should any difficulty be encountered in the effort
at enucleation, which is scarcely possible, the same precaution in securing all bleeding points should be exercised in
removing the tourniquet, and enucleation done with the
tourniquet out of the way.

4. The closure of the wound with the usual precaution of
drainage remains.   I prefer silk-worm gut for suture material, and one good-sized rubber drain from the acetabulum
out at the most dependent part of the wound.

When, by reason of the proximity of a neoplasm, or the
destruction of the parts by accident or disease, this ideal
method is not practicable, any modification may be practised, preference being given to that incision which keeps
farthest from the tumor or gives the healthiest flaps.   When
there is not sufficient material for perfect closure, it is even
safer to err on the side of an unclosed wound and trust to
granulations or grafting for ultimate closing of the wound.

Before concluding the technique, I wish to emphasise a
point of great importance.   When, by reason of severe
haemorrhage before operation, or any pathological anaemia or
condition of weakness, the operation should be rapidly completed, and the small amount of blood which of necessity will
be lost from capillary oozing should be saved, sutures of silk-
worm gut should be rapidly introduced, the wound packed

with hot sterilised plain gauze (not iodoform or bichloride gauze), and the sutures temporarily tightened, for snug compression of the wounded surfaces. This packing at once controls all oozing, and can be removed and the sutures firmly tightened in from 24 to 48 hours after reaction.

I have been able to obtain the histories of thirty-nine amputations at the hip by the foregoing method, of which the following brief histories are given :

I. Dr. John A. Wyeth, New York city, 1890.

Rev. J. H. S., 39. Twelve years ago noticed small, hard tumor in popliteal space. This gradually increased to date, when the whole half of femur was involved, forming a large tumor—osteo-sarcoma. February 4, 1890, first step completed by amputation through femur at lesser trochanter. Second step, enucleation of neck and head, February 20. Recovered without interruption. (First case on record.)

II. Dr. John A. Wyeth, 1890.

J. G., male, 34, February 15, 1883. Neuro-sarcoma of internal popliteal nerve below knee, removed by Dr. D. M. Stimson, October 15, 1888. Recurrence in loco, and amputation at middle and lower third thigh by Dr. Wyeth in February, 1889. Growth recurred in stump in winter of 1889-'90, and March, 1890, amputation on hip. Recovered without interruption.

III. Dr. John A. Wyeth, 1892.

Miss J. B., 17 years. Osteo-sarcoma left femur at knee. First noticed October, 1891. Amputation, February 5, 1892, by Dr. Allen, of Cleveland, O., about middle of femur, wound never healed, growth recurring at once. April 22, 1892, I disarticulated at hip-joint. Recovered.

IV. Dr. M. J. Ahearn, Montreal, Can., 1892.

Male, 22 years, osteo-sarcoma of femur. Patient was subject of acute nephritis, passing four and one half grammes of albumen to every litre of urine. Operation practically bloodless. Patient recovered. (L'Union Med. de Montreal, 1892.)

V. Dr. J. B. Murdoch, Pittsburgh, Pa., 1892.

Male, aged 17, osteo-sarcoma of thigh. Patient died from shock twenty-two hours after the operation, which was done February 20, 1892.

VI. Dr. W. W. Keen, Philadelphia, Pa., 1892.

Female, 30. Enormous osteo-sarcoma of left femur, extending from knee to within ten inches of hip. First symptoms of trouble dated back seventeen months. Operation January, 1892. Patient five months pregnant. Recovered uninterruptedly.

VII. Dr. Frank Hartley, New York city, 1892.

Female, 26 years old. March 19, tumor of tibia near ankle-joint incised. Giant-cell sarcoma made out. March 25, amputation at knee, disclosed femur found to be involved. Amputation at hip, done May 14, 1892. No haemorrhage, no shock, primary union, patient discharged cured June 22, 1892.

VIII. Dr. Chas. McBurney, New York city, 1890.

Male, 84 years old. Sarcoma of lower and middle third of right femur, infiltrating the muscles. Amputation at hip, May 3, 1890. Limb elevated to empty it of blood, but Esmarch's bandage not employed. "The haemorrhage was extremely light and estimated as perhaps an ounce of blood in all, and the operation in consequence was finished with great rapidity." Rapid and uninterrupted recovery.

IX. Dr. J. McFadden Gaston, Atlanta, Ga., November, 1890.

Male, age (?). Enormous osteo-sarcoma of left femur (tumor weighed seventy-three pounds). External iliac artery also tied. Profuse diarrhoea twenty-four hours after operation, which continued for ten days. Died on twenty-sixth day after operation, from septicaemia.

X. Dr. A. J. McCosh, New York city, 1892.

Male, 27. Osteo-sarcoma of femur, involving head, neck, and upper one fourth of shaft. Recovered.

XI. Mr. R. L. Swan, Dublin, Ireland, 1892.

Female, 19. Had morbus coxarius from her fifth year. Pathological dislocation of caput femoris. Thigh and leg extensively infiltrated and burrowed by sinuses. Extremely little shock. Good recovery.

XII. Dr. A. M. Phelps, New York city, 1891.

Male, 55 years. Recurrent sarcoma middle third of thigh, clavicle having been removed two years before for sarcoma. Operation concluded in fourteen minutes. Patient was extremely anaemic. Not more than one ounce of blood in all was lost. Recovered uninterruptedly. Done at Charlottesville, Va.

XIII. Dr. A. M. Phelps, December, 1891.

Male, 24 years. Hip-joint disease of long standing. No shock or rise of temperature, and no bleeding. Patient up on crutches in two weeks.

XIV. Dr. A. M. Phelps, 1892.

Male, 16 years old. Extensive osteitis of whole lower extremity, of two years' duration. Patient almost moribund from septic absorption. Portion of the pelvic bones, which were involved, was also removed. No blood was lost. Patient died from exhaustion twelve hours after operation. Dr. Phelps advised against operation in this case, and only did it at urgent solicitation of parents.

XV. Dr. G. A. Baxter, Chattanooga, Tenn., 1891.

Patient, negro lad, 17 years of age. Compound comminuted fracture and pulpification of right leg and foot and left lower extremity as high as the middle of thigh, in railroad accident. He was hauled in a wagon over a rough country road for two miles. Found by Dr. Baxter in profound shock. As soon as reaction set in, amputation of the right leg at the middle, and of left thigh at the hip-joint. Wyeth's technique closely followed. No loss of blood, and disarticulation easily effected. Patient rallied encouragingly, but four hours after the operation, contrary to the directions of the doctor, he raised himself to the sitting posture, and instantly expired. Heart failure was evidently induced by loss of blood prior to the operation, and to profound shock following the injury, to which was added the shock of operation. "The control of haemorrhage by the method employed was perfect."

XVI. Dr. W. B. Johnston, Ellicottville, N. Y., 1892.

Patient, male, 39 years old. Railway injury, in which foot, leg, and thigh, to a point above the middle third, were pulpified and the femur divided near the trochanter minor. "No arterial bleeding whatever, and only slight oozing from muscles." He died from shock and exhaustion ninety hours after operation.

XVII. Dr. J. D. Thomas, Pittsburgh, Pa., 1891.

Patient aged 18 years. July 31, while attempting to grasp with tongs a red-hot bar of iron passing through the rollers, was struck by the rod in the left thigh. It penetrated, searing through the saphenous and femoral veins and femoral artery. The loss of blood was at once almost fatally profuse. Dr. J. M. Duff, who first saw him, placed a compress and bandage over the wound. As the patient rallied slightly, bleeding occurred, chiefly from the proximal end of the divided femoral vein. Wound packed, by Dr. Thomas, with iodoform gauze; over all, cotton bandage. Heat applied locally and stimulants hypodermically. On third day, amputation at hip proposed on account of threatened gangrene, but not permitted. Ligatures applied to the large vessels. On seventh day, amputation done. Patient rallied well for thirty-six hours, then failed rapidly, and died eight and one half days after the injury.

XVIII. Dr. W. F. Fluhrer, New York city, 1890.

Female, 18 years, osteo-sarcoma of left thigh of six months' history. Spontaneous fracture of thigh at middle, April 26, 1890. Amputation at hip, May 2. July 1, patient was up and out on crutches.

XIX. Dr. B. Merrill Ricketts, Cincinnati, O., 1893.

Female, 23 years of age. Osteo-sarcoma of right thigh. February 2, 1893, "operation bloodless." Recovered promptly.

XX. Dr. C. A. White, Atlanta, Ga., 1891.

. Male, 23 years, osteo-sarcoma of left femur, involving whole length of shaft. Tumor four times the size of thigh. Operation, May 26, 1891. Patient recovered rapidly, gained twenty pounds in weight, by June 22 up on crutches. Seized with acute pneumonia on 27th day, and died five days later. The pneumonia was independent of the operation, as the wound was entirely healed a week before the onset of the malady which carried him off.

XXI. Dr. John B. Deaver, Philadelphia, Pa., October, 1890.

Female, 20. Extensive osteo-arthritis of upper end of femur and acetabulum. Excision of head of femur in 1889 by Dr. J. Ewing Mears.

Numerous sinuses and extensive infiltration of soft parts. November 30, " entirely well."

XXII. Dr. John B. Deaver, 1893.

Male, osteo-myelitis of femur. Greatly emaciated and depressed from long septic absorption. Amount of blood lost did not exceed two ounces. The fixation pins were discarded, and the circular constriction at the hip held up by strips of bandage held by assistant. Good recovery.

XXIII. Dr. J. Ewing Mears, Philadelphia, 1892.

Male, 10 years. Chronic osteo-arthritis of hip and femur. Recovered.

XXIV. Dr. Archibald E. Mallock, Hamilton, Ontario, Can., 1892.

Male, 30. Chronic osteo-arthritis of hip, for which excision of head of femur had been done, December 16, 1891. Amputation, March 12, 1892. Lasted thirty-five minutes, including the dissecting out of several deep sinuses. Recovered.

XXV. Dr. Chas. B. Nancrede, Ann Arbor, Mich., 1893.

Male, 31. Tubercular osteitis of femur as high as the trochanter, with general infiltration of the soft parts. Operation, May 1, 1893. Uninterrupted recovery.

XXVI. Dr. Chas. B. Nancrede, 1892.

Male, 32 years of age. History of injury, L thigh several years before operation. Osteo-sarcoma developed for ten months. Operation, November, 1892. The disease involved the soft structures close to the joint level. Haemorrhage quite free after tube was removed. Recovered.

XXVII. Dr. Emory Lanphear, Kansas City, Mo., 1890.

Male, 9 years, coloured, osteo-myelitis of shaft of femur. Excision of knee, October 21, 1890. October 24, the condition of the patient was so desperate that longer delay meant death. Amputation at the hip was done. Scarcely an ounce of blood was lost. Uninterrupted recovery.

XXVIII. Dr. Emory Lanphear, 1892.

Male, 15 years, "osteo-myelitis of entire shaft of femur, with profound septicaemia." Operation completed in twenty-nine minutes. "Not more than two ounces of blood could have been lost, and this was from parenchymatous oozing." Patient died from septicaemia.

XXIX. Dr. Emory Lanphear, 1892.

Female, 28 years old. Severe neuralgic pain in great toe, for which, in 1888, her physician amputated this member. No relief followed, and Chopart's amputation was done by another operator. Subsequently amputation just above the ankle, then just below the knee; again, through the condyles of the femur; the middle of the thigh. August 28, 1892, Dr. Lanphear amputated at the hip. A sharp process of bone was found developed from the femur near the trochanter. This had penetrated the sciatic nerve, and caused the severe pains. Patient recovered, and was relieved.

XXX. Dr. Emory Lanphear, 1893.

Male, aged 28 years. Osteo-myelitis of shaft of femur, occurring after amputation, at junction of lower and middle third. Operation, February 24, 1893. Recovered without interruption.

XXXI. Dr. Samuel H. Pinkerton, Salt Lake City, Utah Ty., 1892.

Male, 6 years. Compound comminuted gun-shot fracture of femur. Died two hours after operation, from shock.

XXXII. Dr. Samuel H. Pinkerton, 1892.

Male, 17. Extensive tubercular osteitis of femur. Disease in progress many years. Recovery slow. Subsequent curetting of acetabulum.

XXXIII. Dr. Samuel H. Pinkerton, 1892.

Male, 17. Tubercular osteitis of upper end of femur and acetabulum. Recovery. Healed by granulation.

XXXIV. Dr. Samuel H. Pinkerton, 1892.

Male, 17. Osteo-arthritis of femur. Recovered.

XXXV. Dr. Samuel H. Pinkerton, 1892.

Male, 43. Necrosis of femur. Spontaneous fracture. Died ten hours later from shock.

XXXVI. Dr. Samuel H. Pinkerton, 1892.

Male, 42. Extensive necrosis of femur. Recovery. Healed by granulation.

XXXVII. Dr. H. O. Walker, Detroit, Mich., 1892.

Boy, 14. Seven months previous kicked by horse. Osteo-sarcoma at middle of femur. Amputation, September 27, 1892. Recovered.

XXXVIII. Dr. H. O. Walker, 1893.

Male, 21. Six years ago hip-joint disease developed. Joint exsected, August 11, 1892. Amputation, August, 1893. Recovered.

XXXIX. Dr. H. O. Walker, March, 1893.

Young man. Chronic tubercular osteo-arthritis of hip. Operation undertaken with but little hope of success, as he was in very low condition—temperature ranging from 102° to 105°. Died four days after operation.

XL. Dr. F. W. Parham, New Orleans, 1893.

Child, male, 3 years old. Sarcoma of thigh. Recovered.

SYNOPSIS OF FORTY CASES.

No.	Operator.	Date.	Sex.	Age.	Cause of Operation.	Remarks.
1	John A. Wyeth	1890	Male	39	Osteo-sarcoma	First step, divided femur at lesser trochanter. Sixteen days later enucleated remainder of femur.
2	John A. Wyeth	1890	Male	34	Neuro-sarcoma of popliteal nerve, internal	Tumor of internal popliteal extirpated in February, 1888. Recurrence and amputation at lower third thigh, October, 1888. Recurrence in stump and amputation at hip.
3	John A. Wyeth	1892	Female.	17	Osteo-sarcoma of femur at knee, recurrence	Amputation through middle of femur by Dr. Allen of Cleveland, Feb. 5, 1892.
18	William F. Fluhrer	1890	Female.	18	Osteo-sarcoma femur	Spontaneous fracture at middle of thigh, April 26, 1890.
8	Charles McBurney	1890	Male	34	Osteo-sarcoma femur	
7	Frank Hartley	1892	Female.	26	Osteo-sarcoma femur	
19	B. Merrill Ricketts	1883	Female.	23	Osteo-sarcoma femur	
20	C. A. White	1891	Male	23	Osteo-sarcoma femur	Patient was up and about. On 27th day after operation was seized with pneumonia, and died five days later.
12	A. M. Phelps	1891	Male	55	Osteo-sarcoma femur	
6	W. W. Keen	1892	Female.	30	Osteo-sarcoma femur	Patient pregnant five months at date of operation,
4	M. J. Ahearn	1892	Male	22	Osteo-sarcoma femur	

5	J. B. Murdoch	1892	Male	17	Osteo-sarcoma femur	Shock twenty-two hours after operation. Died.
26	Charles B. Nancrede	1892	Male	32	Osteo-sarcoma femur	
9	J. McFadden Gaston	1890	Male	....	Osteo-sarcoma femur	Died on 28th day from septicaemia.
10	A. J. McCosh	1892	Male	27	Osteo-sarcoma femur	
13	A. M. Phelps	1891	Male	24	Distinctive osteo-arthritis of hip, long standing	
14	A. M. Phelps	1892	Male	16	Osteo-myelitis of entire femur	Twelve hours after operation, exhaustion. Patient's condition was so bad advised against operation, but patient insisted. Died.
27	Emory Lanphear	1890	Male	9	Osteo-myelitis of femur	
28	Emory Lanphear	1892	Male	15	Osteo-myelitis of femur	
29	Emory Lanphear	1893	Male	28	Osteo-myelitis of femur	
25	Charles B. Nancrede	1893	Male	31	Osteo-myelitis of femur	
32	Samuel H. Pinkerton	1892	Male	17	Tubercular osteitis femur	
34	Samuel H. Pinkerton	1892	Male	10	Tubercular osteitis femur	
36	Samuel H. Pinkerton	1892	Male	42	Extensive necrosis femur	
35	Samuel H. Pinkerton	1892	Male	43	Extensive necrosis femur	Shock ten hours later. Died.
33	Samuel H. Pinkerton	1892	Male	17	Osteitis of femur	
28	J. Ewing Mears	1892	Male	10	Chronic osteo-arthritis of hip	
24	Archibald E. Mallock	1892	Male	80	Chronic osteo-arthritis of hip	Operation lasted thirty-five minutes.

SYNOPSIS OF FORTY CASES.—*Continued.*

No.	Operator.	Date.	Sex.	Age.	Cause of Operation.	Remarks.
21	John B. Deaver....	1890	Female.	20	Chronic osteo-arthritis of hip..	
22	John B. Deaver....	1868	Male....	....	Osteo-myelitis..........	
11	R. L. Swan..........	1892	Female.	19	Chronic osteo-arthritis....	
15	G. A. Baxter........	1891	Male....	17	Railroad pulpification of right leg and foot, and lower extremity as high as middle of thigh....	Patient rallied well. Four hours later raised himself in bed and reached for cup of water, and instantly expired.
16	W. B. Johnston....	1892	Male....	39	Railroad pulpification of foot, leg, and up to middle of thigh..	Exhaustion, and shock ninety hours later. Died.
17	J. D. Thomas........	1891	Male....	18	Division of femoral vessel in Scarpa's span by red-hot bar. Impending gangrene.	Profuse hemorrhage at accident. Seventh day after injury, amputation. Died in thirty-six hours.
31	Samuel H. Pinkerton	1892	Male....	6	Compound comminuted gun-shot fracture femur......	Shock two hours after operation. Died.
30	Emory Lanphear....	1892	Female.	28	Osteoma of femur penetrating sciatic nerve.........	
37	H. O. Walker........	1892	Male....	14	Osteo-sarcoma of femur......	
38	H. O. Walker........	1868	Male....	21	Chronic osteo-arthritis of hip..	
39	H. O. Walker........	1868	Male....	....	Chronic osteo-arthritis of hip..	Exhaustion in four days. Died.
40	F. W. Parham........	1868	Male....	8	Sarcoma of thigh.............	

This limited number of cases—40 in all—gives a death rate of 22.05 per cent.

Sarcoma,	17 cases,	2 deaths,	11.75	per cent.
Inflammatory bone disease,	18 "	3 "	16.6	"
Violence,	4 "	4 "	100.	"
Nerve injury,	1 ,		——	

For disease,	36 cases,	5 deaths,	13.88	per cent.
For injury,	4 "	4 "	100.	

Ashurst's table of 633 cases gives a total mortality of 64.1 per cent.

For disease,	276 cases;	death-rate,	40.2	per cent.
For injury,	309 "	"	82.4	"

Luming gives,—

Gunshot wounds,	289 cases;	death-rate,	98	per cent.
Disease,	153 "	"	42	"

Without discussing statistics, I claim it safe to conclude that, by the method given, bleeding after hip-joint amputation is as safely and securely controlled as for an amputation of the thigh lower down.

In no single case has it failed, and it has been employed now by operators of all grades of experience.

Prof. W. W. Keen, who employed this operation successfully at Jefferson hospital, Philadelphia, in January, 1892, for an enormous sarcoma of the thigh (the patient being five months pregnant), in reviewing all the methods of controlling haemorrhage, said,[1] "It was reserved for an American surgeon to devise what is undoubtedly the best method, and, in fact, what I think we may call now the only method of haemostasis in amputation at the hip-joint."

Prof. J. B. Murdoch, of Pittsburgh, who has four times performed hip-joint amputation, and once by my method, says,[2]

[1] Medical News, March 26, 1892.
[2] Annals of Surgery, January, 1893.

"I believe this method to be the best, and the one destined to supersede all other methods for the temporary arrest of haemorrhage."

Prof. W. F. Fluhrer[1] emphasised—what was evident to all —that as little blood had been lost as in an ordinary amputation at the middle of the thigh.

Professor McBurney[2] expressed the opinion that no other appliance that had been suggested for the purpose could in any way compare in utility with that of Dr. Wyeth.

Prof. Emory Lanphear, of Kansas City, who has four times amputated at the hip by this method, says,[3] "This operation (Senn's)[4] is certainly better than any other yet devised, save that which is known as the 'Wyeth bloodless method,' by which method failure to control haemorrhage seems to me to be impossible."

Prof. McFadden Gaston, of Atlanta,[5] says, "There was absolutely no trouble from haemorrhage . . . and I feel satisfied that with this process all bleeding may be prevented in amputation at the hip-joint."

Dr. B. Merrill Ricketts, of Cincinnati, writes me that "The operation was entirely bloodless."

Dr. W. B. Johnston, of Ellicottsville, N. Y., writes, "There was not one drop of arterial blood, and only a slight venous oozing from the muscular tissue."

Prof. H. O. Walker says, "We have in this a safe and reliable method for controlling haemorrhage, which, in my judgment, is superior to any yet offered."   ·

[1] International Journal of Surgery, 1890.
[2] Ibid.
[3] Kansas City Medical Journal, May, 1893.
[4] The method devised by Prof. N. Senn requires an incision eight inches in length, commencing three inches above the trochanter. The capsule, trochanter, and upper portion of shaft are exposed, the trochanteric muscular attachments severed, the digital fossa emptied, the capsule divided, and the head of the femur dislocated, before any constriction for the control of haemorrhage is attempted. I do not think the method will be received with favour by surgeons. The only instance in which it has been applied, to my knowledge, was by Dr. W. D. Foster, of Kansas City. "The patient was the subject of chronic coxitis, was much emaciated, and very weak. The operation was tedious, protracted, and bloody, and the patient survived between three and four hours."—Private Communication.
[5] Transactions Alabama State Medical Association, 1892.

By personal communication, Professors McCosh, Baxter, A. M. Phelps, and Hartley have expressed themselves that the method met every requirement in the prevention of loss of blood.

The question of *shock* is very important in this major operation. It is strongly brought out by Professor Murdoch, who insists that "the greatest care must be exercised to maintain the vital forces, by the moderate use of stimulants before the operation, and the protection of the surface of the body from cold and exposure during its performance." To this should be added the minimum of anaesthetic and the maximum of rapidity in technique consistent with thoroughness and the prevention of bleeding. When ether is employed, the Ormsby inhaler secures the safest narcosis, with the smallest amount of ether.

DISCUSSION.

Dr. JOSEPH D. BRYANT, of New York county, thought there was but little to be said about the paper itself, for the statistics presented sufficiently emphasised the value of this method of amputation. The operation speaks for itself, and the profession owes its thanks to Dr. Wyeth, who has so fortunately combined the use of the skewer with that of the elastic pressure.

Dr. D. McLEAN of Detroit, Mich., said he had listened to the paper with very great pleasure, and he was sure he voiced the sentiment of every member present when he said we were very much indebted to the author for his presentation of the subject. Yet, with all honesty, he felt compelled to say that he thought there was a better method still: he referred to compression of the abdominal aorta, which, he held, could be done without the slightest danger to any organ or the slightest uncertainty as to the control of haemorrhage. Even though the parts be unusually vascular, the abdominal tourniquet may be adjusted with the utmost nicety. He would speak more in detail when he read his paper.

Dr. REGINALD H. SAYRE, of New York, said he had not had any personal experience with Wyeth's method, but it seemed to him that in the majority of cases it would be most advantageous. Nevertheless, he thought at times the elastic ligature would come unpleasantly close to the upper end of the femur, so that very little room would be left for enucleation of the femur. He had done amputation at the hip in two instances,—one for sarcoma, and the other for osteo-myelitis. In the one case, he used Trendelenburg's needles, with a figure-8 in front and behind the thigh, and in that case the haemorrhage was perfectly controlled at the time of removing the bone, although there was considerable capillary oozing after the removal of the constricting band. In the second case, he used the Jordan-Lord method of controlling the haemorrhage. Here, too, the haemorrhage was well controlled, and there was more space for operating. Both cases recovered. Dr. Wyeth had not published his description at that time, or he would have tried it.

Dr. WYETH, in closing the discussion, said that he did not place much value on the statistics based on such a small number of cases: it was, rather, an endorsement of the technique. The mortality had been reduced from sixty-four per cent. to twenty-two per cent., but, of course, this was partly due to the improved technique of modern surgeons. The four cases of injury, it was true, yielded one hundred per cent. mortality, but all of them were very severe injuries. He did not think the abdominal tourniquet would ever hold out in the race with direct compression. The little constricting band holds all the vessels which pass out from the body into the thigh, and he could not imagine a condition in which it could not be applied without interfering with the operation.

THE TREATMENT OF ANGULAR DEFORMITIES AT THE HIP-JOINT.

By Reginald H. Sayre, M. D., of New York County.

October 10, 1893.

Like a very large proportion of the cases which come to the orthopedic surgeon for treatment, the best thing to do for angular deformities at the hip-joint is to prevent their occurrence by proper treatment in the first place, and I hold that any patient who has sufficient recuperative power to recover from an inflammation in the hip-joint should do so with the legs practically parallel and in a straight line with the body. But it very frequently happens that cases are so treated that they do not recover in this favourable position, but, when the symptoms of active inflammation have all passed by, the limb is left in a practically useless condition from the amount of deformity present.

The treatment to be adopted in these cases varies with the nature of the disease which produced the deformity, and with the condition of the joint at the time the patient comes under observation, and these conditions differ so widely that very different means must be adopted in different instances to secure a favourable result. Perhaps I can best make this clear by detailing the history of a few cases of different classes of injuries at the hip, accompanied by subsequent distortion.

CASE I. D. D., Salt Lake City, Utah, a miner, about forty-five years of age, stout, thick-set man, was seen in August, 1886. Nine months previously, while working in a coal mine, the ground gave way and fell upon him, burying him out of sight. It was estimated there were about five tons of earth in the mass which covered him. When dug out, the left femur was found to be broken just above the knee, and the right hip injured. He was stooping when injured, and received the blow on the small of the back and buttocks. Was confined to bed for two months,

13

and did not know whether his right hip was broken or not. Bed-sores formed in less than two weeks and the catheter was necessary part of the time, so that it is probable that his spinal cord was injured. When he finally got out of bed and moved about on crutches he could not move his right hip or knee, and his right leg seemed short to him. After consultation with various physicians, who decided nothing could be done, he was sent to New York. He was a large, healthy-looking man, and when first seen walked with a very marked limp, using a cane to support himself, and stooping a great deal. Had marked difficulty in removing his clothes, as his right hip and knee were ankylosed and the thigh flexed on the body at an angle of thirty degrees and strongly adducted. Measurement of the limbs, as accurately as could be done in their distorted position, seemed to show that the shortening of the right leg was due simply to flexion and adduction. The left knee could be flexed to a right angle, and no more on account of the callus formed by the old fracture just above the knee. The right hip and knee seemed to be firmly ankylosed, but on attempting to move the joint violently (while an assistant held the pelvis securely) more or less pain was caused, and I therefore concluded that the ankylosis was not bony. My experience in these cases is, that if the ankylosis is bony, efforts to move the joint are not attended by pain in the joint at the time or subsequently, and that if your efforts at movement are followed by pain it is very certain proof that it is simply strong fibrous ankylosis, and that your efforts have caused more or less irritation.

Concluding in this case, therefore, that the ankylosis was only fibrous, I referred the patient to a friend for treatment, but he returned in a few days saying that the doctor had advised him not to undergo operation, as the risk was more than the probable benefit. I decided in this case to use massage daily, and active and passive movements rather than to attempt to break up the joints by force. Slight movements were given to the knee and hip every day after the tissues in the neighbourhood of these joints had been thoroughly massaged, and in the course of a month I was able to bend the right knee to a right angle, and move the hip somewhat. The motions became freer and freer in these joints until, in two months from the time when the patient was put under treatment, he could stand on either leg and put the other foot on the seat of a chair in front of him, and could abduct his legs sufficiently wide to ride on horseback, and could cross one leg over the other, bringing the thighs close against the chest, and rise again without assistance.

From contraction of the psoas and iliacus muscles of the right side, which had not yet entirely relaxed, the right limb was a quarter of an inch shorter than the left, but with this amount of elevation on the sole and heel of his shoe he walked with hardly any limp, and returned to work. The photographs which will be passed around show the degree of movement.

CASE II. G. M., North Carolina, age twenty-three, had typhoid fever in the spring of 1893, and after the fever had apparently passed by, was attacked with acute synovitis in the left hip, knee, and ankle. His famlly physician thought the joints would suppurate, but the inflammation eventually subsided without formation of any abscess. When seen by me, in September, 1898, he was in a very emaciated condition, had marks of numerous old bed-sores on his body, and walked with great difficulty by the aid of two crutches. His left thigh was rotated so far inward that the head of the femur could be distinctly felt posterior to the trochanter major. His excessive emaciation allowed the limb to be rotated inward almost as far as it is possible on a skeleton, bringing the left knee behind the right, the left foot being turned at right angles to its normal position. There was marked varus of the foot, very limited motion in the ankle-joint, and limited motion in the knee. The adductor tendons in this case were not tense, as in the preceding instance, the joint being held in its position apparently by thickening of the capsular ligament and adjacent structures. After handling and massaging the joint for a few days, having been able to satisfy myself that there was no bony ankylosis in the hip, I felt a slight movement and yielding of the bands that held the joint in its distorted position while I was manipulating the limb one day, and feeling the joint thus yielding, applied immediate force and brought the limb into a normal position, the movement being accompanied by a loud report, like a pistol shot, caused by the rupture of some of the tight adhesions surrounding the capsule. I should have used an anaesthetic on this patient, but under the circumstances, when I felt part of the resistance yield, I preferred to break the joint completely at once and then immobilise it rather than to run the risk of setting up a fresh inflammation by irritating it slightly and subsequently irritating it still further by divided attempts at reduction, which would have been the case had I ceased at this time and completed the operation under anaesthesia at a subsequent time. As soon as I had brought the leg into a straight line with its fellow and in a straight line with the body, I applied a hoop-iron splint of the Thomas pattern, as well as an anterior wire splint to prevent, as far as possible, any movement in the joint. These cases of *brisement forcé* require absolute rest of the joint for ten days to a fortnight after the operation, and sometimes the addition of ice bags to prevent subsequent inflammation.

The patient's joint was intensely painful for a couple of days following the operation; but inside of two weeks the pain had disappeared, and gradual motions were begun for the purpose of restoring the joint to its normal function, which are at the present time being continued.

CASE III. W. H., North Carolina, age twelve, had hip disease between three and four years of age; was treated in a haphazard fashion with a long traction splint improperly applied, and finally recovered in the position shown in photographs which I exhibit, the left thigh being flexed on the body at an angle of fifty degrees, adducted strongly as far as his flesh would permit, and apparently ankylosed. Examining the boy without an anaesthetic, I thought I detected slight motion in the hip, and proceeded therefore to make a section of the adductor muscles and of the psoas and iliacus through an anterior incision, but found that I was unable (with any force which I felt justified in using) to break up the adhesions between the femur and acetabulum. I accordingly attempted to chisel the femur through just below the lesser trochanter, making use of the anterior incision which I had made for the purpose of cutting the psoas and iliacus muscles. When I had cut part way through the bone, very violent haemorrhage commenced from a point a little below and close to the under surface of the femur, which I was able to arrest only after tedious effort, the bleeding point having been caught by forceps passed down very deep in the wound, and which I was obliged to leave fastened to the vessel, as I was unable to pass a ligature around their point. I presume that the edge of the chisel must have projected slightly from the bone and cut the internal circumflex artery or some branch of it. The wound was packed, leaving the forceps in position, and the boy rallied well from the operation; and some weeks later, when the wound had healed, I did a subcutaneous osteotomy of the left femur just below the trochanter minor, brought the leg into as nearly a normal position as possible, and applied a plaster of Paris dressing from the toes to the arm-pits, strengthening it in front with a wire splint. By means of this plaster splint the hip-joint was kept as nearly at rest as possible, while it was very easy to change the boy's position by means of a couple of swings passed around his body and attached to a block and tackle which hung from a wooden frame over the bed. His recovery was uneventful, and in two months' time he was walking about on both legs, with a very trifling limp, in erect position, as shown in photographs.

CASE IV. Miss Z., Wisconsin, age twenty-three, when about twelve years old, had what was called an attack of rheumatism, and which she attributed to getting wet by wading in a brook in the late fall. Severe inflammation of both her hips, her right knee, and both ankles followed. The right ankle suppurated, and bone was discharged from the sinuses. When seen by me, there were large scars on the sacrum and near the left hip. Whether these were the result of old bed-sores, or an inflammation of the bone, I was unable to determine from the history. She had bony ankylosis of both hip-joints, both thighs being flexed on the body at about fifty degrees, the right one adducted and the left strongly adducted, very much in the position she would assume if riding on a side-saddle. The motion in the right ankle was quite limited, a large bony deposit in front of the astragalus preventing the foot from coming to a right angle with the leg. The motions in the right knee were also slightly limited; she walked with great difficulty, by means of canes, and presented a very distorted appearance. After unsuccessfully attempting to break up the ankylosis at the hips, the pelvis at this time being firmly secured to a table by large clamps, I made an incision over the left trochanter major, as if to perform excision, thinking that it might be possible to chisel the head of the femur loose from its attachments, and make a movable joint by digging out a new acetabulum; but found the two bones united by so thick and extensive a deposit of new bone that this was impracticable, and I therefore chiselled through the femur just below the smaller trochanter, brought the leg in straight line with the body, and secured it temporarily with a wire splint. Having sewed up the incision tightly and painted it with iodoform collodion, I then turned her on the other side and did a subcutaneous osteotomy, also below the smaller trochanter, without attempting to form a false joint, as I had proposed to do on the other side. This wound was also closed, and sealed with iodoform collodion. The patient was then incased in plaster of Paris bandages, from the arm-pits to the toes of both feet, the plaster being reinforced by iron-wire splints laid on the front of each thigh and running up over the thorax and secured by additional layers of plaster bandages. A strip of corn-plaster felt was placed along the back for protection before applying the elastic bandages.

I cannot too highly recommend this means of putting up osteotomies of the femur, and also fractures of the femur high up, the ease with which patients can be shifted from one position to another, and their necessary wants attended to, being altogether greater than by means of any other dressings which I have tried; and when the patient is an adult, and weighing perhaps one hundred and fifty pounds, it is very difficult for them to be moved except by means of a block and tackle attached to a stout beam over the bed. Unless a very rigid splint is applied, there is almost certain to be movement at the hips when the patient's weight hangs suspended by means of straps passing under the body and lower extremities; and in these cases it is of the utmost importance that the dressing should be sufficiently secure not to require new adjustment until the fractured bone shall have had a chance to become consolidated.

At the end of two weeks I cut the dressing in two on the right femur, at the point where the hip and body join, adjusted the position of the limb slightly, and rejoined the portions of this splint by new bandages and wire. The patient made an uneventful recovery, and her position before and after the operation is shown in the photographs which I pass around.

From my experience in various cases of ankylosis about the hip, I have found that many of the distortions following hip disease, which are supposed to be due to contraction of the tendons around the joint, are in reality retained in place much more by the adhesions about the capsule and between the bones, and that in many cases the cutting of the tendons alone will be insufficient to allow reduction of the deformity. I believe it is a simpler and safer operation, in many instances, to do a subcutaneous osteotomy below the trochanter minor than to endeavour to cut, either subcutaneously or through an open incision, the adhesions which retain the joint in its distorted position. I have also learned that it is very easy to be mistaken in regard to the presence of movement in a joint, and that we very frequently imagine we feel a slight amount of motion in ankylosed hips, whereas the motion is really between the flesh and the bone, or in the sacro-iliac synchondrosis; and even in joints which are more easily accessible (as the knee and elbow), I have seen men of large experience deceived in supposing that movement was present, when subsequent operation showed firm, bony ankylosis.

In regard to the choice between osteotomy or *brisement forcé*, a good deal must be left to the judgment of the operator and determined by the conditions of each individual case, and there are certain cases where I believe the dangers of reëxciting inflammation in the joint by *brisement forcé* are so great that I think it is safer to do an osteotomy. If the joint is to be broken up, I believe in making section of all constricting bands which can be safely cut, breaking up the adhesions thoroughly under an anaesthetic, placing the limb at once in the required position, and then keeping the part absolutely at rest until all pain, swelling, and tenderness has subsided; and I find benefit in many instances by diminishing the blood-supply to the joint by means of moderate compression over the artery which supplies it. After the joint is completely free from pain, slight motions should be given every day to restore its function, but never carried to the point of producing pain or tenderness which will last as long as twenty-four hours. If your efforts to restore functions are followed by increased heat or tenderness, cease your manipulations, and be content with the improved position and a stiff joint. If, however, as in Case I, there is slight motion in the joint, and the employment of gradual manipulation and massage is not followed by inflammatory reaction, continue the procedures daily, increasing in force and frequency as experience warrants, and in many instances you will be able to cause absorption of inflammatory deposits, break down old adhesions, and restore excellent motion in joints which have been considered useless for months, and sometimes for years.

TREATMENT OFTEN INDICATED AFTER TRA-CHELORRHAPHY.

By W. H. Robb, M. D., of Montgomery County.

October 12, 1893.

If the treatment of diseases of women was always successful and satisfactory; if the complications associated with
laceration of the cervix could be removed before the operation, as first suggested by Dr. T. A. Emmet; if no inflammatory disease was excited or rekindled by the operation itself,
and if complete union of the torn surfaces always followed
trachelorrhaphy, there would be but little, if any, excuse for
presenting the following paper. These results in the majority of patients are obtained. The treatment proves satisfactory, and the results of the operation are all that could be
desired. The womb is restored to its normal condition, and
the woman to her former health. In a few these happy results are not secured. The womb is not restored to its normal condition, neither is the woman restored to usefulness.
It has been my misfortune to have had a few of the latter
class of patients. Complications were found in a few women
who had received both their treatment and operation at the
hands of one of the most experienced surgeons in New York
city. They have also followed my own operations. They
have been in my hands the most obstinate and unsatisfactory
cases that I have had to treat. It is for this reason that I
ask your attention to "Treatment often Indicated after
Trachelorrhaphy."

It is with deep feelings of regret that I frankly acknowledge that after long, faithful, and persistent treatment, a few
of these women have been but little benefited. They remain
in much the same condition as before the operation. To
fully appreciate the condition of the woman who needs treat-

ment after trachelorrhaphy, we must inquire into the anatomy of those organs that are most concerned in keeping up
pelvic disease; their location in the pelvis; the changes
brought about in the uterus by operation; the process of
involution; with the complications resulting from laceration
of the cervix. The uterus is located between the bladder
and rectum, the base resting on a line below the brim of the
pelvis. It is retained in its position by the broad and round
ligaments on either side. In the virgin state the uterus
measures three inches in length, two in breadth, and one
inch in thickness, and weighs from an ounce to an ounce
and a half. Its blood-supply is derived from the uterine
artery, a branch of the internal iliac, and the ovarian, from
the aorta. They are remarkable for their tortuous course in
the substance of the organ, and for their frequent anasto-
moses. The veins are of large size, and correspond with the
arteries. In the impregnated uterus these vessels form the
uterine sinuses. They terminate in the uterine plexuses.
The lymphatics are of large size, and terminate in the pelvic
and lumbar glands. The nerves are derived from the inferior hypogastric and spermatic plexuses, and from the third
and fourth sacral nerves. As the greater bulk of the uterus
is composed of muscular tissue, we may consider the whole
organ as a hollow muscle. The posterior and superior surfaces, and two thirds of its anterior surface, are covered with
peritonaeum. Its cavity is lined with mucous membrane,
which extends out through the Fallopian tube to the fimbriated extremities. The Fallopian tube, on either side, takes
its origin from the superior angle of the uterus, and is about
four inches in length. The canal through the inner half of
the tube is very small. The tube terminates in a dilated and
fringed extremity, the fringes being called fimbriae. The
tube lies in the free margin of the broad ligament, and extends from the fundus of the uterus to the side of the pelvis.
The ovary, on either side of the uterus, lies below the tube,
in the posterior part of the broad ligament. It is oval and
elongated in shape, an inch and a half in length, three quar-

ters of an inch in width, and a third of an inch thick. It is attached to the uterus by a ligament, and by a ligamentous cord to the fimbriated extremity of the tube.

The changes that occur in the different structures of the uterus during gestation, and that begin immediately after conception, are described by Lusk as follows: "The uterus from the inception of pregnancy increases in vascularity. Its mucous membrane becomes soft and thickened. The muscular fibres are increased seven to eleven times in length, and three to five times in width. During the first five months new muscular fibres are developed, especially upon the inner layer of the uterus. The delicate connective-tissue processes between the muscular fibres become more abundant, and toward the termination of pregnancy display distinct fibril- lae. The vessels increase in number, length, and circumfer- ence. The arteries, as we have noticed, assume a spiral course, and in places communicate directly with the veins. The veins are dilated, and form—especially in the placental region—wide-meshed net-work. The walls of the veins are intimately united with the muscular walls of the uterus, and form, when divided, open-mouthed canals. The lymphatics, starting from the spongy tissues of the lining mucous mem- brane, traverse the muscular structures, and are gathered up by abundant plexuses, which are distributed especially over the fundus and sides of the womb. The nerves increase in length and thickness, and grow inward toward the uterine cavity. Upon the inner surface of the uterus ganglia may be found. The bulk of the uterus is greatly increased by these textural changes. From an ounce the uterus is in- creased to two and a half to three pounds during gestation. In volume it is proportionately increased. In length it is increased from three inches at the time of conception to twelve inches at the end of the ninth month."

In width it is increased from two to nine inches during gestation. According to Levret, the surface of the virgin uterus measures sixteen square inches, while that of the preg- nant uterus at term measures three hundred and thirty-nine square inches. The uterine cavity is stated by Krause to be enlarged five hundred and nineteen times. Immediately after labour the uterus weighs from two to three pounds; it is from seven to eight inches in length, and four and a half inches broad. The walls of the uterus are from an inch to an inch and a half thick. Involution begins with the first labour pain, and is completed in six or eight weeks after labour. During the first week following labour the uterus loses one pound in weight, and is reduced two inches in length and one in width. At the end of two weeks it is reduced to three fourths of a pound in weight, five inches in length, and its walls to half an inch in thickness. During involution the muscular walls of the uterus undergo fatty degeneration and are absorbed. Through this process the uterus is restored almost to its original condition, both in size and weight.

This is the usual course after normal labour. Either accident or disease may check or prevent involution. Months and years after a complicated labour we may, and often do, find that this process has not been completed; the uterus is still as large and heavy as it should have been at the end of the second week. We have a condition of sub-involution of the womb. This is due to injuries received during labour, or to the complications that immediately follow. Sub-involution is due more frequently to laceration of the cervix than to any other cause. General inertia of the womb, or an excessive loss of blood from a torn vessel, may immediately follow this accident. This is not only a great shock to the nervous system, but it is a powerful factor in establishing the profound anaemia, from which the woman suffers later. The lochia is not only profuse, but the flow continues for days and weeks. Septic poisoning follows, *i. e.*, there is absorption of putrid matter. Slight febrile excitement, lasting for a few days, may result; or we may have a severe or even fatal case of puerperal septicaemia. From the same source we may have phlebitis, lymphangitis, metritis, perimetritis, or endometritis, not only involving the endometrium, but extending out through, and implicating, the tubes and peritonaeum.

If the woman escapes death from one or more of these conditions, and recovers sufficiently to be about on her feet, she soon begins to suffer from other symptoms, very distressing at times, the result of descent or displacement of the uterus. The weight of the organ crowds it down in the pelvis, until the cervix rests against the posterior vaginal wall. In this position, eversion and erosion of the torn surfaces soon follow, as does inflammation of the cervical glands and hypertrophy of the whole neck. From the position and sub-involuted condition of the uterus the circulation of blood in the pelvis is impeded, and a condition of congestion of all the pelvic organs arises. The uterus, left after labour in a condition of sub-involution, is more or less changed in its structure by congestion and repeated attacks of inflammation to which its several structures are exposed. To the condition of fatty degeneration has been added the results from inflammation. In this connection I will quote a single paragraph from Dr. West, who says, "It must, however, be apparent, that after inflammation has passed away its effects may remain in the large size and altered structure of the womb, and that the very nature of these changes will be such as to render the repair of the damaged organ both unlikely to occur and slow to be accomplished, and must leave it in a condition peculiarly liable to be aggravated during the fluctuations of circulation and alterations of activity and repose to which the female sexual system is liable."

This condition has been described by different authors under different titles. Dr. T. G. Thomas describes it under the title of "Areolar Hyperplasia." This would indicate that the enlargement of the uterus is due to increased growth of connective tissue, the result of hyperaemia of the organ. A case beginning as one of sub-involution terminates in hyperplasia. It is in this very condition that trachelorrhaphy is particularly indicated. In the great majority of cases, the operation is followed by the most gratifying results; in a

few, but little, if any, good follows.   In those not benefited,
who have fallen under my care, I have found complications
that seemed sufficient to account for the failure.   That some
of these had existed before the operation I am quite certain.
Others may have been rekindled or excited by the operation,
or been developed later through its failure.   While there is
much in common in the condition of these patients, still
there may not be two suffering from exactly the same complications. Congestion, enlargement, weight, and displacement
are common.   Other conditions complicate individual cases.

The treatment after trachelorrhaphy may be considered as
general and local.   The general treatment requires the careful supervision of the hygienic surroundings of the patient,
the selection of suitable dietetics, and the judicious administration of needful medicine.   Much of our success will
depend on the care with which this part of the treatment is
managed.   The local trouble rarely improves, until the general health of the woman is made better.

I must not omit to mention two drugs from which I have
gotten especially good results.   These are mercury and
iodide of potassium.   The one seems " to unload the portal
circulation," thus relieving pelvic congestion.   The other, by
an alterative action, changes the nutrition of the uterine tissues.   The local treatment must vary, and should be adapted
to meet indications required in individual patients.   Each
complication may require a line of treatment particularly for
its removal.   All are familiar with the benefits derived from
placing the woman in bed and giving her regularly hot vaginal douches, using glycerine tampons, elevating the uterus to
its normal plane in the pelvis by the use of a suitable pessary
or woolen tampon, applying compound tincture of iodine
to the vault of vagina, cervix, and endometrium, taking
blood locally from the cervix, and puncturing the cervical
glands as they become inflamed and distended.   This seems
to be appropriate treatment, and is advised in all cases complicated by any pelvic inflammation.   Three months of such
treatment often originates an improvement that terminates

in recovery. Pelvic cellulitis, pelvic peritonitis, catarrhal endometritis, and salpingitis are often removed by this treatment alone.

In considering the treatment of complications that are found after trachelorrhaphy, I shall refer only to those that have fallen under my own observation. The one I have most frequently met is endometritis, complicated either with catarrhal salpingitis or fungus degeneration of the endometrium. Without treatment, these conditions become chronic. For their relief, I have obtained the best results from dilating the cervix, scraping the entire endometrium with a sharp curette, and from packing and draining the cavity of the uterus with antiseptic gauze.

We sometimes find the uterus tied down by adhesions in either a retroverted or retroflexed position. These adhesive deposits follow attacks of pelvic peritonitis.

I can advise but two remedies for the relief of these conditions. These are Galvanism and abdominal section. The pessary has in these conditions proven a snare and delusion to the physician, and a curse to the woman. The inflammatory deposit is in many cases removed by the use of Galvanism. The electric current seems to dissolve all the deposit, after which it is absorbed and removed. The uterus, thus freed from its abnormal attachments, soon returns to its normal position and mobility in the pelvis. Electricity not only removes the inflammatory deposit, but at the same time reduces the size and weight of the womb. This is probably due to its destructive influence on the formation of new connective tissue, to which the hyperplasia is largely due. If Galvanism is thoroughly used, I am led to believe that but few of these cases will require abdominal section for their relief. If not benefited by this agent, and still suffering severely from either of these conditions, I believe the woman should have an abdominal section, through which the adhesions may be separated, and the uterus elevated and fixed by sutures to the abdominal wall in front, as suggested by Dr. A. Palmer Dudley, of New York.

If laceration of the perinaeum is a complicating factor, it should be repaired, with the hope that it will materially assist in supporting the vagina, bladder, and uterus in their normal positions, and thus assist in restoring the healthy circulation of the blood through the pelvic organs. Inflammatory deposits, the result of cellulitis, are readily removed from the pelvis by Galvanism.

If suppuration exist in either tube, and the condition is not improved by the treatment already suggested,—*i. e.*, dilatation of the cervix, scraping the endometrium, packing and draining the cavity of the uterus with antiseptic gauze—I believe the diseased tube, and the diseased one only, should be removed. If both tubes are diseased, both should be removed by abdominal section.

If disease of either ovary is found, or it is believed to exist, an abdominal opening should be made, and as much of the organ as is diseased should be removed. If the whole of either ovary is diseased, it, with the tube on the corresponding side, should be removed. I have lately had under treatment a case of hyperplasia, that resisted all remedial measures, and was finally relieved by the removal of both tubes and ovaries. In this case, both ovaries and tubes were diseased and required removal. Whether this woman will be as much benefited by the removal of the tubes and ovaries as she would have been if the uterus had also been removed with the appendages, as suggested by Dr. William N. Polk, of New York, is a question for discussion before this Association. As the operation has been but lately made, I shall watch the results with a great deal of anxiety and curiosity. Chronic enlargement of the womb is sometimes due to imperfect union between the freshened surfaces of the torn cervix. It is difficult to say whether this is the fault of the surgeon or the fault of the woman. It may be due to faulty nutrition in the cervix, by which nature fails to throw out enough plastic material with which to bind firmly the parts together. It may be the fault of the surgeon, who fails in securing the properly freshened and coaptated surfaces. Let the fault be where it may, the fact is the same,—the woman has been but little, if any, benefited by the operation. A second and more perfect operation is the only remedy for this condition.

I was told very recently, by one of the most successful surgeons in New York, that most of his operations were now made for the purpose of obtaining better results than had been secured by previous operators. In his own practice he had been obliged to operate three times on the same woman before he secured the desired results.

It is through the removal of these complicating conditions that we succeed in restoring these women to health, usefulness, and happiness.

In conclusion, I wish to say that it has been my experience to find after periods of treatment extending over years of time, during which the most carefully regulated general treatment had been pursued, combined with such medicinal and local treatment as the case seemed to require, that some of my patients had been but little benefited, either by trachelorrhaphy, or by the treatment that had followed the operation. The uterus was still large, dense, and heavy. I have yet to learn whether in this particular class of patients any treatment short of the menopause, the removal of both tubes and ovaries, or the extirpation of the uterus with its appendages, can be offered for their relief.

I hope the conditions alluded to in this paper will be freely discussed by the Fellows of the associations, so that from their combined experience we may learn much to aid us in making our treatment in the future more successful.

DISCUSSION.

Dr. A. PALMER DUDLEY, of New York county, said the title of the paper confused him somewhat; he would rather change it so as to read, "The treatment indicated *before* trachelorrhaphy," for it is well known that many of the conditions demanding treatment after trachelorrhaphy should have been carried out before the operation. Certainly trachelorrhaphy is not a panacea for all the ills of the female pelvis, and it is a fact that in those cases where failure is met with there has been an error in the diagnosis. He was speaking now of cases in general, and not of those described in the paper.

He did not approve of the term "areolar hyperplasia," or "chronic uterine infarct," as it is sometimes called, for the areolar tissue, which is supposed to originate after delivery, he believed was already in the uterus at the time of labour, and that a little sepsis, or a continuation of congestion from some cause or other, retains that cellular tissue in the organ which nature put there during pregnancy. Hence, he believed, the term "subinvolution" is the more appropriate one for this condition.

If, then, we have to treat sub-involution, or the consequences of it, chronic endometrial trouble—not necessarily inflammation, but, for example, a swollen and over-vascular mucous membrane—trachelorrhaphy will not aid us. We really do every such patient an injury by sewing up the cervix, for the reason that free drainage is absolutely necessary, and we really are interfering with nature's efforts to cure. Where there is congestion of the tubes, as indicated by tenderness or irregular menstruation, or tenderness of the cellular tissue not amounting to inflammation, where the mucous membrane bleeds on the slightest touch, and the cervix is scarred, he does not begin by treating the cervical canal, if the patient's circumstances will permit; but by putting the uterus in proper position, and restoring the endometrium to a normal condition. After using a moderately dull curette, and washing out the uterine cavity, he invariably touches it with 95 per cent. carbolic acid. Some may think this application a dangerous remedy, but it is anaesthetic and antiseptic, it coagulates the mucus, and its action is sufficiently deep to insure a thorough cleansing of the mucous membrane. In the next place, he packs the uterus with gauze, not only to assist drainage, but for the purpose of reducing the size of the uterus. This latter object is accomplished by the gauze irritating the uterus and promoting contraction. Even these steps are not sufficient. The cervix is then to be repaired. He denudes the injured surface, and then severs the circular artery, and allows free bleeding,—even four ounces—in order to deplete the uterus; then the main branches of both uterine arteries are ligated, and the uterus is "starved" in this way for about forty days. During this period, the organ may be reduced from three fourths to one and a half inches. He had placed on record a series of cases in which this treatment had been carried out, and in all the uterus was reduced to this extent. Of course, if there are other operations demanded below the uterus, it is customary to perform these operations all at one time. If there be pelvic disease above the vaginal vault, of course abdominal section must be considered.

He recalled a case upon which he operated just before going on his summer vacation. She had been under preparatory treatment for this work for two months previous. Her uterus was retroverted and fixed. When she was on the table, she informed him that she had not menstruated at the last expected period, and that the flow was now ten days overdue. Curettement of the uterus was performed, and the early products of a conception found. Trachelorrhaphy, colporrhaphy, abdominal section, and ventral fixation were successively performed, all within one hour, and the patient stood it well. Her temperature after the operation never rose above 100°; the gauze was removed from the uterus on the third day.

It was his practice in obstetrical cases to inspect the cervix after delivery with the aid of a speculum, and to carefully close with catgut any laceration of the cervix that might be discovered. Eight or ten days ago, as a result of a precipitate labour, a woman was torn through to the sphincter, and the cervix was also badly lacerated. All the lacerations were closed at once, and now an examination does not even show the scar in the cervix. We can, therefore, prevent the ulterior results in many of these cases if we attend to them a little earlier.

Dr. FERGUSON asked if Dr. Dudley experienced any trouble in recognising the extent of a laceration immediately after delivery, and whether he employs any special means for determining in a primipara the extent of the laceration.

Dr. DUDLEY replied that he was only careful to secure good illumination. He had had no experience in primipara on this point. The uterus remains pretty fairly open, and he opens the cervix with a tenaculum to ascertain the existence of any laceration. When this is done, there is almost always some bleeding from the freshly lacerated surface.

Dr. FERGUSON said he had asked this question because in one case such inspection led him to believe there was a laceration, yet, notwithstanding it was not closed by sutures, the examination made a few weeks subsequently showed no trace of any such laceration.

Dr. ROBB, in closing the discussion, said that in many slight lacerations following labour, we find that by cleanliness alone they unite without any operation whatever, so that he did not consider it necessary in many cases to perform such operations immediately after labour.

14

THE VOLUNTARY COMMITMENT OF PATIENTS TO ASYLUMS FOR THE INSANE.

By Wm. D. Granger, M. D., of Westchester County.

October 11, 1893.

There has been a growing and wide-spread demand for some system allowing an easy access to asylums, and also an easy departure,—a demand that they should be, so far as possible, more like hospitals in their reception and discharge of patients. Of course it is still recognised that a large majority of the real insane must be committed by binding legal process, so as to allow those in authority to deprive the individual patient of his liberty, so far as is needed for his own good and the safety of the community. But for a large minority of the insane, such as in incipient cases, border-line cases, cases of neurasthenia, certain epileptics, some mild and harmless cases of delusional insanity, paranoiacs, and some cases of chronic insanity, or some of the more acute type, also in the various forms of "habit," voluntary admission is constantly sought for. Every physician knows of many patients who express themselves willing to go to an asylum for treatment if they could go as voluntary patients—persons who, though insane, fully understand what an asylum is and why they go there,—their motives being desire of friends, confidence in the advice of a physician, a desire for the special treatment afforded, or for rest, and from many other actuating motives. In my experience for eight years in a large state asylum, such application was not infrequently made by the person desiring treatment, and in a number of instances patients so fully made up their minds to come that they secured their own medical examination and came alone to the asylum, bringing their commitment with them.

The history of the commitment of the insane to asylums shows conclusively the preponderance of the legal idea—that there are, and must be, places where persons are deprived of their liberty,—incarceration is the controlling element,—it is a place for the safe-keeping of the dangerously and furiously mad; the main use of asylum superintendents consists in their being legally jailers, and every patient is in duress. So strongly does this old common-law doctrine hold sway that in a writ of habeas corpus, in almost every case, special argument is necessary to convince the judge that the primary idea is treatment, and that the patient, though not dangerous or furious, is rightly held, from the medical point of view, and that the being in duress is entirely secondary, and alone for the purpose of enforcing the major reason.

For this error, the medical profession, and more particularly those who had charge of the insane, are much to blame. A false conception of the nature and character of the disease, and a fatal mistake in conducting these asylums too much like a prison, placed them in the position of false teachers. Bars, bolts and locks, high surrounding walls, forbidding and gloomy buildings, cells and darkness, restraint, seclusion, secretiveness and mystery, jealousy of advice, interference, or inspection, a want of touch with the world or the profession on the part of the medical and lay control of asylums, bred false ideas of the nature of the disease, of the character of the insane, and what an asylum really is. The false legal ruling arose from the false medical views. Enlightened medical views and knowledge are the cause of changes in the public mind, and in legal decisions it is educating to truth as before it had been to error.

One can hardly realise how, within this century, the sunlight of truth has penetrated the barred windows of error and illuminated the imprisoned darkness and driven out the mould and rust of centuries of superstition and ignorance. Certainly where patients were locked in filthy cells, manacled and chained, unclothed and unwashed, when patients were chained to the table at meals, to their seats during the

day, and to their beds at night, asylums were fit only for the
furiously mad, though these were made more furious by
abuse, and were not fit for places of treatment and medical
supervision and care. In 1815, in the principal asylum in
England, a man was found, by a parliamentary committee of
investigation, restrained for years as follows: (1) A collar
about the neck, confined by a chain attached to a pole at the
head of the bed; (2) an iron frame—the lower part encircled the body, the upper part passed over the shoulders, with
an opening for the arms, which, however, encircled them
above the elbow; (3) a chain passing from the ankle to the
foot of the bed. This is the historic case of one Norris.
Many were also found manacled, or chained at the wrist or
the feet. The conception at that time of what use treatment of the insane was, is found in the answer of the apothecary in charge of the institution, who, when asked if a violent patient could be treated when chained by the fist and
wrist, replied, "Then he would be an innoxious animal."
The distance from pole to pole is not greater than the difference between asylum care to-day and the imprisonment of
the insane in old Bethlem, London, in 1815.

The central idea of asylum care to-day is the overpowering
preponderance of medical supervision, with every effort
made to promote the recovery or to ameliorate the condition
of each patient. Individualisation is the key-stone. In the
management of an asylum, the centre of effort is to do away
with everything that is institutional, and to make the life
led by the patients as natural and homelike as possible.
The exercise of liberty, and the consequent self-control required, is conferred upon each patient just so far as it is in
his power to enjoy and profit by it. Under these changed
conditions legal ruling is changing. Under these changed
conditions asylums, becoming hospitals, are desired by physicians for the treatment of certain forms of disease, and
the voluntary wish of the patient requires a voluntary admission. One of the so called "reforms" is, therefore, along
this line. Law and practice have excluded such cases; but

law and practice are changing. It is my province to-day to point out to you how far this change has taken place and along what lines. Several states have enacted laws governing voluntary admission, and by recent enactment in England the same step is taken.

In Pennsylvania, the law permits the admission of voluntary patients into asylums on the patient's signing an application, witnessed by a friend, and approved by a physician of the asylum. This admission, however, is for a period of seven days, but is subject to renewal. It is so limited as not to be much used.

In Connecticut, a person may commit himself upon his own written application to any asylum in the state, but must be discharged upon a written notice within ten days.

In Massachusetts, voluntary patients may be admitted into any public asylum upon their own written application. They must, however, be discharged upon their written application within three days.

The new English lunacy act of 1890 allows voluntary commitment of patients or boarders into licensed asylums, or, as we call them, private asylums.

Written application must be made, and permission must be given, signed either by two justices or by two members of the lunacy commission.

The permission is for a given time, as stated in the certificate. It is, however, subject to renewal. At the end of the time mentioned, if not renewed, the patient must be discharged. If, at any time before that set forth in the permission, the patient makes a written request, he must be discharged within twenty-four hours.

In most cases, when voluntary commitment is allowed, the patient is under the same state supervision as are involuntarily committed patients.

In all these different states and countries the patient is held for a definite time. He is really deprived of his liberty. This he can gain only by the expiration of a certain time set forth in the commitment,—as in Pennsylvania, within seven days, or as in England at the end of a set time, in each case especially mentioned; or he gains his liberty by written application within twenty-four hours, three days in Massachusetts, or ten days in Connecticut. Within that time he is in duress as much as any involuntary patient, can be kept from escape, or returned if he escapes.

In all but England the patient commits himself, and by his own act is deprived of his liberty for a more or less limited period of time, and only gains his liberty by methods pointed out. It is questioned by lawyers if this is constitutional. Can a man deprive himself of his liberty, even for a short time? If the principle is established for twenty-four hours, or three days, or seven days, or ten days, why not for six months, a year, or even longer?

In England, the application is made by the person desiring commitment, but the permission is granted, not by any one connected with the asylum receiving the patient, but by the state lunacy commissioners, or by justices.

In the state of New York, the commissioners in lunacy objected to voluntary commitment, whereby the person was in any way deprived of his liberty, and devised a plan whereby persons could come to asylums as voluntary patients, and yet be able to leave at any time, exactly as they would do in a hospital. The commitment was for no specified time, and if the patient desired to leave, all he had to do was to leave. A patient then would remain in an asylum, exactly as he came, by his own judgment, the wishes of the family, or of his physician, or because of the tact and influence of the head of the institution.

They have granted permission to take voluntary patients to private asylums conducted on the family plan, and ordered that no voluntary patient could be received whose mind is so far impaired as to render him incapable of forming a rational judgment as to the disposition of his person, or whose will is so weak as to render him incapable of resisting undue influences.

The person desiring admission to a private asylum in this

state must sign the following application. This must be signed by two witnesses. A copy of this application is sent to the commission in lunacy :

STATE OF NEW YORK—STATE COMMISSION IN LUNACY.

(Name of asylum [private] ....)

APPLICATION FOR ADMISSION OF VOLUNTARY PATIENT.

I.., hereby request the Physician-in-Charge of the above named Institution to admit me as a voluntary patient. I hereby pledge myself to submit to the regulations thereof, to carry out, or aid in carrying out, all the directions which may be given for my treatment, and that my conduct will not be prejudicial to the good order and discipline of the Institution.

I do hereby declare that I am aware that the above named Institution is licensed by the State Commission in Lunacy to care for and hold in custody insane patients; that the Physician-in-Charge has fully explained to me the character of the Institution, and that I am at liberty to depart therefrom at my pleasure.

I hereby consent that the members of the State Commission in Lunacy may freely visit my apartments on any proper occasion, make such inquiries of me as they may deem necessary, and that I will make truthful answers thereto.

In witness whereof I have hereunto set my hand this..................
day of......................189 , in the.............., of..............
........................., County of ....and State of New York.

....
(Signature of Applicant.)

We,............................, a resident of........................,
County of...................State of New York, and..................,
a resident of..........................., County of...................
and State aforesaid, do severally certify, and each for himself certifies, as follows:

I am a graduate of a legally chartered medical college, and am personally acquainted with the above named applicant for admission to the above named Institution, and am not a committee of the person and estate, nor a relative or guardian of said applicant, nor connected with said Institution. I have read the foregoing application. I believe the statements therein made by the applicant to be true, and in my opinion the applicant is capable of forming a rational judgment as to the disposition of h   person, and is capable of resisting undue influence.

..................................Witness.
..................................Witness.

You will notice that it provides that the patient can depart at his pleasure : there is, therefore, no duress. The question of voluntary admission into state asylums is not considered by the commissioners, because of the already overcrowded condition of these asylums; there is no room for the voluntary class.

My own experience with voluntary patients is limited. I have so far received 15. Of these, 4 were for opium habit, 2 were cases of melancholia, 1 dementia, 2 chronic delusional insanity, 1 partly habit and partly incipient senile dementia, 1 hypochondria (syphilomania), 1 morphine, 1 alcohol, 1 hysteria, 1 neurasthenia, and 1 chronic alcoholism. The case of dementia was considered by the lunacy commissioners to be too weak-minded to decide so momentous a question, and was then regularly committed.

One case of melancholia had cut his throat six weeks previously, and from that moment showed marked mental improvement and was so far recovered when he came to me as to fully understand the character of his commitment, and agreed, should other necessity arise, to allow himself to be regularly committed. His convalescence regularly and rapidly progressed, and it was a source of help to him to realise his form of commitment and to maintain his position, and of pleasure to think he had not been locked up as an insane person. The other case of melancholia was deeply depressed, but without delusions. He visited my home, saw his room, looked over the commitment, and decided to come. He was discharged cured in ten months.

One case of chronic delusional insanity was a harmless species of the so called "crank." He spends his life going from one private institution to another, and is a sort of asylum tramp,—a gentleman, however. He is so used to asylums the question of voluntary commitment was simply one of convenience. The other case of chronic insanity has lately come to me, and would never have consented to enter an asylum except as a voluntary patient. The opium cases were more satisfied, and better subject to my rules than though com-

mitted—at least, this is my judgment. They remained as
long as they agreed to remain, and were less irritated by the
restraint than are patients forcibly committed for habit treatment. In no case has a voluntary patient transgressed any
of the rules or requirements of the place. In each case, except the demented patient, the individual has talked freely
with me upon the subject of coming, learned fully the difference between voluntary and involuntary commitment, read
with care the application, and agreed to abide by my rules.
In no case has the confidence placed in the patient been violated. At the present time I have one engagement of a voluntary patient, an opium case. I have refused to receive
several applications for voluntary patients as not suitable.
The fact being known that voluntary admission is permissible
in some cases, a pressure is brought to bear in almost every
case for such admission. This leads to disappointment, and
brings embarrassment to the asylum physician, and sometimes
to the home physician.

I believe I am not too sanguine and radical on the one
hand, nor too conservative on the other. I do not believe
great things are to be accomplished by voluntary admission,
that insanity will be greatly lessened, or changed or altered
in its character. I do believe some early and border-line
cases will go to asylums, and with benefit; that the more
they receive voluntary cases the more the class of cases coming will require changes in treatment, broadening of ideas
and views of care, and make them in reality more like hospitals and less like asylums and places of mere confinement.
On the other hand, it will change the public conception of
asylums, and make the public more willing to use them, both
for committed and non-committed cases.

Those who have experience in receiving voluntary cases
approve it. The McLean asylum, Boston, receives about
one third of its cases as voluntary. In the report for 1890,
Dr. Cowles, the superintendent, reports 42 such cases admitted. They included melancholia, 21, mania, 3, fixed ideas, 1,
delusional insanity, 4, senile insanity, 1, secondary dementia,

8, paresis, 1, and 6 were not insane. Speaking of an apparent impropriety in admitting so many classes as insane, he says, "The conditions often became apparent upon observation after admission, and they included a more or less doubtful class of cases, for whose commitment attending physicians would not be willing to certify to the insanity;" and then observes most truly, "It is for just such class of cases near the border-line that the system is a great boon."

The experiment in Massachusetts is very interesting and instructive. At the McLean asylum more has been done than anywhere, and with the happiest results. The enlargement of voluntary admission must rest largely with the state authorities. When they look with disfavour, it will be refused or restricted. When favoured, it will grow and increase in use and probably in usefulness. Its administration requires tact, judgment, and justice. Abuses can grow up under it; great good can come from it. The state's position should be to check abuse and encourage in every way the getting of the greatest possible good that can come by its wise laws, administration, and control.

DISCUSSION.

Dr. ELIAS LESTER, of Seneca county, said that the new lunacy law was being made so obnoxious that the press has already begun to condemn it. Judge North recently wrote, a very caustic article, which was published in one of the Rochester papers. It is a very nice point to decide whether or not one is insane; hence, such a law, permitting voluntary commitment, would be very convenient. He had sometimes to stretch his conscience in making out insanity papers in order that patients who evidently needed asylum care might get it. He recalled a case in which an insane patient was driven sixteen miles to an asylum, but was refused admission and sent home simply because he had signed the commitment on one day and the other physician on the next day, instead of both on the same day. The commission in lunacy supported the asylum superintendent in this ruling.

Dr. D. COLVIN, of Wayne county, said that he had had a similar experience with the same asylum. It was not the fault of the law, but was due to the crankiness of this particular superintendent.

Dr. GEORGE DOUGLAS, of Chenango county, said that this trouble was occasioned by the officers of this particular asylum adhering strictly to the letter of the law. Other superintendents had not done so; they had been more liberal in their interpretation of it.

Dr. FERGUSON remarked that law and equity are not always identical. He believed it was a fact that superintendents of asylums may receive patients brought by friends, and hold them for a short time if it is evident that the person would be dangerous if allowed to be at large. There is one provision in the law of this state which seems to be needless, and is liable to cause much inconvenience, and that is the requirement that both physicians signing the commitment shall see the patient on the same day. It is often inconvenient for the two physicians to do this, and some proper interval, for instance twenty-four hours, should be allowed.

The PRESIDENT said that the law permitting the admission of supposed insane persons to a reception asylum, as in New York city, is a great convenience to all concerned. In this city, one can send a patient supposed to be insane to the insane pavilion at Bellevue hospital for five days, during which time the physicians there must decide as to the insanity of the person. We might safely say that some desperate cases of homicide have been encouraged by the various technicalities which prevent the prompt commitment of the insane.

THE TREATMENT OF ENTERIC FEVER.

By GUSTAVUS ELIOT, M. D., of New Haven, Conn.

October 11, 1893.

The great mortality and wide prevalence of enteric, or typhoid, fever, justify frequent discussion of its treatment. It is an important duty of the medical profession to try to discover such principles and methods of treatment as will diminish the severity and fatality of the disease, and to promote their dissemination.

I shall not attempt to bring forward any therapeutic novelties. Every remedial measure of which I shall speak was proposed and tried long ago. It is the modest purpose of this paper simply to discuss those principles and methods of treatment which are in more or less common use, and to point out those whose value has been most thoroughly established, and which seem worthy of general adoption.

The first requisite in the successful treatment of enteric fever is rest. As soon as the physician begins to suspect that his patient has this disease, it is his duty to insist that the sick person should at once go to bed, and should remain there, in the recumbent position, until all doubt in regard to the nature of the disease has been dissipated, or until the patient has entirely recovered. "Every one, unless he is a fool, knows that," you are saying to yourselves. Let me remind you, that a little less than nine years ago Frederic Mahomed, one of the assistant physicians of Guy's hospital, London, died at the age of thirty-five years, of enteric fever, and that a few days before his death, while his temperature was 104°, he left his residence and went to the hospital to see a student ill with rheumatic fever. Certainly this brilliant young Londoner ought to have known, even so long as nine years ago, the importance of rest in the treatment of enteric fever. Let us hear from his own lips the reason why he disregarded this fundamental rule—it was addressed to his wife—"Would you have me stay at home for a bilious attack, when the life of another is in danger?" These words of a young man of extraordinary promise may serve to emphasise a point of the very greatest importance in this connection: it is the necessity of making an early diagnosis, if one wishes to treat enteric fever with the best results. If the brilliant young assistant physician of Guy's hospital had realised that he had this disease, he undoubtedly would have remained in bed, and very likely would have recovered, to continue his investigations in cardiac and renal pathology.

Many reputable physicians have, at some time in their experience, been guilty of this same carelessness in diagnosis, and have allowed patients, whom later developments showed to be suffering from enteric fever, to remain out of bed, or even to continue about their business. And this was permitted, not because the physician did not know that patients with enteric fever must be kept in bed, but because at first he failed to recognise the real nature of the disease. The best results in the treatment of this disease will never be obtained, until the time comes when no physician allows a patient who has any elevation of temperature to remain out of bed, until he has positively and absolutely excluded the possibility that the patient has enteric fever. Every physician ought always to assure himself that his patient has no fever before he ventures to prescribe; and ought always to assure himself that a patient with any elevation of temperature has not enteric fever before he permits him to remain out of bed. The general observance of these simple rules would greatly diminish the mortality from enteric fever.

Immediate rest in bed is entirely inconsistent with a journey by rail, by boat, or by coach. It frequently happens that the victim of enteric fever is taken ill at a distance from home. The first thing such an one wishes to do, when he begins to realise that his illness may prove serious, is to take the first train for home. To travel is one of the most injurious things a man with this disease can do. Probably no one with enteric fever ever took a journey who was not thereby made worse. When these patients refrain from travelling, fewer of them will die.

Rest in bed, furthermore, does not embrace receiving company, transacting business, or conducting correspondence. All must be absolutely forbidden, for either is liable to increase and prolong the fever, or to cause its return if undertaken too early during convalescence.

The patient must not leave the bed for any purpose whatever. He must not go to the water-closet. He must not get out of bed to urinate or defecate, but must use a bedpan. He must not leave the bed to get a drink, or to unlock a door, or to open a window, or to see if the sky is cloudy, or for any other one of the innumerable things which occur to his mind as necessary and desirable things to do.

This complete rest may be most certainly secured, if the patient is early placed in the care of a well trained and faithful nurse. If the case is a severe one, two nurses may be necessary.

The requisite condition of restfulness will be further promoted by the maintenance of an even and agreeable temperature, of an adequate supply of fresh air, and of a moderate amount of natural light. Occasional sponge baths, also, frequently contribute greatly to the comfort of the patient.

This uninterrupted rest in bed must be maintained, until for a week the temperature, both morning and evening, has been below 99° F.

The second point to be considered has reference to diet. This must be such as will necessitate the least possible activity of the organs of digestion and assimilation. Of all food, by far the best in enteric fever is milk. The ordinary duration of the disease is so long that systematic feeding should be continued from the beginning to the end. Milk should be given at regular intervals, in sufficient quantity so that two quarts or more may be taken in twenty-four hours. If intestinal symptoms are severe, the milk should be sterilised.

If, for any reason, raw milk does not seem to agree with the patient, it may be peptonised, or if a mild stimulant is desirable, it may be used in the form of wine whey. A patient who cannot, or will not, take milk is exceedingly difficult to manage. If it is absolutely impossible to nourish him sufficiently with milk, recourse may be had to gruels, and meat soups, broths, and extracts. These, however, are less desirable than milk, because they are likely to ferment in the stomach and intestines with the production of gas, and because they tend to cause or to increase diarrhoea.

Liquid diet, preferably of milk, like rest in the recumbent position, must be maintained, until for a week the temperature, during the entire day, has been below 99° F.

After this period has passed, the patient may be allowed to sit up for a short, and gradually increasing, time each day. He may also be given a somewhat greater variety of food, beginning with gruels, soups, and broths, then eggs, a little later, meat and bread, and last of all, fruits and vegetables. In the mean time, the temperature must be carefully watched and if fever returns, constant rest in bed and a liquid diet must again be enforced.

The general treatment or management of the patient, as already outlined, is applicable to all cases of enteric fever, whether mild or severe, in male or female, in old or young. In fact, this plan of treatment may wisely be followed in the management of any patient who has fever, whatever the cause of it may be. With regard to the rules which have been enumerated, there would be practically no difference of opinion among educated and sensible physicians.

Turning now from the hygienic and dietetic rules, which may be denominated the physiological side of the treatment, we pass to the more strictly therapeutical side of the subject. The measures which have been mentioned promote the normal physiological action of the various organs. Those which remain for discussion are employed to produce modifications of the disease process, or of those disorders of function which it has caused.

If one were to attempt to enumerate all the remedies which have been used with alleged benefit in this disease, the list would be a wearisome one.   On the other hand, some maintain that all drugs are injurious or useless, except as they are used with reference to some special symptom or complication.   Osler, the clinical oracle of three great cities, teaches that enteric fever " is not to be treated by medicines."   Other writers and teachers make equally discouraging statements. Very many believe that it is impossible to shorten the course of the disease, or to diminish its severity by the administration of drugs.   I shall venture to present a somewhat more optimistic view of the subject.

What therapeutical measures should be employed in the treatment of enteric fever?   I reply, It depends entirely at what stage of the patient's illness you commence to treat him, with reference to the fact that he has that disease.   You may feel inclined to sneer at this statement, and to say that it is puerile; but no one who has had much experience in the practice of medicine, if he looks at the matter without prejudice and in a rational way, can fail to realise that, in the case of many a patient who has passed through the course of enteric fever, or who has died before he reached the end of the disease, the physician in attendance has confidently and repeatedly asserted that the patient had malarial fever, or bilious fever, or gastric fever, or typho-malarial fever, or some other disease which he did not have.   Perhaps before the disease has ended, or has destroyed his patient, he has modified his earlier opinion, and has affirmed that the disease has run into enteric fever, or that enteric fever has developed in addition to the earlier condition.   Of course a physician who said anything of this kind, and believed it, would not begin to treat his patient for enteric fever very early in the course of the disease.   You will, I have no doubt, agree with me that such vacillating diagnosis is generally the fruit of ignorance or carelessness.   Intelligent practitioners, who are not so profoundly convinced of their own infallibility as to be unwilling to admit that they ever make a mistake in diagnosis, understand and will agree with me, that while enteric fever may commence insidiously, and may at first be difficult to distinguish with absolute certainty from other affections, it nevertheless, as a rule, runs a definite individual course, and is not, except in very exceptional instances, entangled with other inflammatory or febrile disorders, as a complication or sequel.

But it is not always the fault of the physician that he commences the treatment late in the course of the disease. Often the patient does not seek medical advice until the disease has been pursuing its course for days or even weeks. Often, also, the patient, by choice or necessity, wisely or unwisely, passes from the care of one physician to that of another. To him who sees the case first, at the middle or end of the second week of the disease very different indications for treatment appear from those which are usually observed at the beginning or middle of the first week.

Assuming that the physician sees the patient early in the course of the disease, and is alert to detect its nature, one of the first questions concerning the medicinal treatment which arises has reference to the use of cathartics.

The time was, fifteen or twenty years ago, when medical teachers almost unanimously condemned the use of cathartics in enteric fever. They protested against their use on the ground that, inasmuch as looseness of the bowels was one of the common symptoms, there was no necessity of causing any increased action of the bowels, and, furthermore, that there was danger of increasing the inflammation of the intestinal mucous membrane, and of producing hypercatharsis.

For the last ten or fifteen years there has been a tendency to regard one member of this class of remedies with less disfavour. During the last decade calomel has acquired considerable popularity in the treatment of enteric fever. A considerable proportion of practitioners now approve of giving one or more doses of this drug, when the patient is seen early in the course of the disease, and when the diagnosis is made

15

promptly. The best way to use calomel in this disease is to direct that the patient shall take from seven and one half to ten grains of the drug every other day, until four doses have been taken. The earlier this treatment is commenced the more beneficial results will be observed from it. Occasionally it will cause some griping and a large number of loose movements. Under these circumstances, it may be necessary to give an opiate to relieve the pain and to counteract the hypercatharsis. But, on the other hand, sometimes a dose of the size mentioned fails to produce any action of the bowels. In that case, the patient should be directed to take one drachm of sulphate of magnesia, dissolved in water, every four hours until the bowels move. If, after four doses of calomel have been taken, the bowels show a tendency to constipation, and the condition of the patient does not show positive improvement, a fifth dose may be given with benefit.

Occasionally, signs of commencing salivation are observed. These can generally be relieved by a gargle of chlorate of potash dissolved in water.

The fact that unpleasant symptoms sometimes attend the use of calomel, naturally suggests the criticism that it is wiser not to prescribe the drug at all, if it is likely to occasion symptoms to combat which further treatment may be required, in addition to that which is necessary for the disease itself. In reply to this criticism it may be said, that unpleasant and undesirable effects are of infrequent occurrence. As a rule, these doses of calomel produce a few loose movements, with little or no griping, and very rarely give rise to any signs of salivation. On the contrary, I am able to testify to the positive beneficial effect of this treatment. It is my sincere conviction, that used at the beginning of the illness, in the way which I have described, calomel helps to shorten the duration of the disease and to diminish its severity.

The use of calomel in enteric fever is not a new thing. Formerly its employment was very general. The revival of its popularity was brought about, in part at least, by the teachings of Leibermeister in Germany, and of Bartholow and Wilson in America. A large number of practitioners now use it to a greater or less extent, and bear testimony to its utility. Some give smaller doses, as from one to five grains. Some give a single dose, and others, two or three. Others give minute doses, repeated several times during the day. In no one of these ways is the same favourable action of the drug obtained as when the large doses of from seven and one half to ten grains are given every forty-eight hours until four doses have been taken.

It is difficult to explain positively just how the drug produces a favourable effect upon the disease. It is certain that, as a rule, it removes a large amount of useless, and perhaps injurious, matter from the intestinal canal, including, in addition to faecal matter, bacteria ptomaines and leucomaines. It doubtless, also, relieves to some extent the congestion and inflammation of the intestinal mucous membrane. It very likely, either in its own form, or modified chemically during its passage through the alimentary canal, acts as an antiseptic. It perhaps acts indirectly as an antiseptic by stimulating the secretion of the liver and of the other glands which are concerned with the function of digestion. Possibly it has a sedative action on the entire nervous system. Certain it is, that when used in connection with other remedies, which will be mentioned later, it reduces the temperature so that antipyretics are less urgently demanded, and diminishes the frequency and increases the force of the pulse, so that stimulants are less frequently required.

Rarely vomiting is a prominent symptom at the beginning of enteric fever. If present, it may interfere with the favourable action of the calomel, or may seem to entirely contraindicate its use. But, as a rule, the calomel itself does not cause vomiting, or disturb the stomach in any way. On the contrary, it improves the condition of that organ, and, in fact, of the entire digestive system.

Aloes, podophyllin, and colocynth have justly been banished from the pharmacopoeia of enteric fever. They are likely to aggravate the inflammation of the intestinal mucous membrane.

Sulphate of magnesia may be used with much less danger, and in some cases with considerable benefit.

High injections have been highly commended, and no doubt are sometimes of positive value in clearing the intestines of much useless and deleterious material.

Leaving now remedial measures which promote elimination, we pass next to a class of drugs which are prescribed chiefly with reference to the condition of the alimentary canal. The more prominent members of this group are the mineral acids, pepsin, quinine, salol, turpentine, nitrate of silver, carbolic acid or phenol, and iodine. Most, perhaps all, of these agents may fairly be classed as antiseptics and, for this reason, without doubt have a distinct value.

The mineral acids in particular, and especially hydrochloric acid, have been for a long time in very general use. Their action, although feeble, is distinctly beneficial. They possess antiseptic qualities to a moderate degree. They also aid digestion and improve the condition of the stomach.

Pepsin also assists digestion and promotes assimilation, and is frequently prescribed with benefit.

Quinine, so useful in many other conditions, is of very little use in enteric fever. It rarely, if ever, materially influences the course of the disease, or produces any important modification of its important symptoms. If there is any good reason for suspecting the presence of a malarial element, a few large doses may be given at the beginning. Such cases are rare. In nine cases out of ten—to put the matter conservatively—the patient would be just as well off without quinine as with it. In every case, unless there is a distinct malarial complication, probably something else would do much more good. If no patient with enteric fever were ever given any quinine, probably there would be fewer deaths from the disease, because if physicians gave up the indiscriminate use of quinine, they would be more alert to detect the real nature of diseases presented for treatment, there would not be so many mistakes in diagnosis, and fewer patients who were really suffering from enteric fever would be allowed to walk about while being treated for the results of malarial poisoning.

Salol, although theoretically a valuable antiseptic, especially in affections of the stomach and intestines, has very little influence upon the course or the symptoms of enteric fever.

Turpentine is much used to relieve tympanites, and to strengthen the nervous system. It is a valuable antiseptic, and exercises a favourable influence upon the processes of inflammation and ulceration, as they affect the intestinal mucous membrane.

The value of nitrate of silver in the treatment of inflammations of mucous membranes, and in promoting the healing of ulcers, is universally recognised. Many have testified to its great usefulness in enteric fever, and its employment certainly rests upon a reasonable basis.

Of late years carbolic acid, or phenol, and tincture of iodine have been considerably used, not only separately, but also in combination, and especially in connection with repeated large doses of calomel. This has been called the specific treatment, and has come into considerable popular favour through the writings of Bartholow and Wilson. Carbolic acid and iodine are valuable antiseptics. Both have a sedative action upon the stomach, and are held in some repute as remedies for the relief of nausea and vomiting. Of a mixture containing one drachm of carbolic acid and three drachms of tincture of iodine, four drops may be given, in a wineglassful of cold water, every four hours. Administered in this way, in connection with calomel, the duration of the disease may be shortened, the severity of the fever may be diminished, the tendency to diarrhoea is lessened, the condition of the digestive organs is improved, nervous symptoms do not become so severe, there is less danger of haemorrhage, and convalescence is hastened.

Many of course will say that they do not believe these assertions. Some will say that they have tried this method of treatment, and that it will not do what has been claimed. Others will say that they have seen it tried, with no better results than were obtained from an expectant plan of treatment.

Time permits me to mention only briefly some of the conditions which must be observed in order to secure the most favourable results.

In the first place, the treatment must be commenced early. One might reasonably hesitate to begin the administration of large doses of calomel to a patient who had been sick with enteric fever for two weeks. Carbolic acid and iodine, however, may be advantageously prescribed at any time, and continued until the patient is convalescent. Whenever a patient is sick with enteric fever, his physician ought to remember and suspect the possibility of the existence of that disease the first time he sees the patient. Unless he can, with reasonable confidence, exclude its existence, he may wisely commence the treatment with calomel. It may not be possible to make a correct diagnosis in every case the first time the patient is seen, but it is far safer to treat a doubtful case as if the patient had enteric fever, than to treat him as if he had no serious disease and permit him to remain out of bed.

An assertion of this purport, published in the New York *Medical Journal*, on August 6, 1892, provoked the criticism from an obscure practitioner in a small town somewhere over in New Jersey, that "if one may not be correct every time, it would seem wiser and better for one to be reasonably certain of being correct every time before he begins specific treatment of any kind."

I had endeavoured to make it clear that one ought to commence active treatment even, in some cases, before a positive diagnosis has been made; because, if it subsequently becomes certain that the disease is enteric fever, the patient has been greatly benefited, and, if he has not that disease, he has not been injured in the slightest degree by the specific treatment

Of course every one recognises that physicians differ a great deal in temperament. One man always has a diagnosis ready for every case, and never knows that he is wrong or has made a mistake; another is habitually uncertain about his diagnosis, and rarely feels quite sure that he is absolutely correct. Between these two extremes, there are men who have all degrees of confidence in their own diagnostic ability, and whose faculties of differentiating diseases differ within equally wide limits. The man who is always sure is often wrong, and always dangerous. The one who is cautious is frequently right, and generally safe.

If a man intends to wait until he can make a positive diagnosis—in a case which may possibly prove to be enteric. fever—before commencing treatment, he certainly owes to his patients the duty of perfecting his skill in diagnosis to the very highest possible degree, and of not following the teachings of such writers as encourage delay in making a diagnosis. It is a pity that any man should allow his patients to die because he is not certain what the matter is, and because he is too obstinate to adopt a good plan of treatment as long as there is any uncertainty.

A second condition of success with the specific treatment is, that it should not be abandoned prematurely. After it has been commenced, it should be continued, in the absence of any important contra-indication, until the patient is convalescent. If it is discontinued after a trial of only one or two days, only very little benefit from it will be observed.

If commenced early, and followed up continuously, there is no other treatment now in use which gives so good results in enteric fever.

But there will always be some physicians who will not treat enteric fever in the way described. They will frequently—others, sometimes—find it necessary to resort to other therapeutical measures.

Hyperpyrexia is the most common indication for symptomatic treatment. At present, bathing, according to the method of Brand, is enjoying an enviable popularity as a method of reducing temperature and preventing complications. This may answer very well in hospitals, where it makes no particular difference whether any individual patient dies or gets well, and where there are conveniences for bathing, and plenty of assistants. I venture, however, to predict with considerable confidence that this treatment will never be generally adopted in rural districts, nor in private practice in cities.

Much testimony to its efficacy has been presented, but rarely has any one taken the pains to describe in print the piteous and ineffectual appeals to be spared the distress of further Brand baths of patients who, in spite of a continuance of the baths, died. Such cases never occupy a very conspicuous place in scientific reports on modern antipyretic treatment. The pathetic side of the story never appears in statistics.

Of the drugs which may be used to effect a reduction of temperature, antipyrine, acetanilide, and phenacetine are well known, and are very useful. Given with moderation, and yet with adequate boldness, their effect carefully watched, and unfavourable action guarded against by the use of alcohol, they act with a reasonable degree of certainty, and undoubtedly have been the means of saving the lives of many persons who have suffered from enteric fever.

Stimulants, especially whiskey and brandy, are of great value in many cases. They should not be given as a matter of routine to every patient, and are rarely needed at the beginning of the disease. When the action of the heart begins to become weak, and symptoms relating to the nervous system become conspicuous, the administration of stimulants should be commenced. In some cases large and frequent doses will be found necessary.

If insomnia is a troublesome symptom, the bromide of sodium, morphine, or hydrate of chloral is useful. Their relative value is indicated by the order in which they have been named. Either one of the three may be given separately, or the bromide of sodium may be given with either of the other two, or all three may be prescribed together. These three drugs may also be used if there is much delirium, but morphine will generally be found to act less favourably than either of the others, which, moreover, may often be used together very advantageously. Their action should be supplemented by cold applications to the head.

When diarrhoea is excessive and persistent, bismuth and morphine will in most cases be found useful.

If intestinal haemorrhage occurs, turpentine or ergot will prove most valuable. Their action should be aided and supplemented by the external use of cold compresses.

In conclusion, the following rules may be formulated. They constitute a safe guide in the treatment of enteric fever:

1. Never overlook the disease or forget the possibility of its occurrence in any patient who seeks medical advice.

2. If the symptoms indicate that the patient may be suffering from enteric fever, begin to treat him at once, and follow up the treatment until it is certain that he has not that disease, or until he is well.

3. Commence the treatment by putting the patient to bed, and keeping him there; by forbidding all solid food—limiting him if possible to milk,—and by prohibiting reading, writing, and conversation.

4. Commence at the same time the so called specific treatment, embracing the use of repeated large doses of calomel, in connection with carbolic acid and tincture of iodine. Commence this medicinal treatment early, and continue it until the patient is convalescent.

5. Do not permit the patient to abandon the recumbent position, a liquid diet, and absolute quietude until for a week the temperature, at no time during the twenty-four hours, has been above 99° F.

6. Do not condemn the specific treatment until you have tried it in the way described, and do not attempt to form an opinion in regard to it until you have tried it in a series of cases, and have carefully observed its effects and compared them with those obtained by other methods of treatment.

DISCUSSION.

Dr. GEORGE DOUGLAS, of Chenango county, considered the paper a very valuable one, and especially suggestive as regards the management of the early stage of the disease. He was particularly pleased with the emphasis put upon the importance of absolute rest. Every physician who has had much experience with this disease knows that he has lost patients from the neglect of such rules; yet the laity find it difficult to fully appreciate the necessity of obeying such injunctions. He had been in the practice of medicine for forty-five years, and had had many cases of typhoid fever, especially among summer residents. These were peculiar in that they seemed to be of a malarial type, and the patients particularly liable to have haemorrhages. As a rule, young practitioners err on the side of using medicines too freely, and relying upon them too much. It is useless to administer remedies for the sole purpose of "aborting" or breaking up the fever. In a case of this kind, which he saw in consultation, the attending physician had indeed succeeded, as he expressed it, in "breaking up the fever," but he had broken down his patient, who died the next day. He did not approve of the too early or too free use of alcoholic stimulants. Where there is much tendency to diarrhoea, he had found creosote very useful. A weak alkaline solution—made by dropping the creosote on calcined magnesia, adding water, and filtering—is the best form in which to administer it, and, when given in this way, he had found it superior to nitrate of silver.

In ordinary cases, he had found salicin useful. In the early stage of the disease, where the stools are offensive, he would give ten grains of calomel, but would not repeat it more than three times—as a rule, only twice,—at intervals of forty-eight hours. Sometimes he would substitute a moderate dose of sulphate of magnesia for the third dose of calomel. If the discharges were quite offensive, he gave bismuth with acetate of morphia.

Dr. WILLIAM FINDER, of Rensselaer county, said that while milk may be conceded to be the best diet, of course many patients cannot take milk, and to this class he had found it beneficial to give milk deprived of its fat. As the trouble is well known to be in the small intestine, he thought it was not well to employ cathartics much. The system is unable to digest and assimilate, during the high fever of the early stage, a large quantity of food, and consequently, at this time he gives little food and plenty of water. As a rule, the less medication the better, but the administration of the mineral acids, especially dilute phosphoric acid, is useful, and he had unbounded faith in the sulpho-carbolate of zinc as an antiseptic and astringent. Resorcin is likewise very efficient.

Dr. LESTER said that in his locality malarial diseases are very prevalent, and there are many cases diagnosticated by the physicians there as malarial fever, which, when treated promptly with purgatives and quinine, do not last more than seven days. When these cases are not so actively treated, many of them pass into this typhoid form, and between the twenty-first and twenty-eighth day they will have tympanites, sub-sultus, and delirium. He would like to know whether these cases are really instances of enteric fever, and if the treatment described in the paper is appropriate for them.

The speaker then described the occurrence of three cases of this kind in the family of a physician, a member of this Association. First the son, and then the daughter, were taken ill, and were successfully treated in the manner he had described. Then the father became ill, and the speaker asked for consultation. The consultant insisted that the quinine should be stopped, and it was done. Eight or ten days later the patient had a severe chill during the night, and died in a few hours. He mentioned the case because he thought this was a congestive chill from malaria, and that the quinine should have been continued. If it had been, the patient probably would have recovered. These are the cases which are called typhoid fever in his vicinity. He had never seen in his practice but three cases which had no malarial element.

Dr. JOHN H. MARTIN, of Otsego county, said he could endorse what the author had said about giving calomel; he had given it for the past sixteen years where he had seen the patient before the eighth day. It places the system in a better condition to withstand the disease, and, at the same time, shortens its duration. After the calomel, he gave iodine or spirits of turpentine; the latter he considered a very valuable remedy where the intestinal symptoms are prominent. He did not confine his patients to milk; he fed them from the beginning to the end. He was not frightened by high temperature, and as there is no malaria in his region, he finds no necessity to administer quinine. He had no use at all for alcohol in the treatment of typhoid fever, and, in fact, almost any other disease. He formerly employed it, but where he had pushed stimulants he believed now he had done harm.

Dr. E. R. SQUIBB, of Kings county, said that, under ordinary circumstances, when calomel is taken into the stomach, it is converted into an albuminate of mercury; this passes along the alimentary canal, and small portions of it are probably changed into the more active corrosive chloride. This, he thought, accounted for its antiseptic properties. Its conversion into albuminate prevents its being too rapidly decomposed into the bichloride. This is important to bear in mind. A knowledge of this chemical decomposition of calomel many years ago induced the principal physicians of Philadelphia, notably Dr. Hughson, to always give the calomel dry on the tongue, and let it be washed down by the saliva. It is best given in this way at a time when the stomach is moderately empty, otherwise it is too much diluted. When these precautions are observed, the calomel is most easily and thoroughly converted into the albuminate.

RARE FORMS OF GOUT AND RHEUMATISM.

By SIR JAMES GRANT, M. D., K. C. M. G., of Ottawa, Canada.

October 11, 1893.

MR. PRESIDENT AND GENTLEMEN: This I consider "a red-letter day" in my professional life's work, and more particularly from the very fact of having received so generous an invitation, through the secretary of your Association, to read a paper on this auspicious occasion. We Canadians, as a whole, delight in ·noting the advance of our American neighbours in almost every line of thought in medical and surgical science. The assembled wisdom of this Association from the state of New York, almost a kingdom in itself, is only an index to the intellectual power to-day at work in almost every state of your prosperous Republic. How gratifying it must be to con over such names as Rush, Mott, McDowell, Sims, Gross, Pancoast, Flint, Sayer, Thomas, Emmett, DaCosta, Bowditch, Godell, Pepper, Weir-Mitchell, Bull, McBurney, and a host of others, equally great but too numerous to mention, who by their skill and ability have added lustre to the name of America. To-day I propose offering some observations on rare forms of gout and rheumatism, conditions not by any means frequent, as to their occurrence.

CASE I.—PNEUMONIC GOUT.—The following brief notes are of a pneumonic form of gout, associated with slight hepatic complication. H. V., seventy-eight years of age; stout habit of body; not plethoric, but generally vigourous, and accustomed to long hours of arduous official duty; cannot trace gout to his ancestors, and always lived well and liberally. February 10, 1893, suddenly seized with acute pain in the right side of chest, opposite the middle lobe of lung, with general malaise and rather severe cough; no excessive flushes in the cheeks; the breathing was somewhat hurried, about thirty per minute; temperature, 101.5° to 103° F., and the pulse ranged from 100 to 114. The cough, after the first day, was associated with the expectoration of a thick, tenacious, and rusty-coloured mucus, not uniform, however, in its character, but somewhat patchy as to the distribution of the blood through the tough sputum. The left side moved more freely during the respiratory process than the right, and over and about the seat of pain in the right side there was an evident area of dulness on percussion, and yet the breath sounds were heard with a degree of almost unexpected clearness, with an occasional slight mucous râle. The posterior aspect of the right lung held its ground, kept moderately clear, and in fact the pulmonic trouble was chiefly confined to the lateral and anterior aspect, middle lobe, right lung. Throughout, the sputa presented an unusually tenacious character, and up to February 21 exhibited a patchy, rusty, and most peculiar appearance, after which date it became clear, but retained the sticky, glutinous peculiarity up to February 27, when it subsided. During the entire illness the pain in the side was not of the usual pleuritic type, but more of a burning, throbbing, aching, and piercing pain, and out of all proportion to the ordinary defined pulmonic condition. From his well-known gouty diathesis, I was led to believe the attack was really one gouty in character, and informed the friends that metastasis to the feet of the lung condition was not unlikely. On February 22, both feet became very painful and swollen,—a condition of system (as to his feet) he had experienced several times during the past ten years. Almost immediately the lung improved in every particular, which quite settled the point as to the gouty character of this attack in the lung tissue as a primary development. Throughout, the usual course of treatment was adopted, with the free use of elixir salicylate of lithia, and lithia water as well. During the entire attack I saw no special indications of hepatic trouble, beyond a degree of uneasiness about the liver generally. Four years ago he had a well defined attack of jaundice, unattended by anatomical lesion to account for its development; it was of short duration, and passed off quickly.

CASE II.—PERITYPHLITIC GOUT.—The same individual whose case I have just cited was the subject of the following data: September 10, 1892, aged seventy-seven years. Almost up to the present attack had been enjoying apparently good health; retired to bed this same evening, and in the middle of the night was suddenly seized with a severe pain in and about the region of the appendix vermiformis, attended with a sensation of throbbing, together with a degree of tension in this particular region, which radiated more or less over the entire abdominal walls; considerable heat of skin, with a degree of restlessness, general febrile disturbance, and a sense of uneasiness about the stomach, with occasional vomiting. Temperature, 102° F.; pulse, 116, full and regular. The pain and sensibility of the abdominal wall, chiefly over the ileo-caecal region. The bowels were constipated and the tongue moderately coated with a moist white fur, pointing to evident gastric derangement for a few days. Knowing the gouty history of this patient for some years, although not of an hereditary type, I suspected, from the character of the pain, boring and gnawing, such as I had observed more than once in his feet,

•

that it might prove a case of gout, of which there were well defined results, such as tissue thickening about the tarsus and heels of both feet, owing to the deposition of gouty material during past years. The fingers in both hands showed also evidences of disturbed chemistry in the system, resulting in gouty thickening in and about various joints. The bowels, though at once relieved by an enema, still continued painful. Linseed poultices were freely applied, sprinkled with chloroform liniment, and tablets of sulphate of morphia freely administered, to relieve the intense suffering, which was so acute as to almost prohibit the most moderate bed-clothing. Salicylate of lithia and lithia water were freely given, as soon as admissible, and the bowels were frequently washed out with warm water, which almost played the part of an internal poultice. The pulse and temperature continued high for fully five days, when both gradually lessened in intensity, and about the sixth day pain was complained of in both feet, particularly about the toes, but not by any means as severe as in the marked metastasis after the attack of pneumonic gout.

At this date there was a marked amelioration in the entire character of the symptoms, the abdomen became more flaccid and much less painful on pressure, and the decidedly caky area in the ileo-caecal region gradually parted with its suspicious indications. McBurney's appendix point was for days an interesting and instructive lookout, until rendered less attractive by the evident outcome of metastatic gouty action. Undoubtedly there was well marked and circumscribed induration in the ileo-caecal area. The precise condition or character of this induration was difficult to define, and yet the rapid change consequent on metastatic action pointed to gouty deposition in or about the region of the appendix, so peculiar and transitory in its manifestations. At the end of three weeks an excellent recovery was made, and since that date there has been no recurrence of intestinal trouble.

CASE III.—RHEUMATIC PERITYPHLITIS.—Miss T., twelve years of age, vigourous and robust habit of body, conformation regular, and organs, as a whole, normal prior to the present attack. Of a highly nervous temperament, but usually enjoyed excellent health and spirits. June 1, 1893, complained of pain and sense of uneasiness in her feet, with a general feeling of systemic irritability. June 3, was suddenly seized with severe pain in the bowels, but more particularly in and about the ileo-caecal region, where tenderness on pressure was most marked. Fully two days prior to June 1, a sense of heat and feverishness was experienced, and prior to being under my charge. Temperature, 102.5° F., and pulse, 120. The bowels were at once washed out by a warm-water enema, which afforded much relief. Hot linseed poultices applied, and placed on milk diet and an aconite mixture. From June 2 to 8 the pain experienced over the bowels was very considerable, and the tenderness so severe that coughing or stretching of the legs increased the pain in a most marked manner. Turpentine enemata also afforded considerable relief. June 4, there was a decided hardness on moderate pressure over the ileo-caecal region, which gave one the impression that some tissue change had taken place, and the fact that rigidity in the abdominal walls was more marked on the affected side than on the other led me to view the condition with a degree of suspicion, although the actual position of hardness was a little lower down than McBurney's point. For fully three days the temperature was over 102° F., on which account suppuration would not be an unlikely result. June 7, the right shoulder, elbow, and wrist joints exhibited well defined symptoms of acute articular rheumatism, these parts being painful on pressure, swollen, and moved with difficulty. Just in proportion as these almost outside rheumatic conditions developed, the abdominal symptoms actually lessened in intensity, and on the 10th the entire features of the case evidenced a marked change for the better, no relapse being experienced whatever.

The question very naturally arises, What was the attack, and how developed ? True, the recognition of appendicitis is not all that is needed.

In this case, almost from the first, there was a localised pain, associated with tenderness over the region of the right iliac fossa and ascending colon, with well defined swelling, and for days the pain was so severe that it was increased at once by coughing or deep inspiration, and the almost constant desire was to elevate both knees to relieve suffering. For days, also, there was entire inability to take nourishment, owing to attacks of vomiting. The bowels were frequently injected with warm linseed tea, which afforded a degree of nourishment as well as a clearing of the contents from the canal.

In this case I concluded there was lodgment of undigested material in the caecum, and most likely induced by inability to assimilate the food, owing to deflected nerve-power from over-mental strain, as is frequently the case in our schools and universities at the present day. In the ordinary avocations of life we can trace the operation of like results, interfering seriously with the very principles of sanguinification and blood change.

The next question is, How is rheumatism associated with perityphlitis? True, the essential cause of rheumatism is still a doubted point. Errors in diet, as an aetiological factor, have much to do with the production of both gout and rheumatism, and such strengthen the metabolic theory, that rheumatism depends on a morbific material produced within the system, the result of defective processes of assimilation. True, Prout, Latham, Richardson, Mitchell, and Dr. William H. Porter, of New York, have thrown much light on the subject of rheumatism, and certainly the present case points to rheumatic complication as the outcome of defective assimilation, an important factor in its production. Thus the chemical laboratory of the human system becomes disturbed, resulting in false products, enabling us to establish a connecting link between even perityphlitis and rheumatism. In the structure of the intestinal walls there is undoubtedly a large amount of fibrous tissue, just as in the fascia and tendons of the joints, and it is reasonable to suppose that these structures should be influenced in the same manner; and assuming that the case under consideration was even quasirheumatic in its character, it affords one more illustration as to the importance of giving due consideration to the line of action embraced in medical and surgical treatment under like circumstances.

In a recent paper by A. Haig, M. A., M. D., Metropolitan hospital, London, on gout of the intestines, he states, that his chemical and experimental experience has led him to believe that " a very large number of cases of colic, enteralgia, and enteritis, and cases which are clinically indistinguishable from typhlitis, are neither more nor less than a gout of the walls of the intestinal tube, or a rheumatism," as has just been defined. In Canada, as a whole, gout is almost an unknown quantity, except in occasional cases of an hereditary type. Our people, in the midst of life's pursuits, live in a moderate way, which contributes greatly to the promotion of health. On the other hand, rheumatism is of frequent occurrence. The coldness of our winter climate, the occasional absence of flannel, and excessive exposure contribute to develop rheumatism. After noting the life-history of many thousands of our "lumbermen," I have been amazed at the few attacked by rheumatism. Bread, pork, and strong tea constitute their chief articles of diet, and the general experience is, that the tea enables them to digest the pork with remarkable comfort; and certainly, after a hard winter's work, they return home well nourished and healthy in every particular.

These facts point to simplicity as to diet. Our progenitors frequently attained the age of "three score and ten," nourished by grain ground between two stones. As a rule, the people of the present generation live too fast, resulting in mental strain and the absence of simplicity. With greater attention to diet, which should be simple in its character, in conformity with the normal functions of the alimentary canal, and the avoidance of alcoholic beverages as a whole, I feel confident perityphlitic and appendix troubles, even unconnected with gout and rheumatism, would become less troublesome factors in the line of disease. To avert various irregularities in the alimentary canal, which, if neglected, will undoubtedly lead to trouble in time, is as important as subsequent treatment, when the stage is passed in which the efforts of nature are powerful to afford relief. What active agent in the system is more frequently tampered with than gastric juice, which requires a normal temperature to perform its part in the economy? Ice-water at the commencement, and ice-cream at the end, of a meal, may be fashionable, but certainly not life preserving. Unassimilated food makes its way to parts not designed by nature to transform and absorb. As the result, how frequently, on percussion, we find extensive portions of bowel ballooned by abnormal efforts to accomplish the digestive process. Such conditions result from irregularities in living. No portion of the alimentary canal is more liable to diseased manifestations than in and about the appendix, which is a species of loop line to the digestive tract.

Insurance associations cannot note too carefully the probabilities of life in this connection. There is still much to be accomplished, and let our medical education be so directed as to bring about simplicity in living, as near as possible, to

16

the normal functions of our organs, and our generation will be greatly benefited.

DISCUSSION.

Dr. Cronyn, of Erie county, said he thought the gouty elements underlying various diseased conditions do not usually receive sufficient attention. The author had alluded to Haig; he is evidently an enthusiast on the subject of uric acid and urates. This author claims that collections of urates around the bowel may even explain the symptoms of typhlitis and perityphlitis, and he goes on to describe such a case, and how he effected a cure by medicines administered with the idea of dissolving these deposits. In a very large number of instances it would be exceedingly well for medical men to recollect the relation between diseases of the various structures of the body and the cachexia of gout; it is not necessary that there should be heredity to allow of the development of the various gouty manifestations.

MEMORANDA, SURGICAL AND PATHOLOGICAL.

By DONALD MACLEAN, M. D., of Detroit, Mich.

October 11, 1893.

Certain facts of modern medical history have, perhaps, rendered the expectation not altogether unreasonable, that on the present occasion some new and startling theory, some original method of practice, some new operation, or, at . the least, some special instrument or device, should be offered for your consideration. At all events, it will be conceded, I hope, that the time is past when the East is regarded as the only direction in which it is worth while to look for suggestive ideas which possess at once the advantages of originality and of practical utility.

When the accounts are fully and fairly balanced, my firm conviction is, that so far as the healing art is concerned, the West will be found very little, if at all, below the general average of the various sections of the civilised and scientific world. Having said this much, I desire to lose no time in relieving your minds of any apprehension you may feel that I come here from the West with the intention of trying to disturb your mental equilibrium or "confound the counsel of your philosophy" with some startling novelty, theoretical, practical, or otherwise. Far from it: my simple aim is to present to this distinguished body a brief and fragmentary glimpse of my own surgical practice, together with a brief résumé of some of the principles by which my work is guided.

And first I invite attention to the subject of ununited fractures of the long bones. It so happens that a large number of this unfortunate class of cases has fallen into my hands after the ordinary devices for relief had been tried in vain. My treatment in cases of so long standing has at last become limited to two expedients, viz.: First, the application of an external splint or support; and second, amputation, followed by resort to an artificial limb where such an appliance is feasible.

Not long ago I advised amputation of both legs below the knees of an unfortunate man for this condition, after many months had been spent in vain endeavours to secure union by resection, wiring, ivory pegs, etc. Examination of the amputated limbs demonstrated a condition of atrophy and of fatty degeneration at the points of fracture, which, to my mind, fully justified the radical course resorted to.

In the case of other bones in which the prospect of securing union seemed equally hopeless, I have been able to afford valuable assistance by the application of a well-fitting splint or brace. In this connection, I submit that heretofore surgical writers have failed to recognise the most common, the most efficient, and the most reasonable of all the causes which produce non-union of fractured bones, viz.: *Intense direct violence* in the production of the fracture,—violence so severe that the vitality of the bones and other tissues involved is destroyed or diminished to so great an extent that reparative action is feeble and imperfect, and degenerative processes are set a-going, which are progressive, and in time render union by bone impossible. In all the cases of non-union which have come to my notice, and they have been many, the original injury was *direct* and *severe*. In the case of double amputation of the legs just mentioned, the fractures were caused by sudden contact with the cow-catcher of a rapidly moving train. Confirmation of the views herein expressed is furnished by the clavicle. The clavicle is the bone most seldom affected with non-union, and we know that fractures of this bone are almost invariably caused by indirect violence.

Only two cases of non-union of the clavicle have come to my notice, and both of these were caused by direct and severe violence. One, by the kick of a horse. and the other, by a blow from the wheel of a runaway carriage.

If this view of the causation of non-union be correct, it
follows, as a logical deduction, that Senn's ingenious proposition to treat ununited and compound fractures by ferrules
and splints of bone will apply to compound fractures more
than to ununited fractures, and that in the latter cases, if it
is to be of any use at all, it must be resorted to early, *i. e.,*
before the degenerative processes inseparable from such injuries have advanced too far. Up to the present time, Senn's
method lacks almost entirely the endorsement of actual experience. My belief and sincere hope is that it will prove to
be a real advance in the treatment of a very important class
of cases.

In the second place, permit me to call attention to the
subject of amputation at the hip and shoulder joints. One
case of primary amputation at the hip for a railroad injury,
and three cases of amputation at the shoulder, one primary
for a railroad injury, one for a large sarcomatous tumor,
and one for a very extensive burn many years before, have
recently fallen to my lot.

The injury in the hip case was peculiar. The unfortunate
young man (his age was twenty-three years) was run over
by an engine, by which the entire skin of the left lower extremity was stripped off, and hung in a long flap from the
upper portion of the gluteal region. The lower part of the
abdomen was also denuded, and the testicles exposed. No
bones were broken, but the soft parts throughout the whole
extent of the limb were filled with coal-dust and foreign
matters of various kinds. The great vessels in Scarpa's tri-
angle were exposed as plainly as the most skilful dissection
could have demonstrated them. The patient was cold, pulseless, and seemed to be almost at his last breath when I saw
him at midnight, November 12, 1892. Stimulants were resorted to, heat was applied to the body, and in an hour a
slight improvement was observed, and under the circumstances it seemed proper to remove the limb, if for nothing
else than for the cosmetic effect on the corpse. I first placed
ligatures on the femoral vessels, then pared out a flap from

the loose skin which had been torn from the buttock, and lastly, I disarticulated and removed the limb with one or two sweeps of the knife. The utmost precautions were taken to save blood, and, as a matter of fact, I don't think that the patient lost more than one tablespoonful in the operation. To the surprise of all concerned, this patient made a rapid and complete recovery, and, notwithstanding the fact that a considerable portion of the flap sloughed, the stump finally healed perfectly, and he left the hospital within eight weeks of his admission.

In such an injury as this the primary ligature of the main vessels seemed the most reasonable procedure for the control of haemorrhage. I think it might often be resorted to with advantage, especially in the case of tumors of the thigh, in which the upper limit is imperfectly defined and uncertain. Still, as a rule, Wyeth, Senn, *et al.* to the contrary notwithstanding, I must declare my partiality for Lister's aortic compressor, of which I here exhibit a somewhat primitive looking specimen, which I had made for my own use in an emergency, by a common blacksmith, more than twenty years ago, and which I have repeatedly used for hip amputations, aneurisms of the femoral artery, dissecting out vascular tumors from the thigh, and so forth, and always with the most perfect satisfaction in every respect. It should be applied exactly at the umbilicus, and adjusted so as to absolutely control the arterial circulation in the legs.

Three recent cases of amputation at the shoulder joint have seemed to me worthy of being briefly noticed on the present occasion.

The first was a case of primary amputation, for a general crush of the whole upper extremity, with laceration and destruction of the skin to such an extent as to make the formation of a flap a matter of some little ingenuity. The first step in the operation consisted in the exposure and ligation of the main vessels. The patient had been conveyed many miles from the place of accident, which occurred in a railway collision, and had lost so much blood that every possible precaution was demanded to prevent further loss. My operation was nearly a bloodless one, and still the shock was so great that the most active stimulation, combined with the infusion of sodium chloride solution, barely sufficed to tide him over.

Nevertheless, his wound, with its irregular and erratic flap, healed by first intention, and he was dismissed in excellent condition on the tenth day.

The second was the case of a coloured man with a large tumor in the axilla, filling that space completely, and extending along the muscles and fasciae of the forearm right down to the elbow. The biceps, deltoid, and other muscles were imbedded in the growth. In this case, also, the only efficient method of restraining the bleeding seemed to be the ligation primarily of the main vessels. This was done, and the operation completed without difficulty, and the patient was dismissed cured on the tenth day. Five months have elapsed, and, so far, no sign of return has appeared.

The third and last case in this series presents one or two points of special interest.

Charles Andrews, aged thirty-eight, when a boy of five was severely burned over the right side and shoulder, as a result of which the arm became attached by deep and dense cicatricial tissue to the side, almost down to the elbow. About two years ago the scar tissue on the outside of the arm began to break down, and an obstinate and foul ulcer was established, which refused to heal in spite of innumerable applications which were used for the purpose of inducing healthy action, and the patient's general health began to suffer seriously. The appearance of the ulcer suggested malignant degeneration, and the microscope confirmed this suspicion. Amputation of the arm at the shoulder was recommended, and readily accepted by the patient. In this case, also, the simplest and only efficient method of restraining haemorrhage was by cutting down and ligating the main vessels first. This was done, but not without considerable difficulty, as the cicatricial contraction had imbedded all the axillary structures in one confused mass, and made their isolation a work of time and care. All possible economy was exercised in the way of preserving healthy tissue for a flap, but a large, open sore on the side had to be left to granulate. Grafting was used to aid this process, and at the end of the sixth week the patient was dismissed in perfect health, and with his wound almost completely cicatrised with good sound tissue.

In the next place, let me present a case or two from the domain of the nervous system, in which of late years surgery has done much to shed light and hope, where formerly all was darkness and despair.

Two well marked cases of spina bifida have fallen to me within a year, in both of which amputation by elliptical flap has proved entirely successful. One occurred in the case of a child a year old, and was preceded by injections of iodine into the sac. The other was in a young man, was located just beneath the occipital region, was the size of a large orange, and, as may be supposed, was a source of much irritation as well as mental distress to the patient. It is not claimed here that this method is applicable in all cases of this affection ; but my belief is, that by a judicious combination of injections of iodine solutions and subsequent amputation a very considerable proportion of cases of spina bifida may be safely and effectually disposed of.

Two cases of tumor of the median nerve of the arm have passed through my hands within the space of a year or two. One of them was a solid, apparently fibroid, degeneration of the nerve, the patient being a young woman, who very reluctantly submitted to excision after numerous palliative measures had been tried in vain, and after the pain had become both severe and constant.

The other case occurred in a man aged fifty-eight years, and had also become so painful that the patient was ready to submit to anything that promised relief. Complete excision was performed, and I am able to show the specimen, which will be found to be a cyst over which the nerve fibres are spread out in a strikingly membranous form. Whether a mere coincidence or a logical sequence, the fact remains that in both of these cases, which were operated upon under chloroform, the patients, at the moment of division of the proximal portion of the nerve, became absolutely collapsed, and were resuscitated only after long continued and extremely vigourous efforts, in which all the ordinary methods available in such cases were resorted to. In each case the recovery was ultimately complete, although a slight degree of paralysis remains in the parts supplied by the median nerve.

On August 20, 1882, I amputated the left breast of a lady aged sixty-five, on account of a scirrhous growth, that involved the whole of the gland, which was an unusually large one. Every clinical sign of malignant disease was present, and the microscope fully confirmed the diagnosis. More than eleven years have now passed, and this patient continues alive and well, with no sign of return or of secondary development anywhere. About five years ago this lady's son, a man of forty, came to me with unmistakable carcinoma of the tongue, for which I removed the entire organ after every other conceivable treatment had been tried. He, also, made a good recovery, and has continued well up to the present time.

And now I desire to present briefly another case of carcinoma, in which, if the result is unsatisfactory, the history is interesting and suggestive,—

J. H. R., aged 41, applied to me on November 6, 1890, on account of an ulcer on the palmar surface of the first phalanx of the ring finger of his left hand. According to his statement, the trouble commenced in what seemed to be a common wart, which he tried to eradicate with the aid of his pocket-knife. The result of this treatment was a sore, which obstinately refused to cicatrise in spite of the most earnest efforts of a large number of medical men, who successively undertook the task of inducing it to heal. My diagnosis of epithelioma was quickly made, and in a very few minutes thereafter the ulcerated finger, along with a good full margin of sound tissue, was amputated. The wound healed by the first intention, and in a few days the patient was again at work on his farm. For two years after this he enjoyed excellent health in every respect. At the end of that time, however, he returned to me with a tumor the size of an orange in the axilla. No other evidence of his former trouble could be detected. Without delay I excised the tumor, together with everything of the nature of a gland in the axilla, which was laid freely open for the purpose. From this operation the patient made a good but rather slow recovery, complaining a good deal of a feeling of general debility, loss of appetite, etc. Still he recovered sufficiently to resume active work. Six months afterwards he returned, but now in a perfectly hopeless condition from general infiltration in the axilla, neck, thoracic wall, etc., from which he soon died, exhausted.

Query.—Is it not an assured fact that cases are common in which such irritation as was supplied in this instance by the injudicious use of the pocket-knife is all that is required to wake up such an outbreak of malignancy as occurred in the unfortunate experience here detailed?

One more brief case, and I have done.

I show you here a gold plate with one false tooth attached, the whole thing making a combination of curves, hooks, and angles, extremely unfavourable for passage either upwards or downwards through the oesophagus. A patient of mine, who is a very large, fat, thick-necked man, having forgotten to remove his plate on retiring, was awakened at two o'clock in the morning in a state of great distress, having swallowed his plate while asleep. The most careful and thorough examination with the finger failed to locate the foreign body, but the persistent hoarse cough, dyspnoea, pain, etc., combined to testify to its presence somewhere short of the stomach. Oesophagotomy and gastrotomy in a man of my patient's physique seemed very unpleasant procedures to contemplate. Fortunately, these contingencies were avoided by the safe delivery of the foreign body by means of the forceps which I here show you. For several days afterward the patient complained of uneasy sensations in swallowing, but these soon disappeared, and his recovery was quite complete.

In closing, permit me to express the hope that I have not entirely exhausted the patience of my audience, but that in the somewhat varied selection of personal surgical experiences I have furnished at least a little food for thought, and material for useful discussion. In one respect, at least, I claim for my paper a slight degree of difference from the great majority of latter-day surgical contributions, namely, the abdominal and pelvic cavities have been carefully steered clear of.

DISCUSSION ON THE TREATMENT OF APPENDICITIS.

QUESTION I.

WHAT PROPORTION· OF CASES OF APPENDICITIS END IN RESOLUTION?

QUESTION II.

WHAT CLASS OF CASES REQUIRE IMMEDIATE OPERATION?

QUESTION III.

WHAT CLASS OF CASES DO NOT REQUIRE IMMEDIATE OPERATION?

REMARKS INTRODUCTORY TO THE DISCUSSION.

By FREDERIC S. DENNIS, M. D., of New York County.

October 11, 1893.

To formulate precise and satisfactory answers to these three questions which are presented for discussion this afternoon, is not an easy task. The difficulty arises from the fact, that though much has been done to clear away many doubtful points in relation to the treatment of this affection, there yet remains a good deal that is obscured in a cloud of uncertainty. Among surgeons there is as yet no unanimity of opinion as to the exact time when an operation should be performed. During the past two years the pendulum has swung so far that now it begins to swing in the opposite direction. It is a noteworthy fact that this operation is one

of the very few in surgery where extreme radicalism and
over-cautious conservatism are both observed. It is seldom
in surgical practice that an operation is viewed from such
diametric points. An honest diversity of opinion exists, and
each side is ably supported, and the questions at issue are of
portentous importance, since human life is at stake.

In regard to an answer to the first question, viz., What
proportion of cases of appendicitis end in resolution? it may
be stated that a pretty uniform opinion exists. By appendicitis in the broad sense of the term, including all iliac inflammations in the right iliac fossa, the figures are placed by
nearly all writers at fifty per cent., while by some as high as
even seventy-five per cent. In general, in about a third of
the cases the question of operation arises.

I believe the chief thing that has confused the general surgeon is the acceptance of the pathology which has been
recently introduced, to the effect that all these inflammations
are the primary result of an appendicitis. Now, as a matter
of fact, there are several different varieties of inflammation
in this region, entirely independent of an appendicitis. I
have seen the post-mortem appearance of inflammation of
the caecum, the result of traumatism and of crude ingesta,
and am familiar with one case of the action of corrosive poi-
sons, and the appendix not diseased. I know of four cases of
perforation of the caecum, in which death resulted from this
condition, and the diagnosis of appendicitis was made, but
the appendix was proved to be not involved. When these
facts are considered, it is no longer a question of doubt as to
whether an iliac inflammation can exist without a primary
appendicitis. Thus it is evident that ordinary inflammation
in this region can undergo resolution just as the same process does in other parts of the body.

In this one third of the cases the question of laparotomy
pertains, since in nearly two thirds of the cases resolution is
likely to follow. In the entire number of cases, perforation
is a very unusual event. It has often been urged, that if a
patient has been fortunate enough to recover by a process of

resolution, that even under these circumstances an operation should have been performed; since the first attack predisposes to a second, and then a recurrent appendicitis is established, all the attacks of which would have been avoided by an early operation at the time of the first seizure. To be sure, there is a certain percentage of the cases that become relapsing in character; but it has been demonstrated that eighty-nine per cent. of the cases involve a solitary attack, and that only eleven per cent. of the cases are multiple. In a careful study of the cases it has been proved that after operation and removal of the appendix the attacks still persist, a fact which must not be overlooked.

In regard to an answer to the second question, as to what class of cases require immediate operation, it may be said that only an approximate one can be given. In the future, without doubt, data will be forthcoming which will enable the surgeon to determine with greater precision some diagnostic points which at the present time are unknown. I do not wish to be understood to advise or countenance delay in operative interference in cases of appendicitis, provided urgent symptoms are present and persistent. I am firmly convinced, however, that often an operation is performed too early and without sufficient grounds, and that a short delay would soon make clear the diagnosis and obviate the dangers of an operation which has proved the incorrectness of the diagnosis. If early operation were restricted to those cases where the onset was sudden, where the pain was intense, where a suppurative chart exists, where a rapid pulse is found, and these symptoms show no abatement within forty-eight to seventy-two hours, the number of cases operated upon would be vastly diminished. The primary object of an early operation is to save life; and as perforation is so rare an event, when all the cases of iliac inflammation in this fossa are considered, immediate operation must of necessity apply to a very limited number. In the cases which do not correspond to the above Procrustean rule, delay is admissible; and by this I mean cases where the temperature is not

much above normal, where the pulse is not out of proportion
to the temperature, where the pain is not severe, where the
bowels are freely moved, and where there is a satisfactory
explanation of the cause.   In such cases early operation is
not indicated.

An answer to the third question,—as to what class of cases
do not require immediate operation,—is attended with some
difficulty.   On the one hand the surgeon is confronted with
the possibility of his patient's death, and on the other hand
with the performance of an unnecessary operation, which has,
to his surprise, revealed the fact that the appendix was not
the aetiological factor in the production of the disease, and
that the trouble in the future has not been relieved.   Under
these conditions the circumstances are most trying, and the
surgeon is sorely perplexed as to the right course to pursue.
I believe that unless elevation of temperature, rapid pulse,
great pain, and suppurative chart persist, the patient's best
chances for life are better by delay.   The reasons lie in the
following facts: The danger of an operation to human life,
the errors of diagnosis, and the development of ventral
hernia.

The danger of the operation to human life is not to be
overlooked.   I am well aware that in the hands of a few
skilled surgeons, with properly trained assistants and nurses,
with every aseptic detail at hand, the danger is slight.   But
these are not the conditions or the circumstances that sur-
round the ordinary patient, who is subjected to a great risk,
owing to the absence of every essential antiseptic require
ment.   I believe, besides the ordinary danger of the laparotomy, a new danger is set up in the introduction of the bacilli
communis coli, which has demonstrated its ability to cause
a suppurative peritonitis in consequence of the operation.

Opening the abdomen for the purpose of finding the appendix vermiformis is certainly attended with risk to life.   That
risk increases in accordance with the amount of pathological
change that has taken place.   I must dissent from the view
held by Morton, who speaks of this procedure as a " compara-

tively trivial operation, at a time and under conditions when prompt and permanent relief and recovery can almost invariably be secured." The same opinion is also expressed by Senn, who writes: " Excision of the appendix in cases of simple uncomplicated appendicitis is one of the easiest and safest of all intra-abdominal operations." Such statements are misleading. In May, 1887, I successfully excised the appendix on account of a stab-wound, with no difficulty as regards finding it; but to remove it and to invert the edges and to introduce sutures and to close hermetically the opening into the caecum, is. a delicate operation which requires nicety of technique. It is by no means to be considered a trivial procedure, and upon the result of the operative work of the surgeon depends the life of the patient. The giving way of a stitch, or the sloughing of a small shred, exposes the patient to imminent peril. One bubble of intestinal gas is sufficient to infect the whole peritonaeum, and such a catastrophe will in all probability lead to a fatal termination. The possibilities of haemorrhage, of purulent oedema, of septic peritonitis, of suppression of urine, and of surgical shock, must not be overlooked. These are the dangers to which a patient is subjected in the ordinary cases; but when, from recurrent attacks, adhesions have formed, the connective tissue has undergone pathological changes, the caecum has become dilated, and the anatomical relations are disturbed, excision of the appendix becomes a serious operation. Surgeons have attempted to find an analogy between removal of the appendix and of the ovary. This comparison causes a tendency to attach too little importance to the excision of the appendix. It must be borne in mind that the vermiform is an integral part of the alimentary canal; it often is adherent to the large and important blood-vessels, it may be buried under the caecum, it may be firmly imbedded in inflammatory exudation, the tearing of which may result in a rent in the intestine or ureter, and the sewing up of which requires time and skill. Not so with the ovary, for here the oozing is easily controlled, and if a pus cavity is found the cavity can be washed out easily and rendered aseptic. For these reasons the excision of the appendix cannot be looked upon in any light other than that of an operation attended with considerable risk to human life.

The Errors of Diagnosis.—No surgeon who has seen many cases of abdominal surgery can overlook the fact that the diagnosis is often fraught with the greatest difficulties and with much uncertainty. The more cases examined, the more real becomes this fact. It is often impossible to arrive at a positive and clear diagnosis as to the real condition that has given rise to the attacks. The most skilled diagnosticians and the most experienced surgeons have made errors in diagnosis as regards lesions in this region. It is only necessary to review the list of diseases that already have been mistaken for appendicitis, in order to estimate the weight of this argument against excision of the appendix during a quiescent period.

Among the conditions that have been mistaken for appendcitis may be mentioned the following: General or circumscribed peritonitis, pelvic peritonitis, renal, biliary, and intestinal colic, ovarian and lumbo-abdominal neuralgia. intestinal obstruction, floating kidney, pyelitis, caecitis, internal strangulation, psoas abscess, pelvic cellulitis, rupture of the serratus magnus muscle, suppurative adenitis, typhoid, tubercular, and stercoral ulcers, caries of ilium and of vertebrae, morbus coxarius, suppuration in the retro-peritonaeal and mesenteric glands, traumatic rupture of intestine and right ureter, rupture of the bladder and of the gall-bladder, rupture of an aneurism in the broad ligament, sprain of the iliacus and psoas-muscles, salpingitis of the right tube, abscess of liver, tubal pregnancy, typhlitis, and perityphlitis.

This list does not embrace nearly all the conditions which eminent men in the profession have frankly acknowledged to have mistaken for appendicitis, or vice versa. The list, however, is of sufficient size to impress the important point that errors in diagnosis may occur, and that a laparotomy for supposed appendicitis may be performed and the real pathological condition, which the operation is intended to relieve, be other than a diseased appendix. Finally, it is significant that in some of the cases in which the appendix has been removed during the quiescent period no change sufficient to cause trouble could be found in the appendix.

This condition is likely to follow a laparotomy for excision of the appendix, since the length of the incision is from four to five inches. Many cases of ventral hernia following operations for removal of the appendix have been reported. The special situation of this incision and the peculiar character of the parts divided, and the tendency of the wound to gape, render the development of hernia a most serious complication. There is no doubt that this condition can give rise to strangulation, and even if strangulation does not follow, the presence of the ventral hernia is a source of great discomfort and annoyance to a patient.

In fact, so frequent is this condition that a special truss has been constructed for every patient to wear after the operation, and a prominent instrument maker has informed me that within the last twelve months he has sold over six dozen trusses constructed for the relief of ventral hernia following operation for appendicitis.

To recapitulate : From one half to two thirds of the cases terminate by resolution. The immediate operation is called for where the urgent symptoms continue without any abatement after the third day, and the cases in which an immediate operation is not required are those in which after the second or third day there is a general subsidence of all the symptoms. There is, of course, always the exception to a general rule in surgery, and I can conceive of a case where within twenty-four hours an operation should be performed, and still again, another case where after seventy-two hours, and even after many days, an operation should be performed. The surgeon must always bear in mind the fact that every case of appendicitis is not certain to terminate in perforation, that there are dangers connected with the early operation, that errors of diagnosis are common, and that a ventral her-

17

nia is a serious complication arising from operative interference, and finally, that in the presence of urgent, persistent symptoms the nature of the disease admits of no delay.

GENERAL DISCUSSION.

Dr. JOHN W. S. GOULEY said he fully concurred with the writer in the views he had so well expressed. He could only add a few facts from his own observation, in corroboration of these views.

He had observed twenty-four cases of appendicitis that ended in resolution. This was since the publication of Dr. Willard Parker's paper. There was no doubt in these cases about the diagnosis and the wisdom of the expectant treatment adopted. In the last two years with the same physician he saw six cases of appendicitis. In none of these was there any doubt about the diagnosis: five ended in resolution, and in one an abscess formed and opened spontaneously into the bowels, apparently into the caecum. The patient made a good recovery. Last July he saw, in consultation, a case of appendicitis in a man having advanced cardiac disease, who was in no condition for an operation. He was treated expectantly, and made a perfect recovery. During Dr. Dennis's absence from the city, he saw in St. Vincent's hospital a man with appendicitis. He advised against operation; recovery was rapid. A few days later a woman was sent into the same hospital for operation. A careful examination established the diagnosis, but no operation was performed; yet the patient recovered completely. About fifteen years ago he operated on a gentleman for recurring attacks. At the third attack a large abscess formed, and this was freely opened in the iliac region and a faecal concretion extracted, but the appendix vermiformis was never seen. Healing was prompt.

A year and a half ago he attended a case of appendicitis at St. Vincent's hospital with Dr. Charles Phelps. It had existed for five or six weeks. If he remembered correctly, the man had been on the medical side of the hospital for two weeks before the nature of the trouble was ascertained. There was distinct fluctuation in the lumbo-iliac region, and the question was whether the patient was suffering from a perinephritic or a perityphlitic abscess. An exploratory operation was done, and this revealed the fact that he had both, the former abscess being secondary to the one connected with the caecum or its appendix. The pus had burrowed under the liver and across the vertebral column, posterior to the peritonaeum, and had extended down towards the left iliac region; it was an enormous pus cavity. The wound was thoroughly washed, and among the shreddy masses washed out there was one resembling the appendix vermiformis. The greater part of the wound was stitched, but a drainage tube was left in for several months. He ultimately made a good recovery. He had observed several other cases in which the long delay was fully justified.

A few years ago he saw a young gentleman in collapse. While dancing, five evenings before, he was seized with a sudden pain in the right iliac region, and he felt so faint that he was taken to bed. When first seen by the speaker, on the afternoon of the fifth day, he was moribund; he died two hours later. The autopsy showed general peritonitis and a perforation of the appendix vermiformis. This might have been a fit case for an immediate operation, *i. e.,* one within five or six hours of the accident. There could have been no doubt about the diagnosis in that case, and the man was only about thirty years of age and in excellent physical condition. If the peritonaeal cavity had been thoroughly washed out there would have been a fair chance of recovery. It is in this class of cases that an immediate operation is justified; nevertheless, he fully agreed with Dr. Dennis that in at least half of the cases of appendicitis there is no need of an operation.

Dr. DONALD MACLEAN said that the questions propounded here for discussion had presented themselves to him, and to every operating surgeon, as among the most difficult and momentous they were called upon to answer. If we refuse to operate, disaster may follow; if we operate, we may regret it, for perhaps we may find no justification for the operation.

Some time ago, he was called hastily to a young gentleman in Detroit, whom he knew to have a very delicate constitution. He was taken sick while in the lumber region of Michigan, and came home on a special train. When first seen, he was in bad condition; his pulse was rapid, his complexion sallow, his temperature 100.5°, and there were all the local signs of appendicitis. Arrangements were made for the operation, but it was decided to wait twenty-four hours, unless there were specially urgent symptoms. At the end of this time there was slight improvement, and he gradually recovered completely, without operation. This was one year and nine months ago, and since then he has been in good health. If the doctrine is to hold, that we must operate so as to avoid subsequent operation, then we should establish the rule that the appendix is to be removed from every child soon after its birth.

A young girl of fifteen years suddenly developed the characteristic symptoms of appendicitis, and an eminent consulting surgeon of Detroit pronounced it as his opinion that an operation was the only thing to be done. A homoeopathic so called doctor was called in, and he held up his hands in horror at the thought of an operation. It is hardly necessary to say that the homoeopathic practitioner continued in attendance, and that, after giving some of his little pills, the patient completely recovered.

He was himself called in to a member of a very prominent family in the same city. The patient had had attacks of appendicitis once or twice before. The attending physician agreed with him, that the time had come for an operation, and the operation was performed. Looking back over all the operations he had performed in the course of his life, there was none in which he felt so completely satisfied with his work when it was finished. On opening the abdominal cavity, he found a swollen, inflamed, and adherent appendix; and although there was no pus visible, there were enough adhesions, he thought, to account for the condition. Nothing entered the peritonaeal cavity except his thumb and fore-finger, no sponges and no irrigating fluid. The operation was done under the strictest asepsis; yet the patient woke up in agony, and remained in this condition up to the time of her death, twenty-four hours afterwards. You can easily fancy how these two cases, occurring side by side in the same city, have been utilised by the friends of honest, beneficent surgery. In this case, there probably existed somewhere in that cavity a secondary depot which carried the infection.

It is all very well for surgeons in metropolitan hospitals to lay down the law that Senn has, viz.: that removal of an appendix is a very safe and easy operation, but such operations are often done under much less favourable surroundings, and hence, it is wrong for surgeons to allow such a doctrine to be spread abroad. We are often called upon to operate in the country. It should be remembered that we not only have to contend against difficulties of our own consciences, but also against the prejudice and gossip and ignorance of our neighbours, male and female.

No one physician's experience can justify us in answering these questions positively, and Dr. Dennis has come as nearly as possible to answering them accurately.

At one time, a young girl, sixteen years of age, came to him complaining only of pain in her right side—a very common symptom in young women—but she had lost twenty-eight pounds in weight within a few weeks and there was a slight febrile movement, although her general appearance was favourable. So great was her suffering that she readily gave her consent to an exploratory operation. A small incision was made, but palpation revealed nothing; the right ovary and tube appeared healthy, but on lifting up the *left* ovary, he found to his surprise an appendix eight inches long, which was attached by its mesentery to the left ovary. In examining it, this adhesion was ruptured. The ovary and appendix were removed, and the patient made a good recovery. One can readily see how easy it would be to overlook such a condition; it was most fortunate that he discovered it.

Here is another case. A blacksmith was treated by a competent physician for an acute appendicitis. All the characteristic symptoms were present, but suddenly there was a marked rise of temperature and other constitutional symptoms, and at the same time there was a diminution of the swelling. The speaker was called in at that time, and found him expectorating very freely the most foetid pus. There was dulness over the lungs posteriorly. Apparently, the pus had started from the appendix and burrowed upwards beneath the peritonaeum, and found an exit through the bronchial tubes. A free opening was made between the sixth and seventh ribs on the right side, and an enormous quantity of pus washed out. A drainage tube was inserted. The patient recovered.

He could recall during the past two years quite a large number of cases of appendicitis in which the symptoms were quite urgent, and yet they recovered without operation.

Dr. JOSEPH D. BRYANT said it was indeed a pleasure to hear the remarks that had been made by the preceding speakers, for it afforded one an opportunity to compare one's own lines of thought and practice with those of others, and profit thereby.

He thought the first question could only be properly answered by making a comparison with the results of inflammation of contiguous structures. It has been estimated that forty to fifty per cent. of inflammations of the caput coli and contiguous structures recover by resolution. But what is resolution? He assumed it to mean a complete recovery, within a reasonable time, from all the symptoms of appendicitis. Taking this view for the moment, he would inquire, Can a patient recover by resolution if gangrene of the appendix takes place? Can a case recover by resolution if there is a perforation, or if an abscess follows the inflammation? He thought not. Now in what percentage of these cases do we have perforation, abscess, and gangrene? He would answer, that in seventy per cent. of adult males there is a foreign body in the appendix; this has been proven, not only by the examinations made by others, but by his own observations on one hundred and fifty bodies in the dead-house of Bellevue hospital. This is not pleasant to contemplate, but it is nevertheless true. In not one of the instances have the traditional grape-seeds been found; the foreign substance is usually a faecal concretion. In the female subject, in only about forty per cent. does the appendix contain a foreign body. As the relative frequency of appendicitis in males and females is about the same as the relative frequency of foreign bodies in the appendix, it is reasonable to assume that the faecal concretions have much to do with causing appendicitis.

Fitch has shown that over fifty per cent. of fatal cases which have been examined show perforation of the vermiform appendix; hence, the real question is, Are there any means by which we can determine whether gangrene or perforation has taken place, or if abscess is present? We can only do this by referring to the history of the case; and on this the question of operation should be based. Admitting the difficulty of diagnosis, he held that, given the symptoms indicative of appendicitis and of perforation, if the operation be performed and no evidence of appendicitis be found, he regarded it as good news rather than as an argument against operating.

The first important symptom is excruciating pain, located as a rule at the caecum. In quite a large number of cases, however, the pain is not referred to the seat of the disease. Will such pain occur if there is no perforation and no gangrene? Does the pain occur only at the time of perforation? In his judgment, where there is severe and continuous pain, followed quickly by tympanites, perforation occurs at this time; and that the gangrene, which so frequently follows, may have existed in the lumen of the vermiform or extended to its outer wall. Assuming that perforation has taken place, he believed in immediate operation. The symptoms will be acute in almost every instance. If he were certain that perforation had occurred, he would never wait even three days. Assuming that gangrene or perforation or abscess was present, he would operate at once. Fever is a very dangerous symptom to rely upon. In one of his recent cases, there was a normal temperature and pulse, yet the patient developed septic peritonitis, and died very quickly.

The McBurney point, *i. e.*, a tender point located midway between the anterior superior spinous process of the ilium and the umbilicus, is said to be indicative of appendicitis. This implies that the appendix must be located quite near this point. When it is remembered, however, that the caput coli may occupy all positions in the abdominal cavity, and that in fourteen per cent. of the cases the vermiform appendix extends into the pelvic cavity, and in two per cent. passes up behind the colon, it is evident that the presence of the McBurney point can only be considered as contributive evidence.

In answer to the second question, he would say that any case which, by reason of the severity of the pain, increase of temperature, and shock, led one to believe perforation had taken place, demands immediate operation; at any rate, the operation should be done within the first three days, provided there is evidence of active inflammation taking place.

Is the presence of a tumor any help to us? In fourteen per cent. of the cases, the vermiform appendix extends into the pelvis, and in many cases there will be pelvic abscess as a result of perforation of the appendix. In about twenty per cent. it is behind the caput coli, and in two per cent. it is high up behind the colon; therefore, the tumor cannot be relied upon; but if the fever, tenderness, and tympanites continue after three days, and the rectus muscle is rigid, he would operate, and he would lay more stress on the muscular rigidity and tympanites than on the temperature. He thought we might safely say that no hard and fast rule can be drawn in regard to operating in appendicitis; each case must be decided on its own merits, and we must decide what method is safest and best to recommend to the general profession.

In closing, he would say, that if the six dozen trusses said to have been sold during the past year by one firm for persons who had been operated upon for appendicitis were ordered as a means of preventing the occurrence of ventral hernia, it was most wise; but if for the relief of such hernia, it was most unfortunate.

Dr. J. A. WYETH said he wished to go on record as endorsing most heartily the position taken by Dr. Bryant. If we are in doubt in these cases, it is safer to err on the side of an exploratory operation, if the surgeon be competent to perform it. There are many surgeons outside of metropolitan hospitals who are perfectly able to do these operations. Many of these cases undoubtedly get well by resolution; but suppose one hundred human beings are attacked with appendicitis, and we let them all alone: how many would get well, and how many die? Supposing, again, they were all operated upon by competent surgeons within the first forty-eight hours: how many would die, and how would this mortality compare with that of the non-operative treatment? All the disasters he had seen in the surgery of appendicitis had been due to delay; he could not recall any from too early operation. If the operation be done early, where proper co-aptation with sutures can be obtained, hernia is not likely to occur; it is in the late cases, where a gaping wound must be left, that it is most common.

Dr. E. D. FERGUSON, speaking from the stand-point of one who did not do hospital work, but who had had a certain amount of experience in operative work in private practice, said he saw at least twenty cases of appendicitis annually. The experience of one man is apt to be peculiar. In stating that number of cases, we must necessarily include the errors of diagnosis, but the chance of error must be included in our cases of exploratory operation. Not more than three to four of his cases had required operation each year. Another curious feature in his experience was that recurrent appendicitis had been very rare. In every one of the cases of peritonitis requiring operation the point of rupture in the appendix had been previously protected by adhesions. Had he done the operation to protect his patients from the contingency of diffused peritonitis, he would probably have had more deaths. In his opinion, the cases requiring immediate operation are those in which there is diffused peritonitis, probably due to a rupture of an unprotected appendix. So far, every one of his operative cases had recovered, and the only cases of peritonitis with fatal result were two which declined operation. All the non-operative cases had also recovered.

Regarding the disposition of the appendix in suppurative cases, he would say it is quite generally considered that the appendix is to be sought for, and when found, removed. This is a gross error. If there be already an abscess cavity, it is our duty to protect the remainder of the peritonaeal cavity from this. He had left the appendix in quite a number of cases where he had been unable to find it without too much manipulation, and with one exception there had been no trouble. In this one case there was a sinus which was slow in healing. It is a matter of importance for us to decide how far we are to search for the appendix, remembering that the search that destroys protective adhesions is an added danger. Personally, he believed if it could not be readily found, it will not do any harm in the majority of cases to leave it.

Dr. W. T. LUSK, of New York, said he wished to speak of the ethical side of this question of operation, for it is now in about the same stage as the operation for salpingitis was not long ago. It was believed at one time that every case of gonorrhoeal salpingitis must be promptly operated upon, as they never recovered without operation, and were likely to terminate fatally. After a while, we found that many of our cases apparently recovered, and now there is a revulsion of feeling regarding the operative treatment of these cases.

The speaker then described the tribulations of a certain gentleman who had an attack of what he believed was colic; but the physician who was first summoned thought it was appendicitis, and advised immediate operation. There was no fever and no disturbance of the pulse, and all the pain was in the neighbourhood of the navel; he could bear any amount of weight on his ileocaecal region. This attack passed off spontaneously. Subsequently he consulted Sir Andrew Clarke and other distinguished men in Europe, and they advised against operation. Coming home in the steamer, he met a number of distinguished American surgeons, all but one of whom strongly advised operation to prevent future trouble. After his return he had another attack, the same as before, but it followed a very hearty lunch of lobster salad. Quite recently, a certain Western paper described a remarkable operation for appendicitis, done by a certain surgeon in New York city, and went on to say that if a person has a pain in his side he is in imminent danger of his life, and his appendix should be removed. This ethical side, therefore, should not be ignored by this Association.

Dr. CRONYN referred to an error in diagnosis which had come under his observation. The patient had localised pain in the right iliac fossa, and other symptoms of appendicitis, but there was very great doubt as to the exact nature of the trouble. One physician advised against operation; others advised operation. After two weeks the pain was so great and the swelling so great and hard that a large trocar was plunged into the hard swelling. This test was negative. After a delay of four days, an exploratory incision three inches long was made down to the peritonaeum, but no disintegrated tissue was found; so the wound was packed with iodoform gauze, and a drainage tube inserted. The pain was intense during all this time, and the bowels were obstinately constipated. The fourth day after the operation something white appeared at the bottom of the wound, which was supposed to be pus under the peritonaeum. Poultices were applied. On the following morning, while the wound was being dressed, the patient, with the help of a looking-glass, introduced a forceps and removed this white substance, which proved to be a piece of omentum. Recovery immediately followed. It is well, therefore, to recall that a piece of omentum may be in the inguinal canal, and may give rise to symptoms simulating those of appendicitis. It is an exceptional case, but is worthy of remembrance.

APPENDICITIS.

By R. N. COOLEY, M. D., of Oswego County.

Read by title October 11, 1893.

It is not my purpose to enter into the aetiology, or a particular pathological investigation of the subject of appendicitis, but simply to relate a few purely surgical cases, as taken from my note-book as far back as 1867, and compare the management then and later; and, as you will see by my relation of my earlier cases, only dire disaster was the result in every case upon which I was not permitted to operate. Gentlemen will please understand that this paper only relates to cases where the swelling, inflammation, induration, and pain were confined to the right iliac region, between its antérior superior spinous process and the umbilicus, without any marked symptoms of disease upon the left side. Hence we shall confine ourselves to purely local conditions, where surgical treatment is the only plan that promises any success; and the cases I describe are only the typical ones in which my diagnosis has been verified either by a post-mortem examination or an operation. I have seen many other cases which have been as clearly marked instances of appendicitis as these I am about to relate, which ran a short course and then partially recovered, only to again and again recur, and at last in the end terminate unfavourably. Many cases are undoubtedly caused by inflammation of the mucous coat of the appendix, which, under proper management, make good recoveries. It is not, however, that class of cases to which this paper refers, but to those cases which demand prompt and thorough measures to insure recovery, and in such cases we usually find foreign bodies, which by their presence induce suppurative inflammation, that must be treated surgically to insure permanent recovery.

During my pupilage, while under the instruction of Dr. Corydon L. Ford, and when he was once illustrating the anatomical relations of the abdominal viscera, he found the vermiform appendix enlarged to over one inch in diameter and over four inches in length, perforated in several places, and containing in its cavity several cherry pits, which, he told us, were probably the cause of the man's death. It occurred to me at the time, that if the organ could be removed near its attachment, that troubles of the kind might be successfully treated by the surgeon, and when an opportunity offered, I asked the professor his opinion in regard to the probability of recovery in such cases. He said he could see no reason why such an operation could not be successfully performed and patients saved, as well as in cases of strangulated hernia.

This case, and Professor Ford's conversation with me on the subject, formulated in my own mind a resolution to attempt the operation should I have a well-marked case in my practice and could obtain permission to make the operation. After commencing to practise, I had not long to wait for the case, but the opportunity to apply surgery I could not obtain. I will give a short detailed account of it, taken from notes made at the time.

June 9, 1867, 9 p. m. Called to visit Mr. H. P., farmer, 45 years of age, of slight build and erect figure. Taken at 3 p. m. with a severe chill, which was prolonged until 6 p. m. Said he thought at the time he was going to have ague. Soon after the chill passed off a very severe pain commenced over the right hip, as he described it, but which I found to be about midway between the crest of the ilium and umbilicus, confined entirely to the right side, and circumscribed to the point named. His pulse rate was 111, and his temperature by the crude, crooked fever thermometers of that time was 108½°. Believing I had a case of inflammation of the appendix vermiformis, I gave opium and alterative doses of calomel, alternating with veratrum viride, and hot, moist fomentation locally.

June 10, at 8 a. m. Pulse rate 104, and temperature 108½° (as our thermometers at that time only marked halves), pain not much lessened. Continued same treatment and increased opiate.

June 11, 8 a. m. Pulse rate 106, temperature 108½°. Pain unchanged. Increased opiate and veratrum, continued other treatment, explained the case to the family, and asked to have council, which was immediately summoned. In the meantime I explained the case to the patient and his wife, and told them I believed an operation was the only thing that could possibly save the patient, and he then consented· to have an operation performed when help arrived, and I prepared to do it, pending the arrival of council. Upon the arrival of Dr. Wm. S. Kyle, late of Sterling, N. Y., he tried to discourage me, and did discourage the patient and family, and said such cases often recovered; that such an operation had never been performed and would likely terminate disastrously, but he advised the continuance of the treatment.

June 12. No abatement of the symptoms. More pain and a more tense condition of the parts, which were more than ever circumscribed. Pulse 112, temperature 104°. Obliged to resort to the hypodermic use of morphia to control the pain.

June 13. Symptoms more aggravated. Dr. Stephen Pardee, late of Fulton, N. Y., called. He would not advise an operation, and said he would not discourage one; but did advise injections of warm water, which were of very little benefit. Bowels slightly relieved of some flatus. Pain remained about the same, and could get slight fluctuation at the centre of the tumefied condition. Then I strongly urged the necessity of cutting down into the abscess which I felt sure was forming, and this privilege was also denied me. Pulse rate 115, temperature 104°.

June 14. Patient seems much exhausted, takes less milk and brandy and animal broth, all of which he had been taking during his illness. Fluctuation plainly distinct, pain less, pulse 122, temperature 103. Urged him to have the abscess opened, which was now very plainly marked, but could not prevail upon them to have it done.

Sent for at 3 a. m., June 15. saying the patient was much worse, and found him in a state of collapse, and he soon died, it being about five days from the time of the chill until the time of his death.

June 16, at 12 m., in the presence of Dr. Wm. S. Kyle and others, I made a post-mortem examination, and found, after cutting down midway between the anterior superior spinous process of the ilium and the umbilicus, slight adhesion of peritonaeum and omentum, also adhesions of omentum and caecum and colon. The appendix was quite firmly attached to the colon, and perforated in several places, as we found after sponging away the contents of the large abscess in which it lay. After removing it, we found it to be the repository of a large number of berry seeds, several grape seeds, and an orange or lemon seed partially decomposed.

My next case of appendicitis occurred in 1869.

Was called to see the daughter of Mr. O., farmer. She was 12 years of age, and was taken with a severe chill in school. Saw her the first time on May 14, 1869, at 6 p. m. Pulse rate 120, temperature 103½°, and she complained of very severe pain in the right iliac region, which region seemed tender to the touch, and the skin and tissues subjoined seemed quite tense, with no pain on the left side. I felt sure I had another case of inflammation of the vermiform appendix.

May 15, at 8 a. m. Patient much worse. Pulse 130, temperature 104°. Pain so very severe it seemed impossible to control it with opiates, except when administered hypodermically. Staid nearly the whole time during the twenty-four hours following, or until 8 a. m., May 16. All the symptoms seemed aggravated. Pulse rate at this time 130, temperature 104+°, respiration 30. Continued the same treatment with am. carb. and milk, with moist and hot fomentations, and all without relief, when I asked for council, and the same gentleman that saw the other case was called, who again opposed an operation, which opposition was sustained by the parents, and all my persuasions and entreaties were without avail.

May 17, 9 a. m. Patient much worse. Pulse rate 140, weak, thready, and irregular. Temperature 105°. Respiration irregular and gasping, cyanosis commencing, and everything looking absolutely unfavourable.

Patient died at 2:45 p. m., May 17, living about seventy-two hours after the first chill. I was permitted to make a post-mortem examination twenty-four hours after death. Well marked rigor mortis. Upon section of abdominal wall, midway between the umbilicus and the anterior superior spine of the illum, I came immediately upon a fold of omentum which was slightly adherent to the colon and to the external end of the appendix, but was easily separated from its attachments. Appendix was 5¼ inches long, and its largest diameter was near the middle portion, where it exceeded one inch, and it was perforated by three openings. Upon a close inspection I found in its cavity several raisin seeds, and a small concretion, which was very hard. Several blackish, friable spots appeared on the colon, and all of the tissues immediately surrounding seemed gangrenous.

I omitted to say that in both of the cases described a full dose of Epsom salts had been administered before I saw them.

My next and third case was E. W., 20 years of age, married, farmer, whom I was called to see October 13, 1878. Marked pain in the right side, midway between the umbilicus and the anterior superior spine of the illum. I immediately recognised my old enemy, and told his family my fears and asked for council, which was procured; but all disagreed with my plan for an immediate removal of the óffending organ. Condition, as I quote from my note-book of that date: Pulse rate 127, temperature—by a better thermometer than used in the other cases—102¾°, respiration about 27. Prescription (as by suggestion of council), powd. opium 1 gr., ipec. ¼ gr., calomel 1-10 gr., once in four hours; veratrum viride 3 drops, and more if needed to lessen the heart's action, to be alternated with the powders, and warm, moist heat to be applied over the seat of the pain. Continued the treatment for twenty-four hours, with little or no abatement of any of the grave conditions.

October 14. Pulse 130, temperature 103°, respiration 28, and no abatement of pain. Gave hypodermic of morphia act. gr. ½, which seemed to quiet the pain for twenty-four hours, when the powders were kept up and all the treatment as first agreed upon. At my suggestion other physicians were called in, and only one favoured an operation. The late Dr. Daniel Pardee, of Fulton, was fully in accord with me in thinking an immediate operation the only possible thing to be done; but our plan was again overruled. Blistering was strongly recommended, and, under protest, I placed a canth. plaster three inches square over the tumefied, inflamed, and painful region previously described. In six hours I had a very fine blister, which did not reduce the pain or swelling, but increased, as I then believed, the adhesions between the inflamed bowels and abdominal wall.

October 15, 9 a. m. Patient suffering terribly. Pulse 140, temperature 103½°, respiration 30. Right limb flexed, tumor enlarged, circumscribed, and, after great difficulty in making the examination, I found it slightly fluctuating. Gave ½ gr. act. morph. hypodermically and continued other treatment, with stimulating nourishment, all without any abatement of any of the symptoms.

October 16, 9 a. m. Pulse 140 and feeble, temperature 103°, respiration 31, and patient failing. Tumor soft and fluctuating. Gave 4 oz. brandy and milk, and at 10: 30 a. m. gave ether, and aspirated the abscess and drew off over 8 oz. of very bad smelling pus; introduced a small glass tube and washed out the abscess cavity with water slightly carbolised, as warm as the patient could bear, which seemed to relieve him very much. Continued the irrigation once in six hours during the day and night, and he seemed to be much better until 8: 30 a. m., October 17, when he complained of a very severe pain in the abscess, commenced sinking, with cold perspiration, and the escape of some very offensive gas from the drainage tube. Died in forty minutes thereafter, after an illness of five days.

October 17, 5 p. m., made a post-mortem examination. Rigor mortis well marked. Right limb flexed and very rigid. Upon section of region of disease found every tissue agglutinated and firmly adherent, and almost impossible to separate them. Appendix 3½ inches long, over 1 inch in diameter, with a large slough on the posterior aspect in its centre; also found in it some well bleached cherry pits, three or four in number, as I now recollect it, which seemed to be the cause of the whole trouble.

The three cases briefly described, with one other with about the same history, which terminated fatally on the fourth day, determined me not to treat any more well marked cases, unless I could be permitted to act as my judgment dictated in the matter, and I had not long to wait for Case V.

April 1, 1879. Was called to see a daughter of Mr. S. T., 13 years of age, said to be suffering from "inflammation of the bowels." Found her suffering from very severe pain in right side of abdomen, with very rapid pulse—130—and temperature 102½°. Ordered injection of glycerine and warm water, which moved her bowels well, and prescribed ¼ grain act. morp. for the pain, with warm fomentations to surface.

April 2, 10 a. m. Patient rested a little last night. Pulse 132, temperature 102¾°. Great tenderness, and circumscribed tense condition over what is now known as McBurney's point; and without hesitation I told the parents of what I considered the very grave character of the case, and advised an immediate operation, which they readily consented to, and at 2 p. m., assisted by the late Dr. W. S. Kyle and two students, I proceeded to place the patient under the influence of chloroform, and made an incision four inches in length along the outer border of the right rectus abdominis muscle; dissecting my way carefully down through the peritonaeum, exposing an omental fold, which, carefully crowding aside, fairly and fully exposed the whole appendix vermiformis, which was 3¼ inches long, 1 inch in its largest diameter, very hard to the touch, and of a deep wine colour, almost purple, with a few soft lymph patches on its surface. Passing a strong ligature around near the base, I lifted it out of its bed and removed it by a double flap operation, and proceeded to invert and stitch the edges of the flaps together, leaving a very short umbilicated stump, which was thoroughly cleansed with hot carbolised water and dropped back into its normal position. I placed a perforated rubber drainage tube in the wound and closed the cavity by stitches through the entire wall with silver wire, and flushed it with hot water once in six hours for forty-eight hours, when I removed the tube, as the wound had ceased to discharge and did not discharge any more.

On April 5, removed the wires and straps and placed new straps upon the wound, covering as before with oil silk and carbolised cotton, and over all a thin muslin bandage.

The next day, April 6, after the operation, the pulse was 108, temperature 100½°, both dropping to the normal rate on the morning of the 7th.

April 10. The patient was dressed and in a chair three times during the day.

April 15. Walked out, seeming perfectly well from that time until the present.

CASE VI. Was called into the town of Huron, Wayne county, N. Y., by Dr. F. M. Pasco, June 15, 1886, to see a case said to be perityphlitis, and found, as I supposed I should find, a case represented by the above misnomer, which in plain English meant inflammation of the vermiform appendix, upon which, with the help of a couple of doctors and a Methodist minister, we proceeded to operate in the same manner as in Case V, using full antiseptic measures, shaving the abdomen, washing with bichloride solution, antiseptic sponges, instruments, etc.

Case: Mr. M., farmer, 33 years of age. Had been sick four days, suffering very severe pain in right iliac region. Pulse rate at this date was

129, temperature 102 4-5°, respiration irregular and 30. A careful examination revealed a tumefied condition, extending from the crest of the ilium across nearly to the umbilicus, making a rounded tumor of about four or five inches in diameter, very painful and very sensitive. Administered morphia and atrópia. Gave ether and made the usual incision, about 4½ inches long, and found some very firm adhesions, which I carefully separated, and found the appendix half hidden beneath the omentum and colon, and it was very purple, hard, and swollen. It was nearly 5 inches in length and more than 1 inch in diameter.

After ligating quite a number of vessels torn by breaking up adhesions, I raised up the appendix, removed it as before described, dressed the stump in the same way, placed a glass drainage tube in the wound, after thoroughly cleansing with hot sublimate water, stitching the peritonaeum and then the external tissues, covering the incision with long strips of plaster, then iodoform gauze, sheet rubber, and lastly a gauze bandage. Directing wound to be flushed with hot bichloride water once in six hours, as long as discharge continued, then directing removal of drainage tube, which was done twenty-four hours after the operation. Pulse and temperature came down to normal condition in five days, the patient convalesced rapidly, and in two weeks was around, and is alive and well now.

Tuesday, April 18, 1893, was called to see Case VII, H. V., 19 years old, patient of Dr. D. B. Horton, of Red Creek, N. Y.

Found the patient suffering terribly with severe pain in the right side, extending from the ribs to the crest of the ilium. Taken sick the 14th of April, but did not go to bed until the 15th. After that time was said to grow worse rapidly. Pulse rate, when I first saw him, April 18, at 10 a. m., was 130, and temperature 103°.

Upon close examination found at McBurney's point a tumor, which seemed 4 inches in diameter, with some fluctuation discernable. Was not prepared to operate at that time, on account of help, instruments, etc., but did April 19, with the help of Dr. D. B. Horton, of Red Creek, and Dr. Watkins, of Wolcott, both rendering valuable assistance. We proceeded to anaesthetise the patient, which took a long time, after which I cut down into the fluctuating tumor, which proved to be an abscess, with walls adherent to omentum, colon, appendix, and mesentery, and contained about 8 or 10 ounces of pus, which had been produced by the suppurative inflammation present. Quite a large piece of· omentum seemed almost ready to break down, and when attempting to push it aside, I tore two large places in it, and thereby got some very embarrassing haemorrhages, which gave us some trouble, as the tissue would not hold to ligate.

When I took up the appendix with a pair of wide, flat forceps, it was so far decomposed and gangrenous that it broke off, and we were obliged to place a narrow piece of muslin around it to hold it up long enough to ligate, when it was removed with an umbilicated stump, tying closely to its outer extremity, after inverting its outer wall.

We partly closed up the incision, after carefully sponging with hot, slightly carbolised, bichloride water. Dusted the wound with iatral, covered with sublimate and rubber sheet, straps, and bandage, with directions to wash out once in six hours through the drainage tube.

April 21, the drainage tube became clogged, and dressings were removed, and found a large piece of omentum had sloughed off.

After the first three days his pulse rate and temperature were nearly normal. His bowels, after the eighth day, were moved each morning with enema of glycerine and warm water. His appetite soon became good, and he has now gained ten pounds in weight.

To me the points to observe are,—

1st. Make a very careful diagnosis, and if the disease be appendicitis, operate early before suppurative inflammation is set up.

2d. Operate at any time, if you cannot operate at the proper time.

3d. Always, in fatal cases, if possible, verify the diagnosis by a post-mortem examination.

THE MALE CATHETER, WITH SOME OBSERVATIONS UPON THE PROPER MODE OF INTRODUCTION INTO THE BLADDER.

By Douglas Ayres, M. D., of Montgomery County.

October 12, 1893.

Celsus, who lived before and early in the Christian era, probably during the reigns of Augustus and Tiberius, was the first to describe, in his " Cyclopedia De Artibus," the catheter and the manner of its use ; and the directions there given are still largely the method of procedure of the present. The catheters of his time were composed of copper only ; but as they were so soon and so readily covered with verdigris, they were soon abandoned, as early as the time of the Arabian practitioners, who made use of silver, which is still the standard material. Attempts were made later to invent those that were flexible. Van Helmont suggested those made of horn, which were found not to be sufficiently flexible and quickly coated with deposits from the urine. Fabricius of Aquapendente, an Italian anatomist and sureon, who died in Padua in 1619, suggested and made use of feather ; but they were soon softened by the urine and mucus, when they contracted and became useless. Others were tried, formed of spiral springs of silver covered by the skins of some special kind of animals; but they were soon rendered useless by putrefactive changes, and dangerous on account of separation of the beak while in the bladder. Inflexible catheters were mostly curved. Desault recommended and made use of those slightly curved one third of their length, which began from the straight part and continued to the extreme end of the beak, the curvature being reg-

18

ular, and forming the segment of a circle of six French inches in diameter. Amussat recommended the use of straight ones, which were passed as far as the pubes, while the penis was drawn upward, then brought down between the thighs to lessen the urethral curve, and so passed into the bladder. It was said that its advantages were in the fact that it could be rotated, and thereby made to pass the more easily any obstacle. Such is a somewhat imperfect history of the catheter up to the beginning of the present century, when those made of elastic gum over woven silk tubes were suggested, the honor of which invention has been claimed both by the Germans and the French, for Theden or Pickel, of Wurzburg, of the former, and for Bernard, of Paris, of the latter. They did away with the inconveniences and dangers of all the former inventions, were sufficiently elastic to follow the changeable course of the urethra, were not softened by the urine, and not liable to be soon encrusted by urinary deposits. They were the first offerings to a more scientific, more perfect class of flexible catheters. We have at present silver catheters of various curves and various openings at the beak—tunnelled, vertebrated, and the so-styled vermicular. In the gum elastic we have the prostatic and olivary, the elbowed and double-elbowed of Mercier, and lastly, the more recent vulcanised India rubber catheter with velvet eyes, in their various forms. These are of German, French, English, and American manufacture. The latter, I have recently learned from an interesting article by Dr. Gouley, possess qualities as to tensile strength, resistance to the action of urine, and general wear that are superior to any of the others.

In presenting the subject of catheterisation in the male, I do not expect to lay before you any new facts, or to depart in any way from the old established landmarks of operative procedure, but simply to review with you for a brief time the technique of an operation which so experienced a surgeon as the late Samuel D. Gross declared, that, "although apparently very simple, is one of the nicest and most delicate processes in surgery. It requires skill of the highest order, as well as the most intimate knowledge of the anatomy of the urinary organs. My assertion is, that few men perform the operation well." This, from the pen of one of so large a clinical experience, is an index of the importance of a close study of the operation by those less fortunately favoured.

We will consider for a few minutes the anatomy of the parts through which we may be called upon to pass the catheter, then the best means of passing it, and the kind of instruments I have found most useful, with a few illustrative cases in point. The urethra begins at the termination of the neck of the bladder and ends at the meatus urinarius. In the normal state it is about nine inches in length, and when the penis is flaccid it constitutes a curve, the concavity of which is downward, but in the erect state it forms a curve the concavity of which is upward. It is divided into three portions—the prostatic, membranous, and spongy or penile portion. The prostatic portion is the widest and most dilatable, and passes through the prostate gland from base to apex; is about an inch and a quarter in length, wider in the middle than at either extremity, and narrower where it joins the membranous portion. The membranous portion extends from the apex of the prostate to the bulb of the corpus spongiosum; it is a half to three quarters of an inch in length, and is about one inch below the surface of the symphysis pubis, and is the narrowest portion of the canal excepting the orifice. The spongy portion is about seven inches in length, and extends from the termination of the membranous portion to the meatus; it is about one quarter of an inch in diameter, and quite uniform in size. Such is the tract through which the catheter must pass—a tract lined with delicate membrane, which requires the utmost delicacy of manipulation to guard it from injury; a tract which sometimes may be traversed in its normal state without great difficulty, but at times, from abnormal conditions, presents obstacles that are with great difficulty surmounted by the most skilful manipulators; and I believe that the very familiar anatomical description just given should always be kept in mind during the introduction of the catheter, as we are thereby enabled to know the precise position of the instrument, and to locate definitely (if there be obstruction) its seat and extent.

We now suppose we have a silver catheter (which I prefer in the great majority of cases) of the proper curve and size. The curve should correspond to the majority of adult urethrae, which may be styled a fixed curve, and is that of a circle three and one quarter inches in diameter, and is represented by an arc of such a circle, subtended by a chord two and three quarters inches in length.

As to size, I prefer a No. 9 or 10, American scale, as they correspond most nearly in size to the diameter of the average urethra, and consequently are less liable to be caught in any fold. Undoubtedly the best position for catheterisation is the recumbent, the thighs well separated, and the legs drawn up, shoulders somewhat elevated. We now (standing upon the left side of the patient) hold the penis with the thumb and forefinger of the left hand, putting it gently on the stretch, exercising care to keep it quite straight, to avoid any twist which might prove an obstacle to the passage of the instrument, then engage the beak in the meatus, holding the catheter parallel to the median line of the abdomen and close to the surface. If the patient has a protuberant belly, the shaft at this time should be parallel to the line of the groin, and kept low until the point is about to enter the membranous urethra, to avoid engaging it in the upper wall of the triangular ligament. We now press the instrument downward very lightly, and gradually lower the handle between the thighs of the patient, the slightest pressure at this time being sufficient to effect it. We next carry it forward with a slight rocking motion, guiding its course by pressing with the fingers under the scrotum against the convexity of the catheter, which turns it up as the handle is lowered. This is the most difficult stage of the operation, and in some conditions frequently requires the most delicate touch and perfect knowledge of the exact position of the instrument in order to be successful in its introduction. Sometimes at this point the beak presses before it the urethral walls, completely occluding the opening, and, even though it is carefully withdrawn and manipulated very delicately and intelligently, the same conditions may occur again. The main point in these cases, however, is the full realization of the condition, which will be overcome by careful and repeated trials. The fingers of the left hand here play an important part in its guidance. Sometimes, when the beak is caught in the fold of the upper wall, great assistance may be rendered by gentle manipulation, and by pressing firmly down the soft parts of the pubes, thereby relaxing the suspensary ligament of the penis.

I saw, a few months ago, a case I judged to be of this kind, in consultation.

The patient, a man of forty-eight years of age, who had been an invalid for some weeks from muscular rheumatism and catarrh of the bladder, had been suffering from retention of urine for nearly twenty hours. His physician, a young man of three or four years of experience in the profession, told me that he had made a number of attempts to pass the catheter, but met with some obstruction in the deeper part of the canal that he could not overcome. I found the patient very timid, and the parts quite tender, but I soon succeeded in quieting his fears as to the result. The doctor had been using a small-sized instrument, No. 7, I think, and informed me that he did not think a larger one could be made to enter, as he believed the deeper parts of the canal were very much contracted. I selected from the instruments I had brought with me one of good size (a No. 9), had the patient's hips elevated sufficiently to furnish room to manipulate the instrument, limbs well drawn up, and then, with the catheter well warmed and oiled, I gently began its introduction. It passed very readily through the first portion, but as it entered the second, and began to traverse the curve, it very suddenly stopped. I gently drew it back and tried again, with the same result; the handle could not be readily depressed, but by firm downward pressure over the soft parts of the pubes it moved forward; then, with the fingers of the left hand gently manipulating it through the perinaeum, with a slight rocking motion, depressing at the same time the handle of the instrument, it glided slowly into the bladder. It was necessary to catheterise him for a number of days, the doctor delegating the operation to me, as he declared after subsequent trials that he could not pass the obstruction.

In the last portion of the urethra, enlarged prostate fre-

quently renders it difficult to pass the catheter.   I saw, a few
years ago, an interesting case of this character.

Mr. D. M., aged seventy-eight, had been suffering from retention of
urine for thirty-six hours.   His attending physician had called a consultant, after his first unsuccessful attempt to relieve him, and they were
unsuccessful in their efforts.   I saw him with them some hours later,
and found him with his bladder greatly distended.   I made a careful
examination, and found the prostate very much enlarged.   We placed
the patient in position, elevating the hips, etc.   I then warmed and
oiled a No. 9 silver catheter, and began its introduction.   It passed
fairly easily through the first and second portions, but when the prostatic
was reached there was a temporary blockade.   I then oiled the finger
and carried it into the rectum, and by gentle manipulation upon the
handle with the right hand, the finger in the rectum pressing the catheter point gently against the upper wall, the obstruction was passed, and
I had the satisfaction of relieving the bladder of fully two quarts of
urine.   In a similar case, a few weeks ago, I made use of an elbowed
gum catheter, with an equally satisfactory result.   A few weeks since, a
call was left at my house to come to the office of a neighbouring physician as soon as I could after reaching home.   I did so, and found an old
gentleman there who had ridden a number of miles to be relieved of the
contents of an over-distended bladder.   The doctor's salutation was,—
"Never so glad in my life to see you;" said he had been trying for nearly
two hours to relieve his patient, each effort followed by a very free haemorrhage.   I made use of a good sized silver catheter, introduced it carefully, met with no obstruction until the deeper parts were reached, when
it seemed to be firmly held.   By carefully withdrawing after reaching
the obstruction, and assisting with the left hand on the perinaeum, in
this case depressing the handle rather more than usual, it glided into the
bladder, having evidently been held by the posterior walls of the canal
pushed before the beak.

I have found many times rents of greater or less extent in
the urethral walls, from undue force having been made use
of in the excitement of being foiled in the attempt to reach
the bladder, and sometimes, I fear, from the lack of that
nicety of touch which practice only can perfect us in, and
which should indicate to us the exact amount of force made
use of.   I would not have it understood that I advocate the
use of but one particular kind of catheter, but think the surgeon should be provided with a careful selection of elastic
gum catheters, in their various forms, and with the soft vulcanised India rubber, as well as the metallic, so that he may

take advantage of any form of obstruction that may present itself, his judgment guiding him as to the particular form required, after careful exploration. I would take this position, however, with regard to the use of the silver catheter. It has always been my main reliance, the instrument par excellence in difficult cases. I always feel certain with regard to its position in the urethra, as to its depth, and the relation of its beak to the surrounding parts. I can guide it more accurately and more intelligently. I have many times been foiled in attempting to pass the gum elastic and vulcanised rubber instruments, by the former twisting, and the latter doubling upon itself, so that all knowledge of their exact position was lost.

In prostatic obstruction, with a tortuous canal, the gum catheter, with its pliable extremity and olivary point, will frequently thread its way past the obstruction; so, when there is hypertrophy or interposing bars, the vulcanised India rubber may be made to pass in some cases easily, when the twisting motion we are enabled to give it helps to propel it forward. There are a few points which I wish to emphasise in closing my paper, points which, if sufficient attention be given them, furnish the key to success.

1. A careful study of the anatomy of the parts, and the various diseased conditions which may arise to produce obstruction.

2. Placing the patient in the most favourable position for the operation.

3. Careful exploration, and the selection of a proper instrument for the case in hand.

4. The greatest care as to the use of undue force.

RESEARCHES ON THE EFFICACY OF VACCINIA AFTER TYPHOID FEVER.

By WILLIAM FINDER, JR., M. D., of Rensselaer County.

October 12, 1893.

But a few years more, and our profession will celebrate the centennial of the discovery of vaccination. This preventive of disease was first introduced to the medical world by Edward Jenner, during the last five years of the eighteenth century. Vaccination, or the inoculation of the human body with lymph from an animal's disease, was one of the first steps taken to prevent, rather than to cure, disease. History speaks of the unsuccessful attempts made by the Brahmins, before the Christian era, who, through inoculation, tried to prevent the spread of variola, which had been existing in India from time immemorial. It remained for our century to produce the successful investigator, whose efforts have led to protection from this disease.

The achievement by Jenner, who through his diligent and laborious investigation gave so great a boon to man, cannot be looked upon otherwise than as one of the greatest achievements of this century of progressive medicine. The protection resulting from pure vaccinia is not doubted by the scientific members of our profession. By the almost universal adoption of this preventive, small-pox has become a rarity, in fact, is so seldom met, that even he who is a student of cutaneous diseases may not meet with it for years, unless he should seek for it where it is endemic. When the fact was demonstrated, that vaccinia would prevent the infection of variola, if not in toto, nevertheless would modify it, the assumption was, to have been once inoculated with vaccinia was to possess for a life-time immunity from variola. This was due to imperfect knowledge, and a want of further investigation. There have been a great many contentions, as to the number of years when vaccination should again be performed after a previous successful inoculation. The various theories advanced, as to a set number of years when re-vaccination should take place, have not been verified. Investigators have been trying for many years to separate the seminiferous particles of disease, and have discovered various forms, and have reproduced disease by the germs thus obtained; but thus far the contagious principle of variola has not been discovered, and the bacteria producing vaccinia have not come to light.

It is held by a number of investigators, that the cause of failure to detect the characteristic micro-organism of small-pox is due to the fact of the lateness of the search, and to the alterations of the disease caused by vaccinia. How much truth should be attached to the above statement I will leave to your judgment. Be it altered or not, enough of the poison remains, and variola still claims many victims. Any new facts that may be discovered, to ensure still greater protection, should be brought to our attention.

During the years 1874 and 1880, some of the people of Troy, N. Y., were infected with small-pox. The disease spread rapidly, and twice assumed the proportions of an epidemic. The probable exposure caused those of careful habits to seek the protection afforded by vaccination. But there were so many failures, that repeated inoculations were required. These failures led to two questions: Did we possess pure vaccinia, or were the patients protected by a previous inoculation? The reliability of our vaccine was unquestioned; that a previous protection existed I shall attempt to prove by the following facts:

Among those who were vaccinated during these epidemics were three who in their early years had suffered from a slight attack of small-pox, and though we did not look for any result, we were very much surprised at the beautiful pox they presented for our inspection. Upon inquiring as to what form of disease, if any, they had suffered from since their attack of small-pox, we were informed by them that they had recently suffered from typhoid fever. Reviewing the history of the cases that had failed to become inoculated the second time, I found they had been free from any illness since their first vaccination. A number of patients who had been ill of typhoid fever were again vaccinated, the result being very satisfactory. This led me to think that the protection afforded by vaccination was eliminated by typhoid fever. I was obliged to wait for another epidemic to give me an opportunity to verify the assumption. This came sooner than I had hoped for. The following year, 1881, there was a moderate outbreak of small-pox, and I continued my investigations and re-vaccinated a number who had suffered during the year from typhoid fever with very marked results, they at this time giving ample proof of being unprotected. I may add that typhoid fever was very prevalent in Troy, N. Y., at that time. I have since made it a rule to re-vaccinate all who will permit it after an attack of typhoid fever, and have a number of friends who have done the same with very good success.

I therefore make this claim, that the protection afforded by vaccination is removed by euteric or typhoid fever, and that that fever also removes the immunity afforded by a former slight attack of small-pox. I base my assertions on thirty successful cases.

Therefore, I will ask you to give some of your time and efforts to prove the utility of these studies. If my conclusions are right, so much more the gain for the protection from disease; and if in error, no harm can come because of them. I have tried them for over twelve years with success. Although we are still unable to explain why vaccination protects, let us continue to use it as frequently as our knowledge of its need demands, and until a better mode of protection is discovered, bearing the established fact ever in mind, that for nearly a hundred years it has been the bulwark between us and repeated epidemics of one of the most loathsome and destructive diseases.

DISCUSSION.

Dr. W. H. Robb, of Montgomery county, said he wished to make a single remark on the advantages of using fresh vaccine. In 1881, there was an epidemic of small-pox in Amsterdam, and the vaccinations were very unsatisfactory until the physicians there procured a couple of heifers, vaccinated them, and took one hundred and fifty points. In the following three days, one hundred and fifty vaccinations were made with this vaccine, and only two of these failed. This fact is significant.

Dr. Finder said that this is a new field, and it is possible that he might have to relinquish this theory, but he was satisfied thus far that it was correct, and he hoped others would investigate this subject. He had been very careful to obtain pure vaccine, and to test it very carefully on infants and adults, comparing the results.

REFLECTIONS UPON THE NEED AND THE POWER OF CLOSE OBSERVATION IN THE STUDY OF DISEASED CONDITIONS OF THE HUMAN SYSTEM, AND THE VALUE OF HYGIENIC THERAPEUTICS IN THEIR TREATMENT.

By H. Ernst Schmid, M. D., of Westchester County.

October 12, 1893.

A well chosen and well applied illustration is the most forcible and pointed method of impressing one's hearers with the subject one desires to have especially understood and appreciated. It belongs to that great new feature of modern teaching, the demonstration of object lessons, which has so wonderfully lessened difficulties for the mass of learners.

For this reason, I begin my humble efforts in behalf of the title chosen for my paper with a few incidents taken from ancient and modern stories, which will serve to illustrate the value of a habit of close observation.

Zadig was a young man who lived, *a good while ago*, in the then great city of Babylon. Becoming dissatisfied with his life there, he left the city and retired to a lonely place upon the banks of the Euphrates, where he studied closely plants and animals, and discovered, in consequence, a thousand peculiarities and curious things where others saw nothing unusual. One day one of the queen's eunuchs, with a squad of officials, came to him in great haste and asked,—

"Have you seen the queen's dog? It has run away."

Zadig answered thoughtfully, "A bitch, I think, not a dog."

"You are right," said the eunuch.

"A very small setter," continued Zadig, "which only lately gave birth; lame upon one foot, with very long ears."

"Oh, tell me quickly where you saw her!" exclaimed the eunuch impatiently.

"I have not seen her at all," was Zadig's rejoinder, "and did not even know the queen had any dog."

A short time afterwards a finely bred horse of the same royal lady strayed off, and one of her body servants, in looking for it, likewise went to Zadig for information, who began,—

"A fine runner, five feet high, with small hoofs, a tail three and one-half feet long, carrying a bridle with a bit of gold of twenty-three karats, and shod with shoes of silver?"

"Oh! where has he gone?" excitedly cried out the messenger.

"I have heard or seen nothing of him," quickly replied Zadig.

Of course he was at once suspected of having stolen both dog and horse. The authorities were about ordering him to be executed, when the missing animals were found. Zadig then was asked how it was he could give such accurate descriptions of beasts he had never seen. This was his explanation:

One day he observed in the sand the tracks of an animal, which he easily recognised as those made by a dog. Long, faint traces in the sand between the footprints he as readily interpreted as caused by the teats of a bitch, and, since they must have been in a pendulous condition in order to hang down low enough to produce any marks, this furthermore indicated that she must have given birth quite recently. Other lines in the sand, faint and long, but outside the footprints, convinced him that they could only have been made by the long, hanging ears of the dog. Finally, the impression of one foot being fainter than that from the others, it was easy to conclude the beast which made them must be lame. As to the horse, the tracks of it were all the same long distance apart, which showed he must be a fine runner. Zadig then noticed that in an avenue of trees, through which the horse had passed, the dust had been whipped off by the horse's tail at a distance of three and one half feet from the centre of the footprints, ergo, the tail was three and one half feet long. Broken off branches and leaves at a distance of five feet from the ground, demonstrated the height of the horse to be five feet, for they had been broken off by the animal as it galloped through the avenue. The bit of the horse had been knocked against a rock—used as and called in those days a test-stone—on which it left its marks, which demonstrated to Zadig the quality of the metal. He gained similar information from the impression of the horse's shoes upon other rocks.

Dr. Brunton related, only a year ago, the following account, which had been communicated to him by D. Milner Fothergill:

In Leeds lived a charlatan whose wonderful cures made him famous far and near. But what was even more wonderful in the people's eyes, was the fact that he made very astonishing diagnoses of sick people whom he had never seen, resting, apparently, his opinion solely upon an ocular examination of their urine. A prominent individual, desirous of witnessing his method of investigation, asked permission to do so. This was readily given, the quack feeling highly flattered by the request.

Shortly after the visitor had taken a seat a woman came in with a bottle of urine, which she handed the charlatan.   He looked first at the woman, then at the bottle, held it up to the light, shook it, and said,—

"From your husband?"

"Yes, sir."

"He is somewhat older than you?"

"Yes, sir."

"He is a tailor?"

"Yes, sir."

"He lives at Scarcrost?"

"Yes, sir."

"He suffers from constipation?"

"Yes, sir."

"Here," he continued, giving her a box of pills, "let him take one pill every night for a week and a glass of cold water on rising, and he will soon be well."

As soon as the woman was gone the visitor entreated the quack to explain how he had discovered all these facts.

"Well," said he, "you noticed she was a young, fresh, healthy-looking woman, therefore it was easy to suppose the specimen was not from her. I noticed a wedding ring on her finger, hence I knew she was married, and that most probably the urine was from her husband.   Had he been as young and fresh as she, it was scarcely possible that he should be sick, and hence I concluded rightly he must be older than she.   The bottle was not closed with a cork, but with a rolled-up paper, tied with a string in a manner only used by tailors, ergo I was sure he was a tailor. As such, he lived a very sedentary life, and was in consequence prone to constipation.   You see how correct I was in all my conclusions, founded upon minute observation."

"I comprehend; but how did you know she came from Scarcrost?"

Upon which the quack exclaimed,—"Oh, have you lived so long in Leeds and do not yet know the color of Scarcrost mud?   I saw it on her shoes the moment she entered the room!"

A pupil of Hebra once told me how the old professor made his hearers gaze with amazement when he introduced in his clinic the various types of skin diseases, which were generally taken from the ranks of the artisans.   The patients were all brought in and placed upon the table, entirely nude.   He was able at once to divine their occupation, provided they had followed it for some time, and unhesitatingly addressed them as shoemakers, tailors, etc.

The great Professor Wunderlich, of Leipzig, possessed the gift of close observation to a marvellous degree.   He on one occasion took a class to the bedside of a patient.   Nothing was said. Everybody remained silent. After a little while Wunderlich demanded of one of the students the diagnosis of the case. There was no answer. "You ought to declare with certainty," then said Wunderlich, "that this is a case of acute angina; an angina because the man just now swallowed without having anything to swallow, in other words, he swallowed dry; and an acute angina, because he is feverish, red in the face, and perspires sensibly."

I have selected my first two illustrations simply because the acumen displayed in them is of so high a type that they teach the value of close observation more than any in my memory, and not on account of the worth the actors in them were to the world. The uselessness of a hermit life, given to nothing but solitary reflections, has long been acknowledged by the world and condemned, as no one has a right to withdraw from the commonwealth forces of labour, powers of activity, either of mind or of body, to which society has undisputed claims. The second one needs no comment. The last two are truly legitimate, and speak for themselves in all their bearings. No man is great enough to be infallible, if he become careless or unmindful of little things in making out a diagnosis. I have read of a case where a clinical professor, who pretended before his class that he was able to recognise certain conditions of patients by merely examining their teeth, was sorely ridiculed. The woman under examination innocently took out the set of false teeth, which the examiner had taken for genuine, saying, "I will hand them around, so you can examine them more accurately."

Not less amusing and instructive is the case where a large number of students were examining a man who had a clearly pronounced cardiac murmur, with a decided dilatation of the pupil of one eye. All kinds of theories were ventilated as to the meaning of this incomprehensible combination, when the man said very quietly that he had one glass eye.

Professor Wunderlich, above alluded to on account of his great acumen, also made once a great blunder. He was

demonstrating at the time the intestinal tract of a patient
purporting to have died of typhoid fever. But instead of
the expected ulcerations in Peyer's glands, he found tuberculous lesions with plain indications of general tuberculosis.
Then did the great teacher proceed to prove with wondrous
skill how naturally this could be made to agree with many
of the symptoms and conditions which had been seen in the
case, when, lo! the door opened, and the clinical assistant
came in to say that the specimen had been exchanged by
mistake for one taken from a patient who had died of general tuberculosis.

A case, perhaps well known to you, is that of a Parisian
clinician who had just said that simulated epilepsy could not
impose upon any experienced physician, when his assistant
uttered a cry and fell down in a fit. " Poor young man,"
exclaimed the sympathising lecturer; " he has been over-
worked.   This is a case of actual transfer of disease, of which
I have taught you." " No, Mr. Professor, it is simple simulation," exclaimed the assistant, as he nimbly jumped up
from the floor, to the amusement of the hearers.

It requires the closest observation at times to arrive at
a proper diagnosis. How difficult often, for example, to
demonstrate a pregnancy ! How great the obstacles thrown
in our way in that direction by the women themselves!
How great the difficulty in tumors! Many a mammary
abscess has been pronounced a cancer. Sir Astley Cooper
tells of two cases where fluctuation betrayed the true state
at last, and the knife emptied the cancer.

I have read somewhere of a case which the surgeon (a
professor, too, operating before a class) mistook for cancer,
whereas it was one of obliterated piles. In proceeding to
excise the supposed malignant growth, he caused the death
of the patient from uncontrollable haemorrhage. He acknowledged his great and awful mistake, nay, even criminal carelessness, when he admitted, " Had I examined the case before
the operation—and I should have done so—this would not
have happened."   If it had happened in general private prac-

tice, and not in a clinic, the law would have punished the operator. And yet, it is so easy to make mistakes. Take only the case of a rare disease making its appearance under the likeness of a common one, or of a grave one developing at first only under trifling symptoms; or does every diseased organ give at once, or do some ever give, evidence of altered conditions? Does it not require minutest watching, closest scrutiny, often the aid of chemistry or of the acoustic instruments, or of the microscope and various other physical means, to discern the true character of a diseased condition? It is true, some organs show changes at a glance; others, again, require some one or more of these just mentioned helps, to be understood as to the nature of their altered condition. Other conditions, again, can only be discovered by methods of reasoning and of exclusion, or may remain unrecognised altogether.

To digress for a moment here, since this last statement tempts me too sorely to do so, I would ask, Has it ever occurred to you how inconsistent the laymen are in their opinion about diagnosis and treatment? If a surgical injury has occurred, a tangible disaster—for example, the breaking of a leg,—they are awe-stricken and silent, and have no opinion or suggestion to offer, although often any one could see plainly the character of the damage done; but let any internal difficulty fall upon a man, no matter how obscure, and these same people are full of opinions, suggestions, and criticisms; then they *know* better than the most learned physician. It is rather singular that ours, the only profession that has no legal or other guides to go by, is nevertheless the one that is punished for mistakes. Has ever a lawyer been punished by law, or sued, for having lost a case? There are books published on the mistakes of the law, full of the errors committed by the legal profession—errors which are never thought of as coming within the limit of punishment; yet this very law punishes mistakes of medical men.

To continue a little further in this vein of digressing, Is it not strange that our profession is so often ridiculed because

19

the same diseases are treated in so many different ways? To
get at the truth of things, which is the real object of science,
many different paths and methods are tried, and many different ways prove successful. It is so in questions of law, of
theology, of philosophy, in political and educational problems, and how pronouncedly in the most exact applied
science, that of mechanics. The same results are reached in
the most opposite ways—sometimes by the bodily power of
man, sometimes by running water, again by steam or electricity; and the selection of the best means often depends
only upon minor or extraneous conditions, so that really it
may remain doubtful as to which to give the preference.
Now the same state of things exists of course in the exercise
of the healing art, where complications are greatest, and
where the external and internal conditions of the organs are
most diversified. Every special illness of the human system
is a malady per se, and must be treated as such; for all of
which reasons it is an unassailable fact that many roads in
the domain of therapeutics lead to the same goal, and that to
select the best one requires the greatest amount of judgment,
even after the closest observation has made out a true diagnosis. Many different methods of treatment are the necessary and legitimate consequence of this fact, and every opinion therefor, which is based upon true scientific research, has
its claim to existence.

It is evident, in reflecting upon the growth of the healing
art, that accident and need were the first teachers; therefore,
curing came before prevention, and the most evident—so to
speak, ready-made—means were the first to be used.

How difficult it is, often, to make people understand the
simplest notions and principles of hygiene, and yet it is upon
hygiene and hygienic dietetics, principally, that our whole plan
of general therapeutics should be based. The great attrac-
tion toward the discoveries in bacteriology has, I fear, led us
too often and considerably aside from this true path. I do
not mean that we should not in certain ways follow the indications of its teachings,—not at all. Hygienic tasks are

plainly laid down for us in that direction. We are bound thereby to watch and provide, prophylactically, that disease germs do not enter our bodies, or that those which have entered are removed therefrom. This is really the ideal therapeutics of modern times. Unfortunately, success in a great measure crowned our efforts *only* in the first direction —in the prophylaxis. I allude only to the keeping off of yellow-fever, typhus, variola, and, most recently, of cholera.

It is an encouraging view, held now, I think, by the majority of medical men, that it is not an altogether easy thing for germs to invade and settle in our bodies. The system must first become in a measure depreciated to give microbes a thriving soil. It is an unquestioned fact, that some people are more easily infected by diseases than others, and that even the same people are more readily attacked at one time than at another. A Swedish physician published about four years ago a book, entitled, "On the Dependence of Diseases upon the Weather." This has always been to me a much overlooked factor in disease, for by it the nervous system is greatly influenced, and by the latter in turn all our functions are more or less controlled. To give you an illustration, I would only allude to the experience we have all had, I imagine, in our own persons, that food can be digested easily and perfectly when the mind is in an exhilarated state, which would, perhaps, thoroughly disagree with us during a season of depression or mental discomfort.

To remove the foreign invaders from the system after a thorough occupation, has been attempted in many ways, and with some success. Some writers have even claimed extraordinary results, but should we give them credence? By energetic internal use of drugs they believe the microbes are killed, and the breaches already made by them in the con-stituent parts of the organs healed, provided they have not grown too large. I speak, of course, of the internal asepsis.

It is really amusing, however, to follow the plain aberrations of some of their extravagant enthusiasm. One sensational writer, especially, speaks of creosote, creoline, and

lysol as the great threefold constellation, and asserts that
these articles can be given in such quantities as to cause
entire destruction of the invaders and their progeny, and,
cessante causa cessat effectus, a stopping of cell proliferation,
and a reabsorption of that so far produced.

Sommerbrodt was the first, or at least the one who did
most, to endorse to the fullest extent the use of creosote in
lung tuberculosis. He says the more a patient can take of it,
the surer the success. Small doses are of no value. He
gives from grs. xlv to 3 ii per diem. This is indeed daring
work, and might be death to microbe and patient alike—
fire companies do often more damage than the fire.

A writer, by name Vopelius, finds a germ for everything,
even for the neuroses. He disposes of neurasthenia, nervous
dyspepsia, all neuralgias, and even epilepsy, in the most summary manner. "There is a microbe," he says, "for all these
diseases, and an antidote for them also. Make out a correct
diagnosis, and the treatment is very clear and very successful."

Schuller, as early as 1878, advocated the internal use of
the benzoate of soda on the principles of internal asepsis, giving it in doses of 3 ii to 3 v, with great advantage in car-
buncle, erysipelas, inflammation of the joints with the formation of pus, acute osteomyelitis upon an infectious basis,
diphtheritic affections, scrofulous enlargements, and several
other affections.

It is a wise warning that has been thrown out, namely, to
consider that many diseases are really the effort of the system to get rid of superabundant, and hence dangerous, material. In this view let us remember the rheumatism and gout
of the aged fox-hunters, whose gluttonous habits were balanced by their violent exercise as long as they could keep in
the chase, but who broke down with these affections when
no longer able to follow the hounds. I have watched with
special minuteness many attacks of asthma, and am certain
that they often, very often, are brought on by overloading
the stomach.

Simply to rely, therefore, for advance in methods of treatment upon the discoveries in bacteriology, is extremely foolish. It is in reflecting upon the causations by daily disturbed habits of the people, by errors of diet in its widest sense, by neglect of inexorable laws of nature, by a spendthrift use of the capacities of the body—in one word, by all that the best knowledge of true bodily functions and hygienic necessities shows us to be outraged—that we learn how best to counteract diseased conditions as the evident result of all these acts. It is a sad state of things, that though we understand in our day pretty much all that is hurtful to our bodies, and know that by avoiding it all we can keep well, attain a great age, and finally end in a veritable euthanasia, we do not follow the dictates of this knowledge, and consequently suffer. This aspect of things gives to us, then, a far different rule for our work from the one which the pure bacteriological therapeutist enunciated, as mentioned above. It is this: Find in what the foolish patient has erred, and use all your efforts to dissipate this wrong influence upon the body, and so regulate the external conditions as to create a return to a sound condition—a *restitutio ad integrum ;*—yet this is not done by a routine treatment.

Alexander von Humboldt, in his physical geography, said, "There are no genera and species in nature, only individuals;" and the same can be said of diseases. Each disease is an individual one, and must be treated accordingly; for I am sure that in no two cases of the same disease do we find all symptoms exactly alike, and still we can go too far in this direction.

Beard, for example, maintained, that if two cases of neurasthenia are treated alike from beginning to end, one of them is certain to be treated wrongly. Extremes in anything are dangerous. We must, after all, be guided by general rules. Universal and wide-reaching knowledge alone can raise the practice of medicine—which for a long time was simple empiricism, a mere groping in the dark, resembling a mechanic's work—into the light of a true art.

To thrust aside old methods merely to pose as an independent genius, is dangerous business—dangerous to individual reputation, and, what is far more important, to the welfare of patients. Geniuses are rare in medicine, as elsewhere. The things which, after all, make the real value of a physician, are knowledge, thoroughness, experience, and a boldness which is based upon profound judgment and conscientiousness.

Braun, in his admirable work on balneology, makes the statement that the chronic sick can be divided into two groups, one consisting of those who have strength enough for energetic reaction ; and the other, of those who are weak and need consideration and do not react. For the former he directs exercise, cool rooms, cool bathing, sea bathing, and sea air ; for the latter, ease, warm rooms, a warm climate, warm baths, and mountain air. I mention this here, because it gives hints for a large part of our work. We must study the effect of sunlight upon the well, and apply the knowledge, so gained, in our management of the sick. We are realising more and more the absolute necessity, or great importance, of purity of air in conjunction with other healthful measures in all diseases, and in pulmonary tuberculosis it is, in truth, the first factor in prophylactic and curative treatment. I am sure that the hygieno-dietetic treatment of this dreadful malady is now the best, far in advance of that by purely internal medication, and yet it is exceedingly simple and can be detailed in very few words—the constant breathing of pure air, good and appropriate nourishment, plentiful out-door exercise, and the best care of the skin by hydropathic means.

Ziemssen, in a recent lecture upon the treatment of tuberculosis, stated emphatically that the neglect of just these means favours the colonisation of the bacillus in the lungs, and produces the breaking down into tuberculosis of hitherto well persons. By a persistent devotion to the simple rules laid down above, cases of well established phthisis have been cured.

I met only lately,. at a southern watering-place, an old
gentleman whose lungs demonstrated perfectly a healed cavity. He lost many members of his family by consumption,
and had been terribly reduced through haemorrhages. Sent
to the mountains of western Virginia, about 2,500 feet above
sea-level, he spent his days out-of-doors, on horse-back and
on foot, deer hunting and plant seeking ad infinitum. Gradually the consuming fever left him; his appetite, with the
decline of the fever and the allurements of a delicious table,
returned; the general state of nutrition improved visibly,
bodily weight increased, cough and expectoration diminished, the bacilli disappeared from the sputa, and, finally, on
physical examination the lungs were found with the evidence
of a cavity entirely healed.

A proper diet is one of the important points in hygienic
therapeutics. I have come to this one great conclusion: To
lay down cast-iron rules for indigestion is folly. It matters,
on the whole, really very little *what* you eat, as far, namely,
as digestibility is concerned, but *how* you eat it. Eat slowly,
and do not swallow anything till you have reduced it to a
condition resembling that of mush. So properly comminuted
and insalivated, no food will produce indigestion, provided,
of course, that you are moderate in the amount you take and
do not go beyond the needs of your body. An over-amount
of food, even if properly eaten and digested, will nevertheless produce disease, such as mentioned above in the case of
the aged fox-hunter, leading to inflamed states of all kinds.

Much has been accomplished in hygienic therapeutics by
certain peculiar diets. Thus we find a method of cure by
a system of dry diet, by a diet which withdraws watery
effusions, by a milk diet, a skim-milk diet, a grape diet, and
by one of forced feeding, originated by Weir-Mitchell. Add
to this a persistent employment of rest, reclining, exercise—
including home gymnastics, Swedish movement, massage,
etc.,—and finally, one of the most important of all, the various methods of hydrotherapy. This system is of vast importance and of wide range of application, and yet it is taught

but little. Dr. Baruch, in this city, has, to my knowledge, done more for it than anybody else.

In this department, more than in any other, it has been difficult to bring people to the understanding and accepting of its benefits. How impossible is it still, in many places, to induce the use of cold water applications where for ages the unsavory poultice alone ruled, and yet how many indications are easily and efficiently filled by the various ways of applying water. By it can be changed, increased, and depressed at will local and general innervation. Not simply the periphery of the body is affected by it, the very heart itself can be influenced by it. By it you can contract and dilate vessels, you can elevate or depress their tone, you can accelerate or retard, weaken or strengthen cardiac contraction. We may also note its effect upon the bodily temperature and the alterations it works upon tissue change, secretion and excretion, and the intimate cell-life. All this raises hydrotherapeutics to the level of a rational and scientific method of cure. And this, and the various hygienic methods spoken of, open new fields of research and study, and new methods of cure for the enthusiastic and progressive seeker after that which will benefit diseased and suffering humanity.

UNIQUE CASE OF TRAUMATIC TETANUS WITH GENERALISATION AND RECOVERY.

By J. G. ORTON, M. D., of Broome County.

Read by title October 12, 1893.

In reporting the following case of tetanus, I may be allowed to premise that I present it not only as a marked illustration of the pathological reflex state of the disease, having a peripheral irritation for its immediate point of origin, an exaggerated functional activity of the spinal centres for its condition, and muscular contractions for its effects, but as a remarkable instance of the power of endurance of the human body under long continued muscular contortions, accompanied by painful paroxysms of spasms involving such important parts as the diaphragm and muscles of the larynx, and yet followed by complete recovery.

I. D., aged nine years, of slight build, light brown hair, blue eyes, fair complexion, received a contused wound of his left fore-finger, at the distal end, which was not thought at the time of sufficiently serious character to call for surgical care.

On the fifth day from the accident the boy was seized with symptoms of trismus, at which time I was called to attend him. The jaws could only be partially opened. The injured finger presented the usual appearance of a neglected contused wound, unhealthy pus surrounding a denuded and dead portion of bone. I removed the diseased portions, and gave the parts suitable antiseptic dressing, and I may here say, it rapidly took on a healthy character and fully healed in due time.

The second day thereafter the muscles of the face became involved, giving the characteristic expression of the risus sardonicus.

The third day found an invasion of the muscles of the pharynx, exhibiting the dysphagic form of tetanus.

Fourth day, extensors of the neck contracted, the lower limbs stiff, abducted, and extended.

Fifth day, unyielding contractions of the muscles of both arms and the fingers.

Sixth day, generalisation fully established; during a painful paroxysmal spasm, involving the whole body, opisthotonos was produced to a remarkable degree, and remained for hours before any relaxation occurred. Besides this continued and powerful contraction of the muscles, painful paroxysms frequently supervened under the slightest external excitation, such as a jar of the bed, or walking in the room. Complete remission never occurred. The generalisation was so thorough at times as to involve the integrity of the diaphragm and muscles of the larynx; the patient apparently ceasing to breathe and becoming as one asphyxiated, and finally, at one time during these paroxysms, simulated the act of dying, became pulseless, pale, and ghastly in the extreme. Out of this critical condition he would gradually rally, only to have it repeated for many days in succession.

The spasms of the jaws and pharynx were for a long time so uninterrupted that he was unable to swallow even liquids, and became extremely emaciated.

The deviation of temperature did not assume any definite cycle, and ranged from 101° to 105°; pulse 110 to 150. No evening increase was observed, but the pulse kept quite a close parallel to that of the temperature. During the exacerbation of temperature delirium was always present, otherwise intelligence remained perfect. After generalisation became fully established, on the sixth day after the first symptoms of tetanus appeared, there was not a moment when complete relaxation of the contracted muscles occurred during a period of forty-five days. When resolution commenced to take place, it was in the order in which the several parts of the body had become involved by the disease, and assured convalescence was established sixty days from the time of the accident to the finger. Complete recovery followed.

As to the line of treatment pursued in this unique case, I will only briefly allude to it, for I am far from sanguine that the various measures resorted to, save one, had any special controlling influence over the disease. The amputation of the diseased bone, and subsequent rapid healing of the parts, did all that could be desired in that direction, but failed to abate the course or severity of the contractions. Ergot, chloral, quinine, Indian hemp, etc., were each given a fair trial, with only temporary effects, if any. The excessive contortions of the body, opisthotonos, and the powerful contractions of the upper extremities, were only mitigated or controlled by the application of the ice bag along the cervical region of the spine. By this means, and this alone, was I able to allay the severity of the contractions, which many times seemed about to terminate the case in death by asphyxia during an attack of the dysphagic form of the disease. For a period of twenty days this application was frequently resorted to, and always gave quite prompt relief from impending danger to life—in fact, it was the only remedy that afforded me any satisfaction in the treatment of this case.

A CASE OF PUERPERAL BLINDNESS.

By DARWIN COLVIN, M. D., of Wayne County.

October 12, 1893.

That I may be in harmony with modern lexicons in expressing the maximum morbid condition of the visual organs in the case which I am about to report imperfectly, I have used the word blindness rather than terms which have been and are now made use of to express the same grade of lesion. Not having had the full care of the case, I know not whether I am justified in reporting it. However, the predilection which I have, until recent years, always had for the care of the pregnant woman, as well as during her puerperium, more especially when assailed by intercurrent maladies, prompts me to do so, as I confess that with cases of this grade I am quite unfamiliar, never having seen one so grave.

• Mrs. W., a robust woman, aged thirty-seven, and the wife of a farmer living in the eastern portion of the county in which I reside, became pregnant in June, 1876, and her confinement was expected in March, 1877. I am unable to report the varying conditions or therapeutic means used in this gestation, as the attending physician, an excellent practitioner in that vicinity, left the locality some years since. This much, however, I have learned, to wit: that six weeks previous to labour, cephalalgia and anasarca were very decided. On the 2d of March, 1877, labour pains came on, and after twelve hours a severe convulsion, followed by coma, occurred. Soon after the convulsion the forceps were applied, and the child delivered, dead. I also learn that venesection was not resorted to. In February, 1878, she again became pregnant. The same ignorance in my report of this gestation and labour prevails as in the first. I can only learn that two months previous oedema was noticed, yet general anasarca was absent. Vertigo was a very annoying symptom from this time up to parturition. She passed through her confinement on November 15, 1878. Child living. In February, 1890, she again became pregnant. During the following August, or early in September, anasarca with impaired vision, together with cephalalgia, became very troublesome. These symptoms beginning about two months before the confinement, and the eye symptom being something new to her, together with the fact that she was not only to be under the care of a strange physician, and one in whom, very naturally, there was less confidence than in the one who had cared for her during the first two labours, led the family to seek my advice and services. Being unable to have the full care of the case, I consented to render all the advice that was possible under the circumstances, being assured that it would be agreeable to the medical gentleman who would otherwise attend her. I asked for specimens of urine, together with a report of the quantity voided during twenty-four hours. They were brought to me by the husband, and I asked him to return in twenty-four hours, which he did. Upon examination, I found a large amount of albumen in each, and was informed the renal secretion in twenty-four hours did not exceed ten ounces. Added to this was decided constipation. I advised the following course to be pursued:

First. Venesection to a liberal amount, believing that not less than twenty-four, and perhaps thirty, ounces would be necessary, and that it be done with the patient in a recumbent position.

Second. That soon after the abstraction of blood a hydragogue cathartic be given. The following was also advised: Squibb's powdered extract of jalap, five grains, combined with super-tartrate of potash, fifty grains,— to be repeated in two or three hours unless satisfactory stools should be produced by the first. After which to keep the bowels in a soluble condition by sulphate of magnesia, or by alternating with the first agents prescribed. I also advised the daily use of Trousseau's diuretic wine in such doses as might be necessary to aid in restoring and keeping up the necessary amount of urine.

Whatever agents for the relief of headache seemed necessary were given, pro re nata. Specimens of urine, and a report of the case in general, were brought to me at proper intervals. The physician postponed the abstraction of blood from day to day, assigning no reason therefor. Finding that, although there was some improvement in the patient's condition, yet not sufficiently satisfactory, I again insisted that blood must be abstracted, and advised that the attending physician should call in for that purpose a prominent though somewhat retired practitioner, a friend of the family, and one who had often witnessed the benefits derived by such a course in similar cases. It was done, but not until the 15th of October, when the woman was totally blind. A large bleeding was the result of my friend's visit, which was followed by great relief to the head symptoms. So urgent did the general symptoms appear to the physician called in (as he has since told me), that he promised another visit, with a view to the loss of more blood, unless it should be contraindicated by as great an improvement of the symptoms as would be possible after that, while gestation continued. Loss of blood was not again induced, as quite unexpectedly parturition took place on the 21st of October, six days after venesection. With the exception of occasional spasmodic twitching of the facial muscles, and the expression, "I begin to feel as I did before my first baby was born" (I infer that she had reference to her feelings before the convulsion, as she was unconscious during the delivery), there was nothing worthy of note during labour. A healthy child was the result. I visited this woman on November 1, eleven days after the confinement. Total blindness was still present; albuminuria was well marked. The urine was below normal in quantity. I continued to prescribe for her, with less trammelling prospects, until the following April, when, from an attack of pneumónia, and my not being able to give her sufficient attention, her physician again took charge, and I met him in consultation. She was then unable to distinguish me at the bedside.

During December, and occasionally throughout the winter, there would be an illusive trace of improvement, but not until March was there positive evidence that a change, however feeble, was beginning. At that time, an object moved between her eyes and a window at the foot of her bed could be faintly perceived, and yet she was unable to tell what it was. Such was her condition at my visit in April. Later on, the improvement was more decided. In a letter received from her not long since, she writes,—" The return of vision was so slow that it required a year, as near as I can get at it, before it was as good as now; and, while I get along very well now, yet my vision is not as good as before my last pregnancy, now three years since."

From my long experience in the varying results of what may be called the albuminuria of some pregnant women, I have been irresistibly drawn to certain conclusions.

With reference to this case, so imperfectly reported, I would say,—

First. That being a multipara, there was greater danger, if possible, with her past record presenting indisputable evidence of a system strongly disposed to certain toxic influences, to be apprehended than though she had been a primipara.

Second. That immediately after oedema, and before anasarca and the eye symptoms were present, she should have been under close surveillance.

Third. When the anasarca and cephalalgia, with or without the amblyopia, were first observed, from twenty-four to thirty ounces of blood should have been drawn, in addition to the other adjuvants, with explicit dietetic rules.

Fourth. Not long before the period for her confinement, if the gravity of the symptoms, more especially the cephalalgia, had not been materially improved, another abstraction of blood would not only have been eminently proper, but in my judgment was imperatively demanded.

Fifth. Had not the free venesection, even though so lately done, been instituted, she would undoubtedly have had eclampsia, and quite probably a more lasting lesion of her visual organs.

Sixth. The different grades of the eye lesions in this case are due to the same cause as is eclampsia.

I do not report this case and imperfectly carried out treatment for the purpose of inviting, nor defending it against, criticism, as previous papers read by me before this Association on kindred subjects and their treatment have been through that ordeal. Only, so far as is possible, I wish to sustain a position which I have long since assumed, and one which the results, in very many cases, from analogous causes, have fully corroborated.

DISCUSSION.

Dr. T. J. McGILLICUDDY, of New York county, said that he had seen five cases of blindness occurring with puerperal eclampsia. None were bled, but all recovered perfectly after delivery. The most important point in the treatment was to treat the nephritis by dietetic and hygienic measures, using chloroform and other narcotics for the eclampsia. These five cases all occurred in young women, just prior to the convulsions. One woman remained blind for two or three days, and then recovered her vision. In one case, Dr. C. H. May examined the eyes, but could find nothing except a slight cloudiness of the disc. It seemed to him that there must be a severe congestion of the retinal blood vessels, sufficient to obscure vision. The other cases all occurred during the convulsions. He had at present under his care a woman who is recovering satisfactorily from her blindness, and also from puerperal mania.

A NEW AND NON-OPERATIVE METHOD OF TREATING DYSMENORRHOEA, PELVIC INFLAMMATION, AND PELVIC ABSCESS.

By T. J. McGILLICUDDY, M. D., of New York County.

October 12, 1893.

Not only less and better surgery, but more radical therapeutics, should be the aim of all modern gynaecologists. The therapeutics of gynaecology is practically limited to the application of boroglyceride tampons and the ordering of hot vaginal douches, along with a few other minor measures; and standard works on medical gynaecology are comparatively few in number and rather disappointing in their contents. They seem to be seldom utilised by the profession, and are probably relegated to the top shelf of the library. The so called conservatives, while decrying excessive zeal in surgical interference, seem to have done little or nothing to offset it, but have simply taken their fees, in many cases, without giving the patients much, if any, appreciable benefit.

This subject of medical gynaecology is revived for the purpose of bringing forward and emphasising the importance of a therapeutical resource that has hitherto, so far as I am aware, been unknown or entirely neglected, viz., the depletion of the vessels of the pelvis in inflammatory conditions,—first, by the stimulating action of hot water taken in rather large quantities on an empty stomach, and secondly, by the ingestion of a large amount of properly prepared and easily digested nitrogenous food, with a partial abstention from that which is starchy and saccharine. This might be termed the dietetic treatment of pelvic disease; but it is more than that.

I also give, in the subacute and chronic cases, when indicated, the citrate of iron and quinine, and sometimes Fowler's solution. The Fowler's solution I find here of especial benefit as a strong nerve tonic. It gives tone to the arteries of the uterus, a lack of tone being often a great factor in producing the original disease. Where the appetite and digestion are poor, I order a dozen drops of dilute hydrochloric acid in a glass of water, immediately before meals.

The effect of the hot water is to stimulate not only the portal and systemic veins, but also the lymphatic system, and by absorption and endosmosis cause the removal of congestions and inflammations within the pelvis. Exudates, and lymph before its organisation, are absorbed by this process; and if the inflammation is plastic, and not suppurative, the absorption goes on very rapidly. The pus corpuscles, when present, become granular, disintegrate, and are, I believe, absorbed; at any rate, they disappear, in most cases, along with the inflammation. The improvement in the venous and lymphatic circulation produces a continuous beneficial effect, which is, in these cases, a great advantage over the intermittent and astringent action of hot vaginal douching and boroglyceride tampons. These local measures may be combined with the hot water treatment, if it is thought necessary.

The effect of a proper nitrogenous diet is to feed and strengthen the heart muscle (which here, indeed, acts as a pump to the congestion) as well as the muscular fibres of the blood vessels and viscera; and, as a consequence, the circulation in the systemic venous system and its appendage, the portal vein, is stimulated. Sometimes, as an intestinal antiseptic, tablets of 1-100th of a grain of the bichloride of mercury are very useful, and bitter tonics should also be given if indicated. If there exists, as is usual, stomach and intestinal catarrh, with fermentative dyspepsia, rhubarb and soda mixture, in teaspoonful doses, should be given two hours after meals. Before meals, taken in water, it is an excellent detergent, and acts as an artificial bile to the irri-

20

tated mucous membrane. A few drops of the fluid extract
of hydrastis Canadensis in water are also beneficial. As a
vaginal astringent, the white extract of pinus Canadensis
should also be used on tampons, or a solution containing five
grains each of alum and sulphate of zinc to the ounce of
water, with a little glycerine added.

A very advantageous supplementary measure consists in
douching the whole of the colon twice daily with a very
large quantity of hot water. It is administered from a foun-
tain syringe while the patient lies quietly on her back, resting on an inflated surgical cushion that drains the water
off one side into a receptacle. These colonic flushings are
also exceedingly useful in nephritic colic, threatening appendicitis, and many other abdominal diseases.

This flushing not only promotes cleanliness by its mechanical effect, but acts as a stimulant by increasing the volume
of the circulating fluid, and hence the general vascular tension, and at the same time excites the emunctories to greater
activity. If the intestine be flushed with a bland fluid, such
as water, most of it is eliminated from the system by the
kidneys, as is shown by the increased frequency of urination
after such injections. When water is taken by the mouth,
if it be not saline, it is almost entirely absorbed.

This method of relieving pelvic congestions has other
great advantages: it often removes with remarkable rapidity morbid conditions of the blood, and actual structural disease of important organs, such as the stomach, kidneys, heart,
and lungs. Many persons are in a state of apparent health,
and yet the blood may be so vitiated and full of morbific
materials that they are at any minute liable to serious acute
disease, and to the development of chronic visceral disease.
Those who are overloaded with degenerate fat are typical of
this class; and here, especially, this method is of advantage.
To women, otherwise of sound constitution and good habits,
whose diet and hygienic surroundings are of the best, this
treatment, properly given, will certainly do no harm, if it
does not always remove the local disease. To those whose

physical powers have been impaired by excesses, or exhausted by labour and anxiety, or by scanty and improper diet, and whose nervous systems have been irritated by an excess of stimulating food and drinks, it is of the greatest value. After a course of this treatment, under proper hygienic conditions and a freedom from the anxiety of a struggle for daily bread, the pelvic disease rapidly disappears, unless the case is one where an operation is absolutely necessary. In that event, the patient is in good condition to undergo even the most serious operation, with the best prospect of rapid wound healing and freedom from complications.

Let the reader remember the vascular supply and the physiology of the liver and the pelvic organs, especially the entero-hepatic circulation or the portal system; it is then easy to see how the greater number of diseases of the uterus, tubes, and ovaries can be relieved in this way. Other means, however, as adjuvants, should not be neglected; and to accomplish these results, time, skill, and patience are requisite. Its field of application is in those border-line cases now so frequently operated upon, such as dysmenorrhoea, salpingitis, ovaritis, ovarian and hysteric epilepsy, ovarian neuralgia, pelvic cellulitis, pelvic abscess; cases of large cystic or fibroid tumors, and cancer, are not of course in any way benefited.

No one, who has not tried this method correctly and faithfully, can have any idea of its value in chronic disease, and, like the great painter who mixed his paints "with brains, sir," one must bring his common-sense to bear strongly on the subject, and be free from prejudice, which is generally begotten of ignorance. I have absolutely demonstrated its great value by a long series of clinical cases. The whole method simply consists in assisting nature to perform the cure physiologically, *i. e.*, by pelvic venous absorption.

Every physician is, or ought to be, familiar with the extremely intimate relationship of the digestive and pelvic organs, and their mutual inter-dependence. There is every reason why the gynaecologist should be a well seasoned phy-

sician, and that the intimate connection between internal
medicine and pelvic disease should be thoroughly appreciated
by him. It sometimes seems almost as though medicine has
been divided into too many specialties. The true specialist
must, above all, be a first-class general practitioner; if he is
not, he may be well termed a pseudo-specialist.

The fact that the body should always be treated as a
whole, is shown when we know that all the internal organs
in the abdominal and pelvic cavity have a common vascular
and nervous supply, so that when one of these organs is diseased, those that are intimately connected with it suffer at
the same time. If one will but think of the intimate connection of digestion with pregnancy and menstruation, and
the great influence that disturbances of the stomach and
liver have upon the uterus and its adnexae, and that we
never have weakness of one organ without weakness of all
when that weakness is due to deranged nutrition, we can
then readily see the intimate connection between the uterus
and the digestive system. We should also remember that
the blood-supply of all these organs, being more or less a
common one, venous congestion in all of them generally
depends upon obstructions in the portal circulation. This is
proved clinically in a great variety of instances. Take, for
example, a young girl with anaemic dysmenorrhoea. This is
wholly dependent on improper assimilation of healthful food,
and, in the majority of cases, the diet and digestive organs
are at fault. In cases of hepatic obstruction, there is always
portal congestion with accompanying chronic metritis,
endometritis, pelvic congestions, and leucorrhoea. The same
condition may take place when the heart muscle is weak,
from lack of nourishing nitrogenous food to strengthen it.
The digestive tube, with its twenty-seven feet of length, is
by far the most important organ in the body, and the minute
it becomes irritated and coated with catarrhal mucus the
patient begins to suffer.

These catarrhal states of the gastro-intestinal tube are
probably the most common pathological condition existing.

Catarrh seldom limits itself to one portion of the tract alone; it generally extends, by continuity, from the stomach upwards to all parts of the nasal and pharyngeal mucous membrane, and downwards through the intestines to the rectum, and yet often giving but slight warnings of its presence. The common term for it is chronic gastro-intestinal catarrh; but a far better one, because truer and more comprehensive, is the old-fashioned one of catarrhal diathesis.

Most cases of dysmenorrhoea in young girls are dependent on portal congestion and anaemia. Some noted gynaecologists deny that endometritis occurs in young virgins from flexions and stenoses retaining the secretions and causing their decomposition, thus inflaming the lining mucous membrane. They are undoubtedly correct, as there is nothing to prevent the liquid blood flowing away, and there is in reality no cavity to retain it.

We must not forget that the liver, which is a most elastic organ, can also be utilised as a muscular pump to draw up the blood through the portal system from the whole pelvic region; and while we are using astringents, or applying tampons soaked with glycerine, for its hygroscopic effect, we should also remember that we can get a similar result in the opposite direction, by draining the serum and blood from the affected parts through the agency of the intestines and the portal circulation. In these conditions the injection of a small quantity of sulphate of magnesia into the rectum is sometimes very useful. In most cases of chronic metritis and endometritis the condition is very much like that in the rectum when piles exist, and the treatment may be to a certain extent the same or similar.

I am not a believer in the treatment of uterine diseases by excessive drugging; still, I am thoroughly convinced that medical gynaecology has been neglected sadly for some years past, and that our next great advances in medical science will include this department.

The uterus is a sensitive organ, and the over-distension of it by dilators for a stenosis which never existed except in

the mind of the operator and the correction of flexions which
are normal, the application of strong acids to the interior of
the uterus, inflaming its delicate membrane and sealing up
the utricular glands, do a good deal towards the production
of disease and sterility. Endometritis existing alone is a
rather rare condition ; it is generally accompanied by salpingitis, pelvic cellulitis, or metritis. If these are removed, the
endometrium generally takes care of itself without any local
applications. Where the endometritis depends upon vaginitis, this must first be removed before the endometritis will
disappear. Unnecessary and unskilful treatment of the
endometrium has been the cause of some abdominal sections.
We should look at endometritis from above, and consider the
portal circulation, and see if some of the congestion and
inflammation and drainage cannot be diverted in that direction and removed through that channel.

Almost all ovaries on the post-mortem table look more or
less diseased. Of this I have had abundant evidence in the
dead-house on Blackwell's island. Although simple serous
cysts are of extreme frequency, there is still always plenty of
sound tissue remaining, showing how the organ could still
perform its function normally.

When the operation for the removal of a diseased organ is
a dangerous one, as coeliotomy certainly is always, in spite
of good statistics and brilliant operators, the disease should
be incurable by ordinary means, and the patient a chronic
invalid, before the operation should be performed.

The following case is typical, and interesting in this connection :

Mrs. L. M., twenty-eight years of age. Pelvic disease came on with
a severe chill and fever after her first labour, which was tedious and
instrumental. I first saw her several months after this. She was then
extremely enfeebled, emaciated, anaemic, and nervous, and had about
lost all hope of recovery. She was suffering from frequent attacks of
very severe pelvic pain, requiring repeated hypodermics of morphia.
Menstruation was absent.

On digital examination, a very tender, throbbing, and boggy tumor was
found to the left of the uterus. It was larger than an orange, and fluctuation could be distinctly felt. It could be easily examined through the

abdominal wall, and caused great irritation and depression. ,The result of the treatment by the hot water and diet, no colonic flushings being given, was to completely relieve the pain and inflammation, and to cause absorption of the pus and exudation with the exception of some slight thickening. What gave her the most joy, after the removal of the painful attacks, was the painless return of her menses after a period of seventeen months, although her baby had always been bottle-fed.

Her recovery was rapid and complete, she being under treatment for less than three weeks. Her physical condition became entirely changed. She had been told by two surgeons that only an operation would relieve her condition, but she declined operative interference.

There can be no question in the mind of any thoughtful physician that Galvanism, as recommended by Dr. E. Sanders, for the indurations following pelvic cellulitis, is an efficient means of treatment. For that condition, his valuable contribution on this subject can be found in the *American Journal of Obstetrics* for March, 1892.

Our advances in abdominal surgery have been marvellous, but we should be careful not to step too far. For the benefit of any who may have forgotten some of their pathology learned in college days, I would remind them that there is such a thing as the physiological reabsorption of pus. This may be incomplete by a cheesy change or inspissation; and this is a common process, pus being more watery than blood. When complete, the pus entirely disappears, after undergoing a fatty metamorphosis or emulsion. Pus is never reabsorbed as pus, but is broken up first into water, salts, and fat, thus becoming completely transformed. This is a matter of vital importance. Prevent the pus from forming, if you can; but when formed, properly remove it. The knife is not always necessary for this purpose. Surgical treatment has here trenched, in some instances, upon the domain of medicine. The advantage of this method over the knife can be actually seen in abscesses of the lymphatics of the neck, occurring in young patients who have been living on such food as jam, jellies, fresh bread, cake, fruit, and ice-cream.

I have also used this method on patients with pelvic abscess and high fever due to septic absorption. They were so emaciated that one could almost encircle the calf of the leg with the thumb and finger; they suffered agonising pains, and probably could not have stood the shock of an abdominal operation. Their recovery under this treatment was, however, rapid and complete.

The ingestion of an excess of carbo-hydrate food, I believe, tends to the development of bacteria in the digestive tract and wherever pus is present.

In these cases of chronic sepsis, there is a great strain upon the kidneys, and hence, the water taken is of great benefit. In cases of pyosalpinx, with operative interference alone, the results are not at all so gratifying as where this method of treatment is employed. When a writer says, in speaking of salpingitis, "If there is suppuration, there should be no question as to the propriety of an operation," I disagree with him decidedly. This same writer then goes on to show the advantage of operating in all cases, by saying, "To ascertain the real benefits of operation for this disease, one must not decide until quite a long period of time has elapsed." No one can say that abdominal section is a perfectly safe operation, as it is common for patients to die under it; nor does it always remove the disease along with the tubes and ovaries.

If a patient dies from an operation, where proper medical treatment would have readily cured her, what does the white sheet cover? Nothing more or less than a case of scientific murder; but then, ignorance excuses a great deal. While we should be conservative, we must not be cowardly.

In the cases of ulcerating appendicitis and other conditions, which we find impossible to resolve and which demand operation, temporising often leads to a fatal issue. When procrastination is indulged in without reason, after proper treatment has failed, the delay probably kills even more in this department than elsewhere. This is notably seen in cases of hernia, where stercoraceous vomiting and collapse are sometimes seen before an operation is advised.

FIFTY OPERATIONS ON THE UTERINE CERVIX FOR LACERATION.

By John B. Harvie, M. D., of Rensselaer County.

Read by title October 12, 1893.

This condition is one which is often overlooked, and even when diagnosticated, is frequently regarded as a state which requires no attention further than local treatment. On this account, the general impression seems to prevail that operation directed toward the repair of this lesion is unnecessary, and that improvement in health, as a rule, does not follow. At one time I was among those who favoured the non-operative treatment; but since I have done the operation a sufficient number of times, and have been able to follow the subsequent history (in a large percentage of the cases), and notice the improvement which generally takes place in health, I regard it as one of the most serviceable and satisfactory operations within the scope of the gynaecologist.

When the uterine cervix is torn during parturition, convalescence is generally protracted, unquestionably due to the fact that a surface is exposed which refuses to heal properly, delaying the ordinary physiological process of involution. The more or less continued presence of this condition may cause innumerable reflex disturbances.

It seldom, if ever, happens that repair will come about without special interference, and then immediate operation will necessitate too much uncertainty and too much risk to ever become popular. When a cervix is torn, as a rule the edges become everted, and the mucous membrane, to a certain extent, beyond the laceration together with the lacerated surface takes part in an inflammatory process. The influence extends almost invariably to the endometrium, setting up an endometritis. The lacerated surface usually bleeds easily, and secretes copiously together with the discharge from the interior of the uterus caused by the endometritis. Those are the cases which require attention, and those cases go on indefinitely in spite of anything which may be done in the shape of local treatment. When one notes the condition of such a cervix before and after operation, it must be very evident that repair is exceedingly desirable.

The secreting surface is gotten rid of, and the general inflammation of the interior of the uterus, which resulted in consequence of the lesion, naturally enough subsides. In instances where the trouble has been long-standing, it almost invariably happens that difficulty to a greater or less extent exists in connection with the appendages, notably salpingitis, and that is one principal reason why the pelvic distress, so common in those cases, takes often many months to subside after operation. The practice of insisting on absolute quiet for a length of time, so that resolution of the inflamed adjacent parts may take place, is very often an imperative necessity. Until Emmet made his operation known, patients suffering from this injury were invariably called upon to endure all manner of routine treatment, usually with the effect of irritating the patient considerably, and certainly doing no good.

In dealing with cervical lacerations, I think, when the patient is young and is likely to bear more children, the best operation is to remove a large portion of the cervix, after the method of Schröder; or, if the patient has nearly approached the limit of the child-bearing period, simply bringing the parts together according to Emmet will be sufficient; but no single operation will meet all requirements. I have had an opportunity to attend two cases of labour in which I had done Emmet's operation,—in one instance eighteen months, and in the other fifteen months, prior to delivery. The cervix acted in a perfectly natural way, dilated without difficulty, and labour terminated in both instances without recurrence of the former lesion. In another instance, in which a patient of mine, on whom I did an Emmet operation, was delivered, the laceration recurred on one side. The labour, however, progressed very rapidly, and the patient scarcely had time to get to bed when the baby was born. Escape in this instance was scarcely to be expected.

This has led me to incline rather favourably toward the operation of Emmet, as it leaves the cervix in its original state more closely than any of the other operations, and in my experience is followed by equally brilliant results. Generally speaking, after repair of the parts considerable shrinking will take place as a natural course of events, and a cervix which seemed much elongated and hypertrophied will return to almost its original size. I think a mistake which is often made, and one which I committed myself a number of times at the outset, is the neglect to thoroughly curette the uterus prior to repairing the cervix.

It is very wonderful the amount of benefit which that proceeding alone will bring about in an enlarged organ which is the seat of endometrial inflammation. The subject of drainage under those circumstances is of paramount importance, and to close up a cervix without first going over the interior of the uterus with a sharp curette would certainly be very bad neglect of duty. Repair of the lacerated parts is deferred for a time by some operators after curetting, so that the subject of drainage may have thorough attention. I think myself, the result is ordinarily just as good if we go over the ground thoroughly with the sharp curette until the application of the instrument may be heard and felt on the healthy muscular wall of the uterus, at the same time washing out the cavity carefully. The discharge subsequent to this is largely sanguineous, and will very readily escape through the cervical opening. In instances where subinvolution exists, together with diffuse endometritis, it is possible that recovery will be more perfect and rapid if a curettage be done together with intra-uterine irrigation and intra-uterine packing of sterilised iodoform gauze prior to repairing the laceration. It will, however, only be necessary in cases of enlarged uterus, or in prominent inflammatory lesions of adnexa, to subject the patient to a second operation, as in both instances the administration of an anaesthetic is necessary. There is no danger in doing an operation on the cervix, the only difficulty which may be encountered at the time being haemorrhage. Rapid work will of course prevent against any serious loss of blood. There is no use endeavouring to stop bleeding as we go along, as the blood comes from all parts denuded, and is in the form of a very free general oozing. In paring the surfaces, the most inferior parts should be taken care of first, so that the field of operation will be obscured as little as possible.

The instruments needed in this operation are a thin, narrow-bladed scalpel, a good tissue forceps, two tenaculum forceps (preferably Skene's), uterine dilator, sharp and blunt curettes, Sim's speculum, scissors, and, of course, needles and needle-holder.

There is no instrument, so far as I know, which has been devised that will take the place of the scalpel in preparing the cervical edges for being brought together. The Wathen dilator, on account of its simplicity of construction, cleanliness, and efficiency, is perhaps to be preferred. The same may be said of the very ingenious needle-holder recently devised by Dr. Williams, of the Johns Hopkins hospital, a description of which appeared in the New York *Journal of Obstetrics and Diseases of Women*, June, 1893, by Dr. Howard A. Kelley.

A preliminary usually adopted is to cut well up into the angle of the laceration with straight scissors, and complete the denudation with the scalpel. The uterus is held in place and drawn well down by inserting into each opposing lip of the cervix (the patient being in the dorsal position) a tenaculum forceps.

In regard to the material for suturing, I have used wire, silk-worm gut, and catgut, and have had good results with all of them; but I must confess a certain lack of confidence in catgut. I have had no serious accidents from its use except in one instance, where the sutures gave way, giving rise to secondary haemorrhage on the third day. This accident might have been more or less serious in private practice, but as it occurred in a hospital the patient's life was not jeopardised in any way. In private practice I always use silk-worm gut, knowing that when once introduced no accident can come about, the only objection I can see to its use being the possibility of its cutting through the tissues before union has taken place perfectly. However, if the parts are shaped properly, very little traction is necessary to hold the flaps in apposition, and that objection is consequently reduced to a minimum. The silk-worm gut possesses all the good properties of wire, and is much easier of manipulation and less likely to break, and will create much less disturbance in its removal. Catgut, of course, possesses the advantage of becoming dissolved, and, consequently, not necessitating removal, which is somewhat of an advantage, especially if the perinaeum has, been operated upon at the same sitting; but its occasional weakness and premature disappearance render it more or less unreliable; besides, any agent which acts on the principle of catgut will attract septic material, and may spoil a result which would otherwise have been satisfactory. I think there is no doubt but catgut may be made absolutely aseptic, but its strong absorptive properties will attract objectionable agents which may cause stitch-hole abscesses and inflammatory action in the line of union. This might occur very readily in the utero-vaginal tract, which is more or less difficult to maintain in a rigid state of cleanliness. Silk possesses all the vices of catgut except its occasional giving way, and none of its virtues.

The treatment of the patient prior to operation is the same as for other plastic operations in this neighbourhood—the thorough evacuation of the bowels the day before, and an enema the morning of the operation. The vagina should be irrigated by a nurse two or three times before the operation with a sublimate solution (1 : 1,000) followed by plain water. In using a vaginal douche, two fingers should be introduced so as to distend the channel, that every part may be brought in contact with the irrigating fluid. If this precaution is not adopted, many parts of the vaginal folds will escape contact with the liquid, and subsequently infect the wound. If this preliminary precaution be adopted, the tract will remain practically aseptic for two or three days, and little danger of wound infection will follow.

In my last half-dozen cases I have packed the vagina with iodoform gauze for twenty-four hours prior to operation, and am inclined to regard it as a very safe proceeding.

The bladder should be emptied just before the operation. The vagina is loosely packed with sterilised iodoform gauze, and removed at the end of two days. No further packing is required—in fact, the less that is done subsequent to this, except a plain-water irrigation once each day, the better will be the result.

The patient is allowed to pass urine from the commencement, in a bed pan ; catheterisation in a small proportion of the cases may be necessary for a day or so. The stitches are removed at the end of one week except in the case of catgut, which does not require removal. I have left silk-worm gut a much longer time without causing any disturbance, its non-absorption properties rendering it very well tolerated and non-irritating.

CASE I.—Aged thirty-three, married ; one child when twenty-seven years of age. Labour instrumental, no miscarriages. Headache, back-ache, and general pelvic discomfort, loss of flesh. Bowel and urinary disturbance absent. Menses recur every two or three weeks, and flow continues for seven or eight days ; is decidedly neurasthenic. Was under treatment by different physicians, who made use of local applications and supports. An Emmet's modification of an Albert Smith was removed on examination. Perinaeum lacerated through first degree, moisture increased. External os in axis of vagina and cervix bilaterally lacerated. Uterus retroverted. Erosion and eversion of cervix with endometritis. Uterus movable, depth increased. Moderate thickening of the tubes with tenderness. Uterus was lifted into place by glycerine tamponade. This routine treatment was continued sometime without benefit, and she was taken into the hospital and Emmet's trachelorrhaphy done. The result was all that could be desired. Silver wire was used in suturing. The pelvic distress, however, did not clear up as rapidly as was hoped for, and she contracted the idea that an oophorectomy should be done, which I refused. She went to New York and saw Dr. T. A. Emmet, who advised her to return home and wait at least one year, which she did; but before the alloted time she was perfectly well. A recent examination shows the uterus to be in a normal position.

CASE II.—Aged thirty-nine; married; one child when seventeen years of age; never pregnant since. Labour not instrumental. Complains of backache and constant bearing-down pains, frequent and painful urination. Very slight laceration of perinaeum, atony of vaginal wall, cervix in axis of vagina, and bilaterally lacerated; uterus low down in vagina. The torn lips of the cervix eroded and everted, bleed easily; presents almost an epitheliomatous appearance. Copious discharge from interior of uterus and torn cervix, uterus three and one half inches in depth. Emmet's trachelorrhaphy; silver wire for sutures. Patient remained in bed four weeks, subinvolution cleared up as well as the pelvic distress.

CASE III.—Aged thirty-one, married; four children; never attended by a physician. Constant bearing-down pains; inability to retain urine, and profuse leucorrhoea. Examination shows a large cystocele, prolapsed uterus, and lacerated perinaeum. The parts are excoriated in consequence of rubbing on her clothing, the cervix is much elongated and hypertrophied and unilaterally lacerated. In this case I did Schröder's operation, which really amounts to an amputation of the cervix. The cystocele was taken care of by denuding the mucous surface, commencing a short distance posterior to the meatus urinarius and extending back almost to the utero-vaginal fold, and going wide on each side of the median line so that when the surface was bared it was elliptical in form; then, by a series of overlapping buried catgut sutures, the parts were gradually rolled in, and, finally, the mucous edges approximated by interrupted sutures of strong catgut. The perinaeum was taken care of two weeks later, result perfect; complete relief, no return of prolapsus nor cystocele at the end of two years.

CASE IV.—Widow, aged forty-eight; has had seven children, all easy labours; no instruments. Severe pain left side low down, and profuse leucorrhoea; says, "womb falls down, and comes out;" has dysuria and frequent urination with more or less incontinence. Examination reveals a large cystocele with uterine procidentia and laceration of perinaeum extending back to the sphincter, also an extensive bilateral laceration of the cervix. Uterus curetted, and Emmet's trachelorrhaphy, anterior colporrhaphy, and perineorrhaphy. This operation was completed at one sitting, result good, relief perfect.

CASE V.—Aged forty-one, married; three children; never attended by a physician; menstruates every three weeks; headache, backache, and general pelvic uneasiness, unilateral femoral neuralgia, leucorrhoea. Perinaeum lacerated to the sphincter, cervix enlarged and irregularly lacerated. Copious discharge from cervix and interior of uterus. Curettement, and large portion of cervix removed and perinaeum repaired. Result good; health much improved.

CASE VI.—Aged thirty-three, married; five children, always attended by a physician. First labour instrumental; no miscarriages. Complains of backache and general pelvic discomfort, leucorrhoea. Perinaeum lacerated second degree, rectocele. Very copious discharge from vaginal mucous membrane. Cervix bilaterally lacerated, torn edges everted and eroded, uterus retroverted, and profuse discharge from its interior. Curettement, Emmet's trachelorrhaphy, perineorrhaphy, silk-worm gut for suture; patient did well in all respects.

CASE VII.—Aged twenty-three, unmarried; one child when eighteen; delivery instrumental; convalescence protracted; patient anaemic, and general health much impaired; suffers constantly from headache, backache, and pelvic tenesmus, occasional dysuria, intermittent leucorrhoea, and constipation. Perinaeum lacerated second degree, with rectocele, atony of vaginal wall. Cervix bilaterally lacerated with ectropium and cystic degeneration, endometritis; uterus sensitive and anteflexed. Divulsion, curettage, and intra-uterine irrigation, Schröder's amputation of the cervix. Very great improvement.

CASE VIII.—Aged twenty-six, two children, both instrumental. Protracted convalescence. Thinks she had "inflammation of the bowels" after second child; much run down in general health; has lost considerable flesh; menorrhagia and profuse leucorrhoea. Perinaeum slightly lacerated, and moisture of vagina increased; stellate laceration of cervix with endometritis; cervix bleeds easily when touched; curettement, irrigation, Schröder's operation; rapid gain in health.

CASE IX.—Aged forty-three, married; six children, all labours easy, and convalescence rapid. Complains of constant pelvic discomfort; is only easy in recumbent position. Vaginal outlet much relaxed, uterus low down in the vagina, cervix unilaterally lacerated and hypertrophied. Copious discharge from interior of uterus with subinvolution. Thorough dilatation, curetting, and intra-uterine tampon with iodoform gauze; tampon reinserted every other day for one week, when Schröder's operation was done, and perineorrhaphy. The patient did well. In this case, much good resulted from the iodoform packing.

CASE X.—Aged forty-eight, married; one child at thirty, instrumental delivery; convalescence uneventful; menstruation irregular, flows three to four days; leucorrhoea, backache, constipation, frequent urination. Laceration of perinaeum first degree, vaginal mucous membrane normal. Cervix bilaterally lacerated with erosion and ectropium. Copious secretion, external os in axis of vagina, hard masses in rectum, caruncles of urethra. Divulsion, curettage, and Emmet's trachelorrhaphy; urethra dilated and caruncles removed, and ten per cent. nitrate silver solution applied. Improvement very marked.

CASE XI.—Aged twenty-eight, married; one child at twenty-five; attended by a midwife; convalescence slow. Profuse leucorrhoea and menorrhagia; is decidedly neurasthenic; severe headache, and insomnia. Relaxed outlet, copious discharge from vaginal mucous membrane and increased heat, bilateral laceration of cervix with erosion and endometritis, uterus retroverted. Dilatation, curettement, and Emmet's trachelorrhaphy. Very rapid return of health. Has had a child since operation without recurrence of laceration.

CASE XII.—Aged thirty-three, married; two children, both easy labours. Has had continuous pelvic discomfort since birth of last child. Very copious leucorrhoea at times, with backache and pains extending down the legs. Perinaeum lacerated first degree, vaginal mucous membrane healthy, uterus in axis of vagina, but slight descent. Stellate laceration of cervix with cystic degeneration. Divulsion, curetting, Schröder's operation. Very great relief. Has miscarried, at third month, since operation.

CASE XIII.—Aged forty-four, married; seven children; two miscarriages; chronic invalidism, pelvic tenesmus, frequent painful urination and leucorrhoea. Vaginal outlet very relaxed, cervix bilaterally lacerated, and slimy mucus escaping from interior of uterus; cystic degeneration of cervix, and dense cicatricial thickening in angles of laceration. Divulsion, curettage, amputation of cervix by double flaps (Simons's operation, which consists in the removal of wedge-shaped pieces from anterior and posterior lips, denudation of lateral angles, and total removal of all cicatricial tissue). The mucous surfaces, after the removal of wedge-shaped portions, brought together by means of catgut sutures, and the operation completed in the same way as in Emmet's operation; perineorrhaphy. Result perfect; patient regained health after several months.

CASE XIV.—Aged forty-one, married; one child at thirty-four, labour difficult and instrumental; menorrhagia during last four years, leucorrhoea, backache, pain extending down limbs, dysuria, and constipation. Perinaeum lacerated to sphincter, rectocele, cervix unilaterally lacerated and elongated. Uterus in axis of vagina, but low down; cervical catarrh. Curetting, and Schröder's operation, perineorrhaphy. Result good; improvement fairly satisfactory.

CASE XV.—Aged fifty-seven, married; six children, labours moderately tedious, first two deliveries instrumental; no miscarriages. Has been an invalid since menopause at forty-eight. Perinaeum lacerated second degree. Rectocele, cystocele, complete uterine procidentia, unilateral laceration of cervix extending beyond utero-vaginal junction. Simons's operation, anterior colporrhaphy, perineorrhaphy. Good result; improvement in health more than satisfactory.

CASE XVI.—Aged thirty-nine, married; five children, never attended by a physician; regular menstruation not painful, profuse leucorrhoea and backache, vaginitis, cervix bilaterally lacerated, endometritis, thickening and tenderness of tubes. Divulsion and irrigation of uterine cavity, 1 : 1,000 bichloride, followed by sterilised water, curettage, Emmet's trachelorrhaphy. Slow recovery; pelvic distress, although abating, still occasions much discomfort.

CASE XVII.—Aged twenty-seven, married; three children, no instruments; no miscarriages. Regular menstruation, dysmenorrhoea, headache, backache, leucorrhoea, general pelvic discomfort, health much impaired. Perinaeum intact, vagina sensitive, bilateral laceration of

21

cervix, endometritis, divulsion, curetting, and Emmet's trachelorrhaphy. This patient made a good recovery, and is very comfortable.

CASE XVIII.—Aged twenty-four, married; one child; two miscarriages; metrorrhagia, constant bearing-down pain, unable to stand for any length of time, neuralgic pains extending down front of both legs, backache, leucorrhoea, loss of flesh. Perinaeum lacerated to sphincter, atony of vaginal wall, cervix incompletely and bilaterally lacerated, copious muco-purulent discharge from interior of uterus. Divulsion, curetting, complete division of mucous surface and thin wall remaining unbroken, Emmet's trachelorrhaphy, perineorrhaphy; good result. This patient has since borne a child, and no accident further than a rent in the perinaeum, which was immediately closed. Health at present good.

CASE XIX.—Aged forty, married; four children, natural delivery; one miscarriage; menstruates profusely every three weeks; urination frequent and at times painful, backache, pain in both iliac fossae extending down limbs, frequent headache. Perinaeum lacerated first degree, vaginal moisture increased, uterus in axis of vagina, cervix lacerated on left side with erosion and eversion, uterus sensitive, and tubes thickened and tender. Divulsion, curettage, packing with iodoform gauze, Emmet's operation after one week; recovery slow.

CASE XX.—Aged thirty-nine; one child, premature at eight months. In labour many hours; delivery instrumental; convalescence slow; irregular and painful menstruation; anaemic, and easily fatigued. Pelvic discomfort, and pain extending through to both iliac fossae; leucorrhoea; perinaeum intact; vaginal mucous membrane sensitive; heat and moisture increased; stellate laceration of the cervix, endometritis, uterus anteflexed, no tubal swelling. Divulsion, curettage, Simons's operation; result good. Improved in health, and continuing to feel better.

CASE XXI.—Aged thirty-eight; married; one child; attended by midwife; menstruation regular, lasts eight to ten days. Is easily fatigued; anaemic; has lost considerable flesh; backache, leucorrhoea, bilateral laceration of cervix, endometritis, uterus retroflexed. Divulsion, curetting, Emmet's trachelorrhaphy. Improved very decidedly for a time, but returned to hospital after one year complaining of general weakness, backache, very obstinate constipation, and insomnia. Hysterorrhaphy was advised on account of the very great retroflexion of the uterus; patient submitted; uterus was bound down firmly by adhesions in Douglas's fossa, which were separated, and the uterus attached to the anterior abdominal wall by buried silk sutures. Recovery rapid, and, so far, very great relief.

CASE XXII.—Aged twenty-four; married; first delivery instrumental; headache, dizziness, and sick stomach; poor appetite, diarrhoea alternating with constipation, leucorrhoea profuse, general pelvic discomfort, frequent urination; is decidedly neurasthenic; perinaeum lacerated, first degree; bilateral laceration of cervix, with erosion and eversion; endometritis. Divulsion, curetting, Emmet's trachelorrhaphy. Very great improvement while under observation.

CASE XXIII.—Aged thirty-three; four children, first instrumental; complains when she stands up that womb comes down; wears a perinaeal bandage continuously for support. Uterine procidentia, laceration of perinaeum to sphincter, unilateral laceration of cervix. Anterior colporrhaphy, double flap amputation of cervix, perineorrhaphy. No return of prolapse.

CASE XXIV.—Aged twenty-six; one child, tedious labour, but not instrumental; one miscarriage; menstruates regularly; backache not relieved when lying down; leucorrhoea, pelvic tenesmus, pain in right iliac region, very obstinate constipation, stomach frequently out of order. Perinaeum intact, vaginal mucous membrane healthy, unilateral laceration of cervix, torn edges very much indurated and secreting copiously; endometritis, uterus sharply anteflexed. Divulsion, curetting, intra-uterine packing with sterilised iodoform gauze. The laceration in this case was not very extensive, and nothing was done beyond the curetting. Very much improved.

CASE XXV.—Aged thirty-one; one child, easy labour; regular menstruation, pain in left side, extending down the limb, with pelvic tenesmus; backache, leucorrhoea, poor appetite; perinaeum lacerated first degree, vagina healthy; bilateral laceration of the cervix and endometritis; uterus increased in depth and anteflexed, no tubal trouble. Divulsion, curetting, Emmet's trachelorrhaphy; good result, marked improvement in health.

CASE XXVI.—Aged forty, married; five children, all easy labours; one miscarriage; menstruates regularly. Has lost flesh and strength in last two years; headache, poor appetite, food causes distress and gaseous distension; pain in back relieved when lying down; pain in both iliac fossae, extending down thighs; leucorrhoea is profuse and occasionally tinged with blood and offensive in odour; pressure of clothing causes discomfort; bladder irritable, vaginal heat and sensibility increased, outlet relaxed. Stellate laceration of cervix, uterus anteflexed and fixed, copious secretion from interior of uterus, salpingitis on both sides. Divulsion, curettage, intra-uterine irrigation, 1 : 2,000 sublimate, followed by sterilised water and cavity packed with sterilised iodoform gauze; health very much improved for a time, but return of former trouble in a milder degree.

CASE XXVII.—Aged twenty-four, one child; natural delivery; one miscarriage; complains of headache, nausea, and frequent attacks of vomiting; backache much relieved by lying down; pelvic discomfort, leucorrhoea, constant desire to urinate day and night, perinaeum lacerated first degree, vagina sensitive, caruncles around orifice of urethra, cervix unilaterally lacerated, edges eroded and bleed easily, uterus anteflexed, endometritis. Divulsion, curetting, Emmet's operation; divulsion of urethra, removal of vegetations, five per cent. nitrate of silver applied every week until disappearance; complete relief.

CASE XXVIII.—Aged twenty-seven, married; one child, labour difficult and instrumental; complains of rectal tenesmus with occasional mucous discharge; backache, pain in iliac regions, extending down the thighs; tires easily, occasional leucorrhoea, frequent urination; slight laceration of perinaeum, haemorrhoids, cervix bilaterally lacerated, edges of cervix eroded and ectropium, endometritis, uterus in axis of vagina. Divulsion of sphincter and ligation of haemorrhoids; divulsion and curetting of uterus, Emmet's operation, rapid and complete recovery. This woman has since borne a child; had only three hard pains; recurrence of the laceration on one side.

Case XXIX.—Aged twenty-nine, married; four children, labours easy, but always had retention of urine after each confinement, requiring to be catheterised for about one week; complains of obstinate constipation, pelvic discomfort, pain in both iliac regions and loins, leucorrhoea. Laceration of perinaeum to sphincter, rectocele and cystocele, cervix bilaterally lacerated, endometritis, uterus low in vagina. Divulsion, curetting, Emmet's operation, anterior colporrhaphy, perineorrhaphy; result good. Relief not as satisfactory as was hoped for, on account of continuance of endometritis; at end of four months dilated cervix and packed with iodoform gauze; local treatment continued some weeks; much improved.

Case XXX.—Aged fifty-three, married; five children, last delivery a transverse presentation; has not menstruated in three years; complains of burning and itching of vulva and falling of womb. Wears a cup pessary supported by a belt around the waist and a perinaeal strap. Examination shows outlet very relaxed; incomplete bilateral laceration of cervix, cystocele and procidentia. Discharge from uterus of slimy mucus. Divulsion, curetting, anterior and posterior colporrhaphy. Health excellent since operation.

Case XXXI.—Aged twenty-two, married; one child, instrumental; dates her trouble from birth of child; severe pain in back, extending down limbs; unable to walk about the house without help; incontinence of urine. Bilateral laceration of cervix, subinvolution of uterus and anteversion, profuse leucorrhoea. Separation of the pubic bones was thought to have taken place during the very difficult extraction of the head, which was large and strangely ossified. The attending physician informs me that she made a very tedious convalescence, was unable to walk for a long time, and was absolutely unable to stand on one foot. The uterus was drawn well down and thoroughly dilated, curettage, Emmet's operation. A large amount of fungoid material was removed; convalescence rapid and uneventful.

Case XXXII.—Aged twenty-nine, married; four children, all easy labours; two miscarriages; menstruated three times in last month, and very profuse at times. Is anaemic; general health poor, easily fatigued; leucorrhoea, backache, and general pelvic discomfort. Perinaeum intact, vagina sensitive, uterus in axis of vagina and somewhat enlarged, cervix bilaterally lacerated; brownish muco-purulent discharge from interior of uterus. Dilatation, curetting, large quantity of fungoid material removed; interior of uterus irrigated with 1 : 2,000 sublimate solution and cavity packed with sterilised iodoform gauze. Emmet's trachelorrhaphy done after one week. Secondary haemorrhage on the third day from catgut giving away; packed with iodoform gauze; sutures replaced after two weeks; good result.

CASE XXXIII.—Aged thirty, three children; first labour very prolonged but not instrumental; one miscarriage; was confined to bed four weeks, and thinks she had "inflammation of the bowels." Complains of backache, bearing-down pains, distress in both iliac fossae, pain extending down limbs, very frequent attacks of headache; perinaeum lacerated first degree; bilateral laceration of cervix, endometritis, retroversion of uterus and slight descent. Divulsion, curettage, Emmet's trachelorrhaphy; very much improved.

CASE XXXIV.—Aged thirty, two children; easy labours; menses regular; complains of leucorrhoea, inability to retain urine, and pelvic discomfort; relaxed outlet, cystocele, rectocele, bilateral laceration of cervix, uterus low down in vagina and glairy mucus escaping from the interior. Divulsion, curetting, and Emmet's trachelorrhaphy; anterior and posterior colporrhaphy; result good, relief absolute.

CASE XXXV.—Aged twenty-three, three children; easy labours, no subsequent trouble; regular menstruation; complains of dizziness, weakness, and is easily fatigued; backache, pain extends down limbs, leucorrhoea, and constipation; perinaeum intact, vaginal heat and sensibility increased, bilateral laceration of cervix with an incomplete laceration of the anterior lip, cystic degeneration of cervix with erosion and eversion of lacerated edges, retroversion of uterus. Divulsion, curetting, and double flap amputation; result good, general health much improved, and has become pregnant.

CASE XXXVI.—Aged thirty-nine, married; one child six years ago, instrumental delivery; convalescence somewhat protracted; pelvic discomfort, dysuria and increased frequency of urination, leucorrhoea, and general health and strength failing; is considerable of a neurasthenic; perinaeum lacerated second degree, extensive bilateral laceration of cervix, copious discharge from interior of the uterus, uterus in normal position. Divulsion, curettage, Emmet's trachelorrhaphy, posterior colporrhaphy. Result good; very decided improvement in general health, and continuing to improve.

CASE XXXVII.—Aged twenty-three, married, two children, natural deliveries, pain in lumbar region, extending down back of left thigh; pelvic pressure, leucorrhoea, frequent urination; has continued to flow for six weeks; is anaemic, and unable to attend to her housework; appetite poor, bowels constipated; perinaeum lacerated first degree, atony of vaginal walls, unilateral laceration of cervix, erosion, eversion, endometritis. Divulsion, curettage, Emmet's operation; a large quantity of material, which looked like retained placental tissue, came away with the curette and irrigator. Result good, convalescence uneventful.

CASE XXXVIII.—Aged thirty-three, married, one child, difficult forceps delivery, was in hard labour many hours when a physician was sent for. Backache, extending down limbs, pain in both sides low down, leucorrhoea; is comfortable when lying down. Perinaeum lacerated second degree, rectocele; stellate laceration of cervix, endometritis, uterus in axis of vagina, both tubes thickened and tender. Divulsion, curettage, double flap amputation of cervix, posterior colporrhaphy. Result good; general condition rapidly improving.

CASE XXXIX.—Aged twenty-seven, married; two children; both forceps deliveries, no miscarriages; has never had any previous illness. Pain in both iliac fossae extending down the thighs, backache, pelvic tenesmus much increased when standing, leucorrhoea, urination frequent; menses regular, always has severe pain first day, flow lasts four to five days; appetite good, bowels regular, suffers from headache during menstruation. Perinaeum intact, vaginal moisture increased, unilateral laceration of cervix with erosion and ectropium, endometritis; uterus anteflexed, left tube sensitive and thickened. Divulsion, curettage, Emmet's trachelorrhaphy. Result good, improvement in health taking place very slowly.

CASE XL.—Aged forty-four, married; two children; twenty years between births, easy labours, miscarriage three years after birth of last child; flowed many weeks after miscarriage, finally had chills and fever and severe pain in lower abdomen, confining her to bed more than one month. Uterus curetted, retention of urine. Has not menstruated in two years, is anaemic. Complains of pelvic tenesmus, severe backache, constipation, frequent urination and pruritus valvae, leucorrhoea. Perinaeum lacerated first degree, vaginitis, bilateral laceration of cervix, endometritis, caruncles of urethra; torn edges of the cervix gape widely and bleed easily, uterus in axis of vagina; no disease of adnexa. Tamponing vagina with iodoform gauze for three days (fresh packing each day) prior to operation, and thorough irrigation with plain water. Divulsion, curettage, Emmet's operation; divulsion of urethra, removal of vegetations, and five per cent. nitrate of silver applied. Good result; improvement in health very great.

CASE XLI.—Aged twenty-nine, married; one child; labour prolonged, but not instrumental; convalescence protracted; always healthy prior to this time. Complains of vertigo, severe headache, backache, pelvic discomfort; frequent urination; menstruates every three weeks, lasts one week, profuse, painful at the onset; leucorrhoea. Perinaeum lacerated second degree; vagina sensitive, and moisture increased; slight prolapsus of bladder, uterus retroverted and somewhat fixed; cervix lacerated irregularly and incompletely, admits first joint of index finger readily; tenderness in right iliac fossa, and thickening of corresponding tube; endometritis. Divulsion, curettage; large amount of cervical tissue removed with sharp spoon; unable to bring uterus down to outlet on account of adhesions; cervical canal packed with iodoform gauze; posterior colporrhaphy. Result good; reflex disturbances have largely disappeared.

CASE XLII.—Aged thirty-six, married; two children; easy labours, convalescence uneventful; no miscarriages. menses regular, painless. Complains of distension of abdomen and colicky pains at times, with occasional vomiting, constipation, backache extending down the thighs, leucorrhoea; vaginal outlet intact, mucous membrane healthy; cervix bilaterally lacerated with erosion and eversion, uterus retroflexed and sensitive. Divulsion, curettage, Emmet's trachelorrhaphy. Result good; uterus replaced, and modification of Albert Smith pessary introduced at end of four weeks. Fails to relieve sufficiently; is, however, more comfortable. Have advised her to accept fixation of uterus to anterior abdominal wall if disability continues.

CASE XLIII.—Aged thirty-five, married; two children; easy labours; convalescence delayed, always hard; retention of urine after delivery; no miscarriages. Began menstruating at fourteen, always regular; was confined to bed six weeks on account of peritonitis three years ago. Headache, backache, pain in right iliac fossa, extending down front of thigh; profuse leucorrhoeal discharge, poor appetite, frequent vomiting, constipation. Vaginal outlet slightly relaxed, vaginal mucous surface healthy, bilateral laceration of cervix, torn edges bleed easily, endometritis; uterus retroverted, prolapse of right ovary. Rectal mucous membrane prolapsed and haemorrhoids. Divulsion of cervix, curettage, Emmet's operation; divulsion of sphincter and ligation of haemorrhoids. Good result; health much improved.

CASE XLIV.—Aged thirty-four, married; one child, difficult forceps delivery. Complains of constant dragging weight in back and limbs, pelvic discomfort, leucorrhoea; says she is not able to attend to her ordinary housework. Perinaeum lacerated second degree. Rectocele, bilateral laceration of cervix with copious discharge from torn edges, and interior of uterus displaced laterally to the right, and fixed adhesions broken down. Divulsion, curetting, all inflammatory tissue of cervix thoroughly scraped away with the sharp spoon, posterior colporrhaphy, intra-uterine packing of iodoform gauze. Result good, improvement in health.

CASE XLV.—Aged thirty-eight, married; five children, labours easy; four miscarriages; prolonged flow after each miscarriage. Easily fatigued, poor appetite, loss of flesh, and constipation; menstruates about every six weeks, flow continues one week. Complains of headache, backache, and general pelvic discomfort; pain referred to left iliac fossa, leucorrhoea, pruritus vulvae. Slight laceration of perinaeum, vaginitis, cervix bilaterally lacerated, endometritis, prolapsus of left ovary, uterus anteflexed. Divulsion, curettage, large quantity of material came away with sharp curette and irrigator, Emmet's operation. Result good, decided improvement.

CASE XLVI.—Aged thirty, married; two children, both instrumental; one miscarriage, convalescence slow. Pain in right side low down, marked pelvic discomfort with frequency of urination, backache, leucorrhoea; menstruates every three weeks; flows five days, no pain but pelvic tenesmus increased during the flow. Perinaeum lacerated first degree, atony of vaginal walls, uterus low down in vagina, cervix unilaterally lacerated, and endometritis. Divulsion, curettage, Emmet's operation, posterior colporrhaphy. Result good, rapid gain in health, pelvic pressure almost absent.

CASE XLVII.—Aged thirty-five, married; three children, all easy labours; one miscarriage at about two months; menses regular, no pain. Complains of headache, insomnia, backache extending down limbs, leucorrhœa, frequent urination. Appetite poor, frequent attacks of vomiting. Perinaeum intact; cervix bilaterally lacerated, with eversion of the segments, endometritis. Divulsion, curetting, Emmet's trachelorrhaphy. Result good; very much improved.

CASE XLVIII.—Aged thirty-seven, married; one child; five miscarriages, menses regular. Complains of profuse leucorrhoea, backache, and pains extending down both limbs, loss of flesh, poor appetite, and constipation. Outlet relaxed, vaginitis, cervix bilaterally lacerated, erosion and ectropium of torn edges, endometritis, tenderness and fulness in right tube and ovary. Vagina douched with sublimate solution (1: 1,000) twice each day for three days, and packed with iodoform gauze. Divulsion, curetting, Emmet's operation. Result good. This patient did not obtain as much relief as was hoped for. Have advised dilatation and intra-uterine packing of iodoform gauze on account of a continuance of the endometritis.

CASE XLIX.—Aged forty, married; nine children, no instruments; two miscarriages; menstruates every three weeks profusely. Complains of leucorrhoea, backache, and constant pelvic discomfort. Is very irritable and melancholy at times. Perinaeum lacerated to the sphincter, cystocele, bilateral laceration of the cervix, endometritis. Divulsion, curetting, Emmet's operation, anterior colporrhaphy, perineorrhaphy. Result good. When last heard from was decidedly neurasthenic, and expressed no special relief from the operation.

CASE L.—Aged thirty-three, married; three children; first delivery instrumental, no miscarriages; menstruates every four weeks, at times quite painful; leucorrhoea, pains in both iliac fossae, anterior femoral neuralgia. Is unable to attend to her work properly on account of the pelvic discomfort. Perinaeum lacerated first degree, vaginal heat and sensibility normal, cervix bilaterally lacerated, endometritis. Divulsion, curetting, Emmet's operation. Good result; very satisfactory return of health.

CURE OF CONSUMPTION AND EMPYEMA WITHOUT A RESORT TO THORACIC SURGERY.

By CHARLES A. LEALE, M. D., of New York County.

October 11, 1893.

Within the past fortnight, I invited two of the members of this Association to an interesting autopsy, demonstrating the advantages of the conservative treatment of far advanced pulmonary and pleural diseases, where a resort to thoracic surgery might have given the physician opportunities for glory and compensation, but could not have resulted in so long continued life. It was as follows:

One of the most prosperous merchants in a rapidly growing and wealthy western city, early in his life, while in perfect health, married a lady who was known to be from consumptive ancestors and then had consumption, to whom marriage had been recommended as a means toward cure. She never had any children. Her wealth gave her many comforts and excellent sanitary surroundings. Her married life was prolonged twenty-six years. After her marriage she at first improved in health and weight, but in a few years she was again an acknowledged invalid, and her disease slowly but steadily advanced until her death. The prolongation of her existence was believed by her friends to have been due to her intercourse with her healthful consort. Her husband's family I traced for five preceding generations, without discovering any hereditary tendency toward tuberculous diseases. About ten years after his marriage and nightly sleeping in the same bed with his wife, he began to cough, but his inherent antagonism to lung disease and his magnificently healthful and capacious thorax and enormous lungs resisted the influence of disease for years; but long before his wife died, tuberculosis was steadily advancing in him, so that, after a quarter of a century of direct contact, he was then pronounced by his physicians to be in the same condition as his feeble wife.   At the end of twenty-six years of married life, with continued cough and profuse expectoration, the wife had become an emaciated skeleton, and died from the effects of general tuberculosis.

The husband's right thorax was then filled with pus and consolidated lung tissue.   He was told that he could never recover, and that it was his duty to retire from business and seek better opportunities to make his life more endurable. He went to Egypt, lived an entire season near the river Nile, and before many weeks had passed found that he was gaining in weight and strength ; had so continued for twenty-five years, and only last summer thumped his thorax while on my physical examination chair, stating how the doctors had been deceived by thinking that he had any disease of the lungs.

He gave his physicians no credit for their correct diagnosis, nor for their influence in prolonging his life.   He stated that they were all wrong, that his consumption was a myth, but his necropsy proved that they were right in every respect except their unfavourable prognosis of a short life, as we found in his lungs all the signs of a cured consumption. There were extensive consolidations of the upper lobe of his right lung, in which were found cheesy and calcareous masses as large as chestnuts, while the pleura was a quarter of an inch in thickness and resembled tough leather.   He had a sufficiency of useful lung tissue to last him for twenty years. Nature had, in her wise way, shut off the diseased upper lobe of the right lung, and had covered his thickened and hardened pleura with a pseudo-serous membrane.   It was plainly seen that no operation could have successfully removed all of his diseased pulmonary tissue, and also that if the pus had been removed from the thorax it would have prevented its desiccation over the dependent portions of the pleura, and thereby prevented such a thick inelastic covering to the diaphragm, which during the whole subsequent course of his life occasionally caused lancinating pains, due to its adhesion to the liver.

The surgeon, if he had opened that thorax during life, could easily have demonstrated to the patient and his friends something wonderful to them, when he had removed three or four pieces of solid chalk the size of chestnuts, and masses of offensive cheesy decompositions, or if attempts had been made to cut away portions of that pathologically thickened and hardened pleural wall, which for years had been so safely guarded. His medical treatment had resulted in giving him an excellent stomach, good appetite, and powerful digestion. By physical exercise he had attained a compensating enlargement of his heart, and his liver had been left in an almost absolutely normal condition. He thereby, with his excellent assimilation of nutritious food, powerful blood, and active glandular secretions, readily overcame all the effects of the other pathological lesions, with the exception of atheromatous changes of the middle coats of the cerebral arteries. Three years before his death I wrote an excuse to the justice to have his name permanently stricken from the roll of jurors, and then wrote that he was in danger of sudden death being induced by either acute indigestion, over fatigue, or undue excitement. His last meal was over two quarts of milk at nearly 32° F., which nature resisted by a violent effort to vomit, causing such pressure as to rupture one of his atheromatous cerebral arteries, immediately followed by paralysis and coma, with death on the third day.

BRIEF COMMENTS ON THE MATERIA MEDICA, PHARMACY, AND THERAPEUTICS OF THE YEAR ENDING OCTOBER 1, 1898, AL- PHABETICALLY ARRANGED.

By E. H. Squibb, M. D., of Kings County.

Read by title October 12, 1898.

The above somewhat lengthy title is sufficiently explicit to describe the purport of the following notes, and those who desire to learn the moderate scope of this digest are referred to the introductory sentences of previous comments, delivered here for the past two years.

Acetanilid (antifebrin) continues to have an extended use, and is now officinal in the new United States Pharmacopoeia of 1890. It is still being carefully studied, and various reports are made from time to time emphasising its benefits as well as cautioning against abuse.

Dr. John Gordon, of Aberdeen, Scotland, reports the results of a series of numerous experiments with some of the recent hypnotics on pancreatic digestion, and concludes that the action of acetanilid, "whether the solution employed was weak, 0.3 cc., or in strengths up to 16 cc. of a 1 : 200 solution, was negative."

Toxic effects had become so frequent with the increasing use of this and some other hypnotics, that the British Medical Association requested its Therapeutic Committee to conduct an inquiry into the frequency and importance of the ill effects, and the honourable secretary, Mr. William Hunter, now reports "that both the frequency and importance of these ill effects have been considerably exaggerated. The predominant opin- ion is, that with due care, especially as regards the initial dosage, ill effects other than those connected with idiosyncrasy, are extremely infrequent, of little or no importance, and are not of such a character as to limit in any material way the usefulness of the drugs. This conclu- sion does not so fully apply to antifebrin, the action of which has been frequently followed by ill effects. In the case of antifebrin the dosage employed has, in the majority of cases, been too large."

It is apparently still the favourite hypnotic to administer to children, and various expedients are adopted to reduce the bulk of the dose in these cases. As considerable quantities of wine, whiskey, or alcohol are necessary to dissolve it, these solvents are objectionable on account of the large bulk of fluid; therefore Dr. J. C. McMechan, of Cincinnati, Ohio, reports that he gives it in mucilage of acacia, according to the following formula, which makes a mixture pleasant to the taste:

Acetanilid......................................	8 grammes.
Mucilage of acacia.............................	40 "
Syrup...	40 "

Take 5 grammes (teaspoonful) every three hours. Be cautious to always keep the amount of mucilage the same, even though the hypnotic may be increased or decreased, but the syrup may be reduced if desired.

Acid Agaricic (laricic acid), spoken of last year as an effective remedy to check sweating, no doubt has been used in the old country fully as much as the year previous, but practically nothing has appeared in print upon it one way or the other, so that the profession at large can hardly judge of its merits at this time.

Acid Arsenous is mentioned here only to call attention to the change in spelling now adopted by the new United States Pharmacopoeia of 1890. The Pharmacopoeias of 1870 and 1880 both called it Arsenious Acid, but now the "i" is dropped in accordance with the most approved etymology.

Acid Boric is mentioned here only to emphasise the fact that this is the approved term by which the commonly called Boracic Acid should be designated.

Acid Camphoric continues to give excellent results in the treatment of sweating from various causes, and one German authority classes it as far superior to all other medicaments in the treatment of night-sweats.

Acid Carbolic (phenol) has received renewed prominence over its great rival, corrosive sublimate, by the declaration of its original noted promoter in surgery, Sir Joseph Lister. In his "Address on the Antiseptic Management of Wounds," delivered in the London Post-Graduate Course at King's College hospital, on January 18 last,[1] he declared his complete abandonment of corrosive sublimate in favour of his first choice. The strength he now adopts is 1 : 20, which he finds to be completely trustworthy for surgical purposes. Its greater efficiency as a germicide is not only established, but he finds it greatly to be preferred in other respects. He writes,—"Carbolic acid has a powerful affinity for the epidermis, penetrating deeply into its substance, and it mingles with fatty materials in any proportion. Corrosive sublimate solution, on the other hand, cannot penetrate in the slightest degree into anything greasy; and therefore, as the skin is greasy, those who use corrosive sublimate require elaborate precautions in the way of cleansing the skin, treating it with oil of turpentine or ether, not to mention soap and water, to remove the grease which they feel it essential to get rid of for the efficient action of the corrosive sublimate. Now all this is unnecessary

[1] Brit. Med. Journal, vol. 1, for 1893, page 161.

care if you use carbolic lotion. I can testify to this from very ample experience. For my part, I do not even use soap and water. I trust to the carbolic acid, which, by its penetrating power and great affinity for organic substances, purifies the integument in a way that inorganic salts, like corrosive sublimate, cannot."

The use of carbolic acid in the treatment of typhoid fever has received some attention during the year, and has brought forth some conflicting testimony as to its merits. Dr. H. Rodger Sloan, M. B., C. M., of Gala-shiels, Scotland, reports having treated during three consecutive years 49 cases—39 by the ordinary method and 10 by the carbolic acid pills containing 162 milligrammes (2½ grains), as recommended by Professor Charteris. He claims that the "carbolic-acid treatment strikes at the root of the fever by the destruction of the micro-organisms which are the cause of the malady. In the cases so treated the fever was cut short, no grave symptoms, as haemorrhage or perforation, ensued, and the process of recovery was quick and attended by no wasting. My opinion is, that the efficacy of the carbolic-acid treatment cannot be questioned, and I am certain, if adopted early, it would prove, in an epidemic of typhoid fever, a preventive as effectual, or more so, than that of vaccination in small-pox."

On the other hand, Dr. J. Leslie Callaghan, of Colyton, Devon, England, writes that he is sorry he cannot agree with Dr. Sloan, as it is his opinion that it "has no power to destroy the bacilli of typhoid—in fact, I am led to believe it has the opposite effect, and that it is useless, if not dangerous, to use carbolic acid as a disinfectant in typhoid fever." Although Dr. Callaghan's statement is rather sweeping and summary under the circumstances, still conservative observers would admit that ten cases, even though all were favourable, were too few to establish the claim of specific action, but surely might be a good basis for more prolonged experience.

At the German Congress of Medicine, held at Wiesbaden from April 12 to 15 last, Professor von Ziemssen reported very satisfactory results from injections of ¼ cc. (about 8 minims) of a 2 per cent. solution of carbolic acid into the substance of the tonsil in many cases of catarrhal inflammation of the throat. The temperature fell almost immediately, and in every case recovery took place rapidly. This method of treatment was also successful, though less constantly, in diphtheria, where its effects were, however, less rapid. In a case of scarlet-fever of a grave character, complicated with erysipelas, which caused a considerable rise of temperature, the desired result was obtained with two injections. In the discussion which followed, Professors Sahli of Berne, and Heubner of Leipsic, corroborated these statements and gave testimony to excellent results, even in diphtheria, and as being well adapted for children on account of giving very little pain.

Dr. Tamamcheff, of Tiflis, Russian Transcaucasia, reports having conducted a series of experiments to ascertain the effects of microbe cultures, to which a sterilised solution of carbolic acid was added, when used as vaccine. The immediate result of the addition of the solution was, "the death of the organisms present in the culture. Guinea-pigs were inoculated with the fluid, and others were treated with the original virus containing the living microbes, in order that a comparison of the effects produced might be made. It was found that the carbolisation, while not in any degree diminishing the immunising value of the vaccine, reduced its toxic effects at least three to six times as compared with the living vaccine."

In this connection, the following incident, reported by Brigade Surgeon Dr. W. Alexander, of Glencorse, Edinburgh, Scotland, is interesting, and may be useful, as he says, in proving the power of carbolic acid as a germicide: "A short time since I had occasion to vaccinate eighteen men; but having only one square of lymph, sufficient for fifteen persons, I proceeded to dilute it by adding three drops of what I considered to be pure water from a vessel placed at hand to receive the points as they were used. On inspecting the arms on the eighth day, I was surprised to find that all had failed with three exceptions, one being a previously unvaccinated person, and each of these presented a single modified pustule.

"On making inquiry as to the possible cause of so many failures, I remembered the incident of diluting the lymph, and learned that what I considered pure water was a very weak solution of carbolic acid, 1 part in 120, thus showing that 1-40th of a drop of carbolic acid was sufficient to render almost innocuous the infecting element of fresh vaccine lymph.

"Sixteen of these men have since been revaccinated, with the following results: eleven perfect, two modified, three failed, two of whom had each had a single modified pustule on the previous vaccination, showing that even these were a sufficient protection."

Acid Cresotic (paracresotic acid) still finds adherents on the other side of the Atlantic, but little has been written upon it during the past year.

Acid Pyroligneous (crude acetic acid), sometimes called Wood Vinegar, is the crude product obtained from the destructive distillation of wood, and the note of last year is repeated here for, owing to the increasing interest in this acid during the year, it will be well to keep in mind what it really is. It is a dark-brown liquid, almost black, the colour depending largely upon the amount of tar contained in it, with a characteristic, not unpleasant, smoky odour. The tar would, of course, be practically insoluble in water alone, but the acetic acid present renders it perfectly soluble, and the whole product will permit of very considerable dilution with water before the tar is precipitated. This solution of the tar no doubt lends additional efficiency to the product. Some attention has now been paid during the past year or more to this acid, with the idea of increasing its use as a disinfectant. From the acetic acid and other antiseptic hydro-carbons which it contains, it should prove of positive value, while from its great abundance, as a by-product, wherever wood is burned for the charcoal and wood spirit, it is everywhere accessible at very low cost. As it can be used with perfect safety, and is always at hand when needed, it will soon be universally acceptable and its efficiency well established. It has been constantly used during the past year in the morgues and hospital wards of more than one city, where it has been found to work admirably. In cases where the proper dilution (according to circumstances and conditions) and proper amount of the solution had been used accidentally or otherwise, it not only masked the prevailing putrid odours but produced the condition of no odour whatever, thus apparently the putrid, and its own peculiar odours masked each other.

In this connection it may well be mentioned that Mr. Charles T. McClintock, A. M., of Ann Arbor, Mich., in some exhaustive and interesting experiments made on "Corrosive Sublimate as a Germicide," found, when he attempted to follow out, as a matter of curiosity, a statement made by Professor Klein in 1884 that corrosive sublimate was of no more germicidal value than vinegar, that such vinegar, containing from 6.3 to 7.0 per cent. of acetic acid, aborted the growth of micro-organisms as much as a 1 : 1,000 solution of the sublimate.[1]

M. Haschimodo reports from Paris, France, that a vinegar containing from 2.2 to 3.2 per cent. of acetic acid, saturated with pure culture of cholera bacillus, can, after an interval of fifteen minutes, be inoculated into animals without danger or be eaten with impunity by human beings. These facts appear to have been confirmed by numerous experiments and are entitled to be followed up pretty vigourously, to either definitely establish the facts or refute them, as it may be easily surmised what inestimable results would follow the thorough confirmation of such a statement.

Acid Salicylic has lately been used endermically with much satisfaction. Professor Bourget, of Lausanne, Switzerland, has made simple applications of an ointment containing this acid to the inflamed joints occurring in rheumatic fever. Friction, apparently, is not necessary, as the close application obtained by wrapping the joint thus treated in flannel, is sufficient to promote absorption and furnish his remarkable results. He tried several excipients: glycerin and starch, vaseline and lard, but the formula giving by far the best results was,—

Salicylic acid	1 part.
Turpentine	1 "
Lanolin	1 "
Lard	8 "

For the last two years every case of acute rheumatism admitted into his wards was treated by the application of this ointment. His results were satisfactory in that the pain disappeared in a few hours after application, the temperature was reduced never later than about the fifth day, and none of the unpleasant features of the internal administration of the salicylates was ever noticed.

Agathin (salicyl-aldehyde-*a*-methyl-phenyl-hydrazone), the new analgesic spoken of last year, had a more extended use during the year just past. Naturally the Germans furnish the largest number of reports, but it was introduced into England during the year, and could be obtained in this country as well.

The doses used ranged from 250 to 500 milligrammes (about 4 to 8 grains) repeated three times a day, but apparently from 2 to 6 grammes (about 30 to 90 grains) had to be given before any effect was produced. In the city of Brooklyn, Dr. Arnold Stub reported last February that he had up to that time used it for three or four weeks with some success in sciatica and neuralgic troubles, but none of the reports from any quarter are very enthusiastic, which would look as if its days were limited as an "anti-neuralgic and anti-rheumatic."

Alumnol is a new astringent and antiseptic salt discovered by Filehne, of Breslau, Prussia, and introduced to the profession for the first time by Drs. R. Heinz and A. Liebrecht at the recent International Congress of Dermatologists at Vienna. It is reported to be an aluminium salt of napthol-sulphonic acid, presented in the form of a nearly white non-hygroscopic powder, with a tendency to a reddish colour, which darkens by age and exposure. It is readily soluble in cold, and to a greater extent in hot, water, and likewise to a less marked degree in glycerine and alcohol —insoluble in ether. It is closely allied to Sozal and Sozo-Iodol, but has more markedly astringent properties than either. Its solutions react acid and it precipitates gelatin or albumin, but such a precipitate is soluble in an excess of gelatin or albumin and thus purulent discharges do not clog up cavities and desirable penetration below the surface is accomplished. This property is invaluable for very obvious reasons, and will be fully appreciated by surgeons in all branches.

Professor J. Eraud, of Paris, France, has used Alumnol with success, both in solution and dry, in simple wound dressings, in specific and non-specific ulcers, and finds that it neither irritates nor gives pain. A 1 to 3 per cent. solution gives satisfaction as a gonorrhoeal injection.

The largest users so far have been the Germans. Chotzen, Wolffberg, Spengler, and others report very gratifying results. Martin Chotzen has employed it in more than three hundred cases—soft chancre, abscesses, erosions, moist eczema, acne of the face, boils, urethritis, urticaria, favus, psoriasis of the head and face, and other affections. He found that it was beneficial in acute superficial inflammatory affections of the skin, as well as in chronic processes where the inflammation was deeper, in parasitic affections, and in acute and chronic inflammations of the mucous membrane.

Wolffberg finds in ophthalmic practice that a 4 per cent. solution is effective in stopping lachrymation.

Dr. Albert Spengler confirms the claim that it does not produce detrimental effects and that it has no poisonous action, but when introduced under the skin in large doses, or into the stomach, it apparently affects the kidneys. He has made extended use of it in throat and nose affections. Aqueous solutions from ¼ to 10 per cent. were employed. Comparing its action with that of 1 to 2 per cent. solution of zinc chloride in pharyngitis, it showed equally favourable results, its advantage, however,

22

being that it was not so unpleasant to the patient; but in laryngeal affections, the cases failing to respond to Alumnol were at once improved by the zinc chloride solution.

In the section in Laryngology and Rhinology of the recent Pan-American Medical congress, Dr. J. Mount Bleyer, of New York city, read a paper on "Alumnol in Diseases of the Nose and Throat," in which he speaks of using it with great benefit in mucous placques of the tongue, showing better results than those usually seen with chromic acid. In the discussion which followed, Dr. D. Bryson Delavan, of New York city, reported having obtained satisfactory results, but could not put it on as high a plane of usefulness as had been claimed for it. He alluded to the fact that the cost stood so much in the way of its more general use in this country, as the price asked here was four times greater than in Germany.

Excellent results have been obtained in gynaecological and otological practice. The insufflated powder used in cases of otitis media purulenta has been of great benefit. It does not clog up the meatus, as most powders do, requiring removal before further treatment, but completely dissolves in the purulent secretion.

It is probably too early yet to hear much from it on this side of the Atlantic, but surely the incentive given by the report in the Pan-American Medical congress will act as a stimulus.

Amido-Eugenol Acetate, the new anaesthetic of last year, has been little heard of this year, and it may be concluded that it did not fill the place which had been selected for it, and therefore it has been dropped out of notice.

Amylene Hydrate (tertiary amyl alcohol) has again to be reported as of decreasing interest. Of course, some observers continue to exalt its usefulness, but they are becoming fewer in number. The only really prominent report of experimental study with it recently was by Peiser, who investigated its influence on the elimination of nitrogen in the urine in comparison with chloral. He found that it diminished the nitrogenous waste, while chloral considerably increased the decomposition of albuminous matter. He concludes that it is the more preferable hypnotic in all cases where long continuous use is indicated, and especially where great nitrogenous waste takes place.

Anaesthetics have been quite the absorbing topic among English practitioners at times during the past year. Commissions continue to be appointed, and bring in unsatisfactory reports, but the whole tendency and purport of the discussion has been very decidedly to elevate ether above chloroform. One of the most recent elaborate reports on this question is that of the commission established by the London *Lancet* to investigate the whole subject of the Administration of Anaesthetics, and Dr. Dudley Buxton draws the following deductions from it:

"1. That the death-rate under anaesthetics heretofore has been unduly high, and may, by improved methods and greater care, be lowered.

"2. That ether when properly given from an inhaler permitting graduation of the strength of the vapour, is the safest anaesthetic in temperate climes for general surgery.

"3. That nitrous oxide gas should be employed for minor surgery, and should replace chloroform in dental surgery.

"4. That chloroform, when given by a carefully trained person, is a comparatively safe body, but is not, in any case, wholly devoid of risk.

"5. That no age or nation is free from danger under anaesthetics.

"6. That the perils of anaesthetics, however slight, demand that the undivided attention of a duly qualified and trained medical man should be given to the administration of the anaesthetic."[1]

After the excitement about the Pictet chloroform had somewhat subsided, Prof. R. Anschütz, of Bonn, Prussia, brought forward what was reported as a great discovery in the form of a solid compound containing chloroform, which was to solve the problem at once of eliminating the objectionable features of the ordinary product. He discovered by accident that chloroform combines with salicylic anhydride (called salicylide) in the form of fine colourless crystals, and in so doing apparently rejects the impurities usually found in it. This was looked upon as a great accomplishment, as now such a compound might be readily carried about and the chloroform eliminated by simply applying the heat of a water bath to split up the combination. This product, however, is now little more than a chemical curiosity, as the details mentioned to produce it are not recognized to be of sufficient value to base any prospect of its being within the limits of a commercial venture.

It may be well to call attention here to the wise decision of the revisers of our new United States Pharmacopoeia of 1890, in dropping entirely the long recognized Chloroformum Venale and altering the title of Chloroformum Purificatum to read simply Chloroformum. The danger is so great in having an authorised impurer article that it is eminently proper to establish only one grade and that a pure one.

Analgen when previously alluded to here was ortho-oxy-ethyl-ana-mono-acetyl-amido-quinoline, but during the past year it has been found that when benzoyl is substituted for the acetyl in its composition it possesses decided therapeutic advantages, and therefore all that is now prepared contains the benzoyl radicle.

It has been used more largely during the past year and its effects have been carefully studied, particularly in the hospital wards of Germany and France. As much as 5 grammes (about 75 grains) have been administered daily. Spiegelberg describes the results of twenty-two successive cases—ten of pure neuralgia with good results in eight, the other two being hysterical; three of hemicrania with one successful case, the remaining two being hysterical; three cases of rheumatic affections with benefit; no effect from two cases herpes zoster, one of tabes dorsalis, and one of gout; one case of bronchial asthma showed good results after six administrations of about 500 milligrammes (7½ grains) every two hours, not having responded previously to potassium iodide and chloral. Headache was noticed in one case, and in some others noises in the ears were found objectionable.

Very few reports have been made from this country as yet.

Antikol (75 per cent. acetanilid, 17.5 per cent. sodium bicarbonate, and 7.5 per cent. tartaric acid) still furnishes no reason whatever for its existence as such, except the very doubtful one claimed by some, of the need of a name for a known mixture to save time and thought in dispensing.

Antinervin (50 per cent. acetanilid, 25 per cent. salicylic acid, and 25 per cent. ammonium bromide), notwithstanding that further apparently favourable reports come from various quarters, has nothing at all to recommend it over its ingredients given separately and in proportions suited to each individual case.

Antipyrin (phenazone) has now become so well established, and its behaviour so well known to the medical profession, that it is rapidly passing beyond the scope of useful comment here. It still has its warm advocates and severe critics. Poisoning cases are still prominent, and promiscuous abuse by too general self-medication among the laity is somewhat on the increase. This bad practice cannot be too strongly condemned, and physicians themselves are largely to be blamed for indifferently lending their aid to establish such a habit.

Antiseptin has now apparently been pretty generally retired from use, as no advantage has been shown to exist for such a mixture of well known ingredients under this special title.

Antiseptol (cinchonine-iodo sulphate), although, no doubt, still used by many, has not been of sufficient merit as a substitute for iodoform to call forth reports during the past year.

Antispasmin is one of the newest sedatives and hypnotics, deriving its name originally from the excellent results reported in relieving cramp.

It is said to consist of one molecule of a combination of sodium with narceine and three molecules of sodium salicylate. It is a whitish, slightly hygroscopic powder, freely soluble in water, and containing 50 per cent. of *pure* narceine, thus apparently freeing the latter from many of its customary unfavourable features.

Unfortunately the late Prof. R. Demme, of Berne, Switzerland, did not live long enough to complete his study of this compound, as he was obtaining gratifying results. There is little or no danger in its use in doses of 7 to 100 milligrammes (about 1-10 to 1½ grains), and it is especially adapted to the treatment of children with spasmodic cough, scarlatina, affections of the larynx, and the like.

It is little known on this side of the Atlantic.

Apiol may still be considered in use by the gynaecologists, but few outside of the manufacturers give much attention to it.

Aristol (annidalin) has received comparatively little attention in print during the year in the way of clinical experience; but this is not because it has diminished in use, for there is abundant other evidence of its varied applications as a more or less effective substitute for iodoform in surgical dressings and ulcerations. It is now more frequently dusted on in the dry powder form, and analgesic effects have been noted. Further observations should now be made in this line, for one can readily appreciate the great benefit derived from these combined properties.

Arsenic was stated in the London *Practitioner*, some ten years ago, to render the taker insusceptible to vaccination; and from this statement Dr. C. F. Bryan, of England, was led to try the drug as a prophylactic in scarlet fever. In his address as president of the Leicester Medical Society, he went so far as to affirm as his belief that a local epidemic in their neighbourhood was checked in 1882, and mentioned that a year later, in a family in which one child had a severe attack, he put the other two on this treatment and they were not attacked, although they remained about the sick child until her death, three weeks after. In a second family, a seven-year-old boy alone was attacked, whereas four other of the children, from three to eleven years old, had no suspicion of the disease, nor did the mother suffer, but·she aborted while she was attending the sick child. His dose was about 0.1 cc. (2 minims) of solution of arsenite of potassium three times daily for the first week and twice daily afterwards. He also suggested, from his observations, that it might be of value in diphtheria and influenza.

Asaprol (B-napthol-a-mono-sulphonate of calcium), the new antiseptic alluded to last year, has had increasing use in France, but has not made much headway here, as far as definite reports go. It has been used in this country, however, during the year; but as far as is known, only one complete report has been made, and that was by Dr. Reynold W. Wilcox, of New York city, before the section on General Medicine of the New York Academy of Medicine, on May 16 last. His report deserves attention by all those who are interested in obtaining a good soluble antiseptic. He used it in his private practice in cases of epidemic influenza, in which it markedly relieved the pain, reduced the fever, produced no prostration or interference with the heart or respiration; in "certain cases of atonic dyspepsia, especially where fermentation alternates with acid eructation," he has "achieved brilliant results;" in "a case of old gastric ulcer, in which, after a period of a year's quiescence, there was recently a recrudescence of symptoms, the pain and dyspeptic symptoms were markedly improvéd," and so on with other cases of a varied nature, showing results of much interest.

Finally he draws the following conclusions:

"1. In chronic rheumatism it is apparently of not much value, except to relieve the pain of an acute exacerbation, but it is better than salophen or salicylate of soda for this purpose. This is only what we might expect, since we believe that chronic rheumatism is a disorder of nutrition.

"2. In gonorrhoeal rheumatism it is not of so much value as the syrup of hydriodic acid.

"3. In acute articular rheumatism its administration does not present the disadvantages of the salicylates, yet it is not so valuable; yet it is of far greater value than either the alkaline or other treatments that were formerly in vogue. So far as we are able to conclude from the cases under observation, the results obtained in this condition with salophen are superior to those obtained by any other so called treatment.

"4. In cases of epidemic influenza, the use of this remedy is to be recommended.

"5. In cases of atonic dyspepsia of the flatulent or acid variety, we may expect to obtain good results. While, on the whole, the results that we have obtained have not been as brilliant as we were led to expect from a careful study of the literature, yet we are of the opinion that in selected cases it is a remedy of value, and its use should be persisted in until its limitations are clearly determined, and the diseases which it may be expected to favourably influence are well known."

Dr. Cyrus J. Strong, of the resident staff of Bellevue hospital, New York city, lends his testimony to its efficiency by reporting cases under his own observation.

Aseptol (ortho-phenyl-sulphonic acid) has not fulfilled its promised mission of supplanting carbolic acid, and may now be considered on the retired list.

Atropine still continues to receive some attention aside from its unique position as a mydriatic. Dr. Lauder Brunton read a communication on its use in cholera, at a meeting of the Royal Medical and Chirurgical Society, on June 13, last. "In 1873 he had drawn attention to the close resemblance between the symptoms of cholera and those of muscarine poisoning. The action of muscarine was almost completely antagonised by atropine, so that the symptoms produced by the former poison were removed by subcutaneous injection of the latter. Dr. Brunton therefore came to the conclusion that good results might be hoped for in cases of cholera poisoning, by the subcutaneous injection of atropine; but the first opportunity he got of testing the supposition occurred a few months ago in the case of a patient who had come across from Hamburg. The father of this child died very shortly after admission into the hospital. The child was collapsed and appeared likely to die, but a subcutaneous injection of atropine revived her for a time. This was followed by a relapse, but another injection was administered with good results, and the child recovered. At no time, either in the child's case or her father's, did the stools present an appearance of rice water, but cholera bacilli were found by Dr. Klein in the intestine of the father. Dr. Brunton suggested that there were various forms of cholera, and that atropine would probably be most useful in cases where cholera appeared to have an action on the circulation, and less useful in those cases where the intestine was chiefly affected, because Dr. Pye-Smith and he did not find in their experiments secretion from the intestine to be arrested by atropine."[1]

Benzanilid (phenyl-benzanide) has been practically unnoticed during the past year. It evidently has not made a place for itself, as its only claim now appears to be that of a simple antipyretic, with nothing in its action to urge its employment rather than that of the almost numberless antipyretics at hand.

Benzol (benzene) is still found useful in the treatment of influenza.

Dr. W. Murrell, of England, has used it not only in several cases of influenza, but in over one hundred cases of chronic bronchitis and winter cough with success, especially in obstinate cases. He employs the formula,—

Pure benzol...............about	6 grammes	(1½ drachms).
Peppermint oil............ "	2	"	(½ ").
Olive oil......sufficient to make 62	"	(2 ounces).

The dose is from 10 to 30 drops on a lump of sugar every three or four hours.

Benzol is still found of use as a parasiticide. Dr. S. I. Snegürsky reports the successful treatment of eight cases of itch complicated with eczema, by inunctions of benzol (benzin), alone or mixed with equal parts of fat. He finds the pure article destroys the parasites best when used alone, but cures an eczema more rapidly when used in the form of an ointment. He directs brisk friction of the skin with a thick cloth until redness is produced, before the benzol itself is applied.

Benzonapthol (*B* napthol benzoate) has apparently shown its reputed superiority over betol (salinaphthol) to be well founded, and reports now come supporting Dr. Gilbert's and Mr. Dominici's conclusions, mentioned here last year. Although the clinical experiments of Dr. Franz Kuhn, of Geissen, Germany, during the past year have led him to conclude that it has no antifermentative action at all in the intestines, still his conclusions seem to be too sweeping. It has never been claimed by the most conservative that it will act beneficially in any but mild cases—best in mild chronic cases—and those where the treatment has been begun early, before the micro-organisms have multiplied to a great extent, or have shown great activity by having become firmly established in a position well suited to their livelihood by being abundantly surrounded with their pabulum and conditions favourable to their exceedingly rapid multiplication.

At the meeting of the Berlin Society of Physicians, on May 29 last, Professor Ewald exhibited two test tubes which he had prepared, each containing some of the same diarrhoeal dejection. To one tube was added a small quantity of benzonaphthol, and the other was left unprotected. The former showed only a trifling evidence of fermentation, while the latter was exceedingly active. This would seem to be pretty conclusive evidence, surely, of some favourable action, and further similar experiments will no doubt show later whether the above theory of excessive numbers, or activity of the micro-organisms alone, is the cause of Dr. Kuhn's unfavourable results.

Dr. Brück, of Buda-Pesth, Hungary, has obtained very beneficial effects in numerous affections of the alimentary tract in children. He finds the best results are obtained after persisting for four or five days. As a rule, the movements became practically odourless, and their character changed for the better. His adaptation of dose to the age of the child is as follows:

Under 6 months, about 200 to 500 milligrammes (3 to 7½ grains).
7 to 12   "   "   400 to 800   "   (6 to 12   "   ).
1 to 3 years   "   1   gramme   (15   "   ).
4 to 7   "   '   1.3   "   (20   "   ).
8 to 14   "   '   2.0   "   (30   "   ).

Benzosol (benzoyl guaiacol) continues to be of service in cases of incipient pulmonary tuberculosis, and, in fact, wherever creosote and guaiacol are applicable. There are poisoning cases on record; but such will always occur with powerful agents, and especially when we know little about their potency. One of the most recent of these unfortunate occurrences was after its administration for diabetes mellitus.

At a meeting of physicians, some months ago, in Prague, Austria, Dr. B. von Jaksch reported that the sugar had disappeared entirely from the urine, after administration of from 1 to nearly 3 grammes (about 15 to 45 grains) of this agent for eight days, in the case of a woman 56 years old, whose urine had 5.7 per cent. of sugar in it, but she died from toxic enteritis with alarming jaundice, which was credited to the use of the benzosol. However, Dr. Marian Piatkowski, of Cracow, Galicia, Austria-Hungary, recommends it as being very useful in the treatment of this trouble. He reports eight cases, showing that the amount of sugar is diminished, whether the case be a chronic one or has been treated previously by other means. In some of his cases the sugar disappeared entirely, and others only partly. The benzosol appeared to act better when a meat diet accompanied it than when a mixed diet was followed.

Betol (napthosalol or *B*-naphthyl salicylate) has no doubt met with increased use during the past two years, but nothing has been reported to show much superiority over its near relative Salol (phenyl salicylate). It continues to be one of the safe remedies in children's bowel complaints.

Bromamide, the new antipyretic of last year, has been very meagrely reported on during the year past, but apparently from no evident disappointment on the part of observers. Dr. Augustus Caillé, whose interesting results were given here a year ago, reports that owing to his failure to procure a sufficient quantity of the agent he has not been able to push his investigations during the year; but he proposes to make more extended trials in different hospitals just as soon as a supply of material is obtained.

Bromides continue to have, and apparently will always have, great prominence in therapeutics. Eulenburg now advocates Erlenmeyer's suggestion to administer them in combination with carbonic acid, and to give the ammonium, potassium, and sodium salts mixed together, as it is apparently considered an established fact that the aggregate dose of the mixed salts is far more active than an equal amount of any one of the salts, and in administering them with carbonic acid—the whole in solution—there is less risk of cumulative or bromism effects, aside from the far greater stability of the solution. He recommends an effervescing draught of a solution in water of the three bromides together with citric acid and sodium bicarbonate. As a rule, the dose for adults should rarely be less than 5 grammes (about 75 grains), and rarely over 10 grammes (about 2½ drachms), per day. Eulenberg would continue the treatment for two or three years after the last seizure. It ought not to be discontinued for slight bromism, as means should be taken to improve the general health in place of a discontinuance on that account. He admits there are cases where the bromides do not suit, but these are comparatively few.

M. Ch. Féré, M. D., of the Bicêtre asylum, firmly believes in the harmlessness and great benefit from large doses of the bromides in epilepsy. He recently reported his results in twenty cases, in which from 16 to 21 grammes (about 4½ to 5½ drachms) of bromide of potassium or strontium were administered per day with the following results: one only lost weight very markedly; nine did lose some weight, but of little importance; four remained stationary, and the remaining six increased in weight. Seven showed temporary improvement, two only no noticeable benefit, while eleven showed permanent improvement. He maintains that doses of 15 to 20 grammes (about 4 to 5 drachms) are harmless if watched, and show improvement where smaller doses have failed. The attention he advises during the course of treatment consists in frequent examination of the condition of the skin, and taking the weight in order to see that the patient is being properly nourished. He claims the strontium salt may be substituted for that of potassium with good results, and that the former is rapidly and completely eliminated by the kidneys. Though this does not occur as early after administration, there is less accumulation in the system than with the potassium salt.

Dr. G. Coronedi, of Florence, Italy, has also tried this strontium salt as an anti-emetic in general, and finds that in every case the vomiting would be checked more or less rapidly. The taste of the salt is so disagreeable that it is best taken in some portion of the food which will mask its taste as much as possible. Often, only one or two doses were required, amounting to about 2 or 3 grammes (30 to 46 grains) per day, taken with the meals.

Dr. John Dougall, of St. Mungo's college, Glasgow, Scotland, confirms these results by actual experience, and considers this salt worthy of trial. Finally, Dr. William Murrell, F. R. C. P., of London, delivered a lecture at the Westminster hospital recently, on "The Therapeutics of Bromide of Strontium," which will be of profit for those to read who are interested in trying this salt. An abstract will be found in *The Medical Week*, vol. 1, 1893, page 401.

The monobromide of camphor is recommended by Dr. Bourneville in epilepsy when complicated by vertigo. He reports the results of five cases in his experience of twenty years. He gave from about 600 milligrammes to 1.4 grammes (9 to 21 grains) per day, in 200 milligramme (3 grain) capsules. The daily dose is increased each week by 200 milligrammes (3 grains)—one capsule—until the 1.4 grammes (21 grains) is reached, when the administration is omitted entirely for one week, then continued in doses of 600 milligrammes (9 grains) per day.

Bromoform has had a very markedly increasing use during the past year, and has proved itself almost a specific in the treatment of pertussis, and of such decided potency that caution must be exercised in its administration.

Dr. F. W. Burton-Fanning, M. B., of Norwich, England,[1] emphasises its value, and states that it is not yet fully appreciated. It has given him far better results "than any of the other treatments usually recommended for whooping-cough." He calls attention to the fact that Stepp not long ago warmly advocated its use and reported one hundred cases treated without a single failure. Dr. Burton-Fanning now reports having treated some thirty cases for ten consecutive months. Their ages ranged from three months to eight years. He finds that the following formula gives a pleasant mixture, with the bromoform well suspended:

Bromoform...................... 1.0 cc. (16 minims).
Powd. Tragacanth Comp......... 80.0 cc. (1 fluid ounce).
Simple Syrup.................... 80.0 cc. (1 fluid ounce).
Water sufficient to make up to.... 240.0 cc. (8 fluid ounces).

(Powd. Tragacanth Comp. of the British Pharmacopoeia consists of one part each of Powd. Tragacanth, Powd. Acacia, and Powd. Starch, and three parts of Powd. Refined Sugar.)

He repeats the caution mentioned here last year, that if bromoform or its mixtures are not *colourless* they must be avoided, as decomposition has started. He cautions attendants to thoroughly shake the bottle before using, and to never give more than a week's supply at a time.

Among his "thirty cases, one death occurred in an infant whose whooping-cough was complicated by capillary bronchitis, its condition being desperate when the treatment was commenced, and only one dose of the medicine being retained." He considers that "the drug is of specific power against the main symptom of whooping-cough—the paroxysmal cough, on which depend the chief dangers of the disease. I cannot satisfy myself that the duration of the illness is materially shortened, the average length of the paroxysmal stage in my cases being thirty-one days. During this time, the patients were free from the characteristic cough and its attendant miseries, though these all returned at once, if the bromoform was discontinued within four weeks." Finally, he points out its value in diagnosis.

Dr. C. W. Dean, L. R. C. P., of Queen-street, Lancaster, England, lends his testimony as to its value in whooping-cough, and relates a case of poisoning.[2] He reports that in "each case the effect of the drug has been most marked, the paroxysmal cough being greatly reduced in violence, and the duration of the disease materially shortened. The form in which we have dispensed the drug is that advised by Dr. Burton-Fanning. My reason for writing this, however, is not so much to extol its

[1] London Practitioner, vol. 50, p. 100.
[2] London Lancet, vol. 1, 1893, p. 1062.

virtues as to point out the necessity for impressing on those in charge of patients that the directions on the bottle must be obeyed implicitly or the results may be the reverse of those desired." The relation of the case of poisoning here follows.

Others in this country speak well of its use and urge all to try it.

Dr. Angrisani, an Italian physician, has obtained gratifying results from the administration of bromoform in cases of cerebral excitement in lunatic asylums. He starts with 0.9 cc. (15 minims) a day, and the dose is gradually increased by 0.3 cc. (5 minims) every second day until over 2 cc. (33 minims) are given in twenty-four hours. In all cases it rapidly produced a decidedly sedative effect, and it was not necessary to continue the drug longer than two weeks.

It would thus seem that bromoform may be given advantageously where bromides are called for, but in which they fail to give benefit. Mr. Thomas Latham, of 1309 Third avenue, New York city, calls attention to the fact that he has previously recommended a much better formula than that of the late Professor Bedford (mentioned here last year), and he takes exception to the latter " as being altogether too pungent to be administered to young children. Something is needed to mask the fiery taste of the bromoform, which certainly is not diminished by adding alcohol, compound tincture of cardamon and glycerin, each of which of itself has a burning taste." His improved formula is,—

> Bromoform............................ 0.9 cc. (15 minims).
> Mucilage of Acacia.................... 45.0 cc. (1½ fluid ounces).
> Syrup of Tolu........................ 15.0 cc. (½ ").

Bromo-Phenol. Ortho-bromo-phenol is stated as being a dull violet-coloured liquid with an odour resembling phenol, and soluble in water, alcohol, ether, and alkalies. It is a derivative of carbolic acid, in which the atoms of hydrogen are replaced by bromine. This compound, together with chloro-phenol, has very recently been used successfully in the treatment of erysipelas. Dr. I. Tchourilow reports excellent results in twenty cases treated at the Alexander hospital, St. Petersburg, when employed in the form of a 1 to 2 per cent. ointment of either agent incorporated with soft paraffin. The ointment was rubbed on the affected part pretty thoroughly twice a day. It produced no irritation whatever, but simply a moderate amount of tingling of short duration.

Remedial action apparently is rapid at times after only two applications, and much more effective than phenol itself. Better results were also attained with bromo-phenol than with phenol simply, in cases of anthrax and tetanus experimentally produced in rabbits.

Butyl-Chloral Hydrate (often called croton-chloral, but now proved not to have any relation to crotonic acid) is not by any means a new preparation, but owing to its slightly increasing use, according to reports, it may be well to recall its composition here. It is produced by passing dry chlorine gas though aldehyde (the oxidation product of alcohol just preceding the formation of acetic acid) at a low temperature. Then, after distillation has produced the colourless oily butyl-chloral in a pure state, the requisite amount of water is added to produce the hydrate.

Its most frequent application has been as an analgesic, but Dr. George Harley, F. R. C. P., of England, finds it applicable in diabetes. In his interesting "Remarks on Diabetes and Gout in their Relationship to Liver Disease, with Hints Regarding their Scientific Treatment,"[1] he says,—"As an example of the good effect it sometimes exercises on a case of diabetes, I may mention that, given in conjunction with opium, ... the quantity of urine was not only reduced from 1¼ gallons to 3¼ pints in the short space of twenty-three days, but at the same time its specific gravity fell from 1.036 to 1.030—a result so favourable that I fancy the reader will ask for a formula, in the hope that he may by its aid be equally successful. To give a single formula that will answer in every case of a Protean disease like diabetes is, however, out of the question; so all I will do is to give the one employed in the case just alluded to. It is the following: ℞ croton-chloral, gr. ¼; opii, gr. j; ext. aloes Barb., gr. 1-6; ext. gentianae, gr. iss. M.; one pill to be taken three times a day."

Dr. Harley uses Barbadoes aloes, and it is doubtful whether this is intentional. In this country it has generally been agreed that this variety of the aloes is entirely too drastic for human beings, and therefore it has been resigned mostly to use on domestic animals. It was not officinal in the last United States Pharmacopoeia of 1880, but is now introduced into the new edition of 1890 to satisfy the veterinary branch of the profession. Dr. Harley may have good reason for the use of this variety in his prescription, but if not, the purified aloes, U. S. P., made from the aloe socotrina, would be preferable.

Butyl-Hypnal is the name given to the new compound formed by the combination of butyl-chloral and antipyrin. Bernin describes it as being in the form of light colourless crystals, with an odour like butyl-chloral, and a bitter taste. It is only soluble in thirty parts of cold, but very soluble in hot, water. Most of the other prominent solvents dissolve it quite readily.

It is analogous to hypnal, but its therapeutic effects are unknown as yet.

Camphoid. Mr. William Martindale has stated since the last comment was made here on this article, that although this camphoid makes a pretty satisfactory film in his experience, still it has never come quite up to his expectations for general use. He, however, desires to correct the published statements made in several journals, including the one made here last year, where his formula was made to read "dilute alcohol" as one of the ingredients, whereas it should have been *absolute alcohol.* The correct formula then should read,—

Pyroxylon (soluble gun cotton).....................	1 part.
Camphor...	20 parts.
Absolute alcohol...................................	20 "

[1] Brit. Med. Jour., vol. 1, 1898, p. 1097.

Mr. Thomas Latham, of 1309 Third avenue, New York city, has made the statement that a similar compound had been patented both in Great Britain and in this country, about a quarter of a century ago, and that a firm here is now manufacturing a " Celluloid Japan Varnish " of very much this composition.

Chloralamid (chloral formamide) is growing rapidly in usefulness. Reports are now numerous, both in the old country and in this, of its beneficial effect in suitable cases. More must not be expected of it than is claimed by conservative observers.

Nothing has been reported to at all alter, but rather to strengthen, the statements made for it here two years ago and confirmed last year, and this is, that its best effects are produced in cases of idiopathic insomnia, cases where the insomnia is not due to either pain or excitement. Although it may succeed in some cases in overcoming slight pains, it cannot be classed as an anodyne. It induces a natural and refreshing sleep, and, as a rule, is not followed by headache on waking the following morning. A sense of well-being is the result of the rest it affords.

During the past year Dr. John Gordon, of Aberdeen, Scotland, has continued the useful study he began in 1891, on the gastric disturbances produced by several hypnotics,—of determining by experiment how they behaved in the economy during pancreatic digestion. He simply attempted to study "one side of the question of pancreatic digestion, namely, that by which this digestive fluid acts on starch, converting it into maltose and dextrin," and he found "chloralamid had no retarding power . . . ." This, of course, is an important point in its favour.

Chloralose is the name given to the newest hypnotic, discovered and introduced by two French physiologists, Mons. M. Hauriot and Dr. Charles Richet. They presented the results of their careful physiological experiments to the Paris Academy of Sciences at the meeting on January 9th last. They apparently went about producing this hypnotic in a very systematic way, to attain very definite properties, the details of which are not called for here, but it will suffice to state simply that it is prepared by the combination of equal parts of anhydrous chloral and dry glucose, heating for one hour at 100°C. (212°F.), adding a small proportion of water and then boiling with ether. Further minor details are followed, resulting in two different products—one inactive, comparatively insoluble pearl-like lamellar crystals and called parachloralose, and the other (about 3 per cent. of the total product) active, comparatively soluble needle-like crystals having superior hypnotic properties and bitter taste and called anhydro-gluco-chloral or chloralose.

A series of careful experiments was tried on animals, and developed the interesting, novel, and contradictory property of acting as a hypnotic and at the same time augmenting the excitability of the spinal cord. They not only tried this agent clinically on patients, but on themselves, and found that its action was not due to the chloral set free in the alimentary canal, as 20 milligrammes (3 grains) cannot yield more than 10 milligrammes (1½ grains) of chloral, and hypnotic effects begin to manifest themselves at the point where 20 milligrammes (3 grains) for every kilogramme (about 2 1-5 pounds) of weight are reached, but such a dose of chloral is ineffective. No toxic effects were noticed, although poison-ous results have been obtained by others. It is well given, especially to children, in milk, but may be administered in capsules—the range of dose being from 200 to 800 milligrammes (about 3 to 12 grains),—although somewhat too large for hysterical patients. MM. L. Landouzy, Paul Marie, R. Montard-Martin, and Charles Ségard, all reported on its supe-riority over chloral and morphine in insomnia in general. No bad after-effects were noticed, but in the insomnia due to alcoholism morphine was preferable. Chloralose appears, however, to be of little use in sub-duing the pains of neuralgia and gout.

Dr. Féré claims that the above doses are too small to produce good results. He would give as high as 1.5 grammes (22 grains) at least, and has already given very much more.

Favourable reports also come from Drs. D'Amore, Lombroso, and Marro, of Italy, and the general conclusion drawn is that it is the least harmful of all the hypnotics in ordinary use, and is surely worthy of further trial.

Sufficient time has not yet elapsed to expect reports of its use in this country.

Chlorobrom is the name given to the mixture,—

Chloralamid..................	1.95 grammes (30 grains);
Potassium bromide...............	1.95 " (");
Water, to make..................	30 cc. (1 fluid ounce)

and flavoured with extract of licorice, to taste.

This is not a new agent by any means, but from reports on the other side of the water it is having an increasing use in the treatment of sea-sickness and insomnia. This compound name simply serves to make a specialty of it, and caters to the too common tendency of the day. Far better write plainly what one is using, as the prevailing inclination is to drift into empiricism by lending oneself to this demoralising propensity. Dr. Hayden Brown, of Hauteville, on the Island of Guernsey, England, quotes in relation to this very compound the wise saying of some great master of his student days: "Learn to make your own prescriptions, and never write two alike." Although to invariably follow the strict letter of this maxim would cause some unnecessary labour, at times, to a hurried practitioner, still the principle is a good one and may well be instilled into the rising generation, as surely the drift is away from this idea about as fast as could ever have been dreamed of.

Dr. John Keay, F. R. C. P., of Edinburgh, Scotland, has obtained some excellent results with this mixture as a hypnotic in melancholia and allied mental conditions, but as a general sedative in various forms of maniacal excitement, in the excitement of general paralysis and of epi-lepsy, he has not obtained sufficiently encouraging results to warrant perseverance.[1]

[1] London Lancet, vol. 1, 1893, p. 587.

Chloro-Phenol (tri-chlor-phenol) is a derivative of carbolic acid in which the atoms of hydrogen are replaced by chlorine, occurring in the form of colourless needle-like crystals with an odour of phenol more strongly marked than its allied product, bromo-phenol. .

With the exception of the slight difference in composition, the remarks made previously upon its ally, bromo-phenol, strictly apply here, as the solubility is the same and its use has been carried along side by side with it.

Cinchona is merely mentioned here to call attention to the fact that the term yellow cinchona of previous editions of the United States Pharmacopoeia has been dropped by the new one of 1890, substituting the term cinchona simply as meaning the calisaya officinalis, and hybrids of these.

The marked improvement, however, in this new edition is shown in the detailed assay process now given for determination of the serviceable alkaloids, by which the quality of bark brought into this market should be improved, for all have it in their power now to demand a rich bark if they will simply take a little trouble to determine exactly what they are buying.

·*Cocaine Phenate* (phenol-cocaine) or so called cocaine carbolate, is apparently rapidly gaining favour outside of the profession of dentistry. Since Dr. von Oefele published his results over two years ago, much good has been accomplished with it, and in Europe it has had an increasing use internally.

Since it was alluded to here two years ago, it has become better known in this country, and favourable reports are now forthcoming. As a fair summary of the good reports of our own practitioners, the results of Dr. C. A. Veasey, of Philadelphia, Penn., may be taken as general. These results appear in a paper on "Experiments with Cocaine Phenate as a Local Anaesthetic."[1] Though his cases there reported were only seven in number, the drug was used in many others of his ophthalomological practice with equally good results. He draws the following justifiable conclusions:

"1. In cocaine phenate we have a drug that can be successfully used without producing systemic effects, in those cases in which there exists an idiosyncrasy to the local use of cocaine hydrochlorate.

"2. As good an anaesthetic effect can be produced with cocaine phenate as with cocaine hydrochlorate, but stronger solutions are required to produce the same degree of anaesthesia.

"3. The anaesthesia does not come on so quickly with the phenate as with the hydrochlorate, but lasts fully as long, if not longer, than the anaesthesia from the latter.

"4. In some cases, though there be no physiologic contra-indication to the use of the hydrochlorate, the phenate is to be preferred on account of its antiseptic properties."

Dr. D. B. Kyle also speaks enthusiastically of it in his nasal and laryngeal practice. He has good records of 150 cases. In none of these were there signs of poisoning, nor were there any after-effects developed. He used solutions varying from 2 to 10 per cent. and an average of seven minutes was required to obtain the anaesthesia.

In Germany local applications in cases of diphtheria have met with good results.

Cocaine hydrochlorate has been added to the new United States Pharmacopoeia of 1890, and a series of good tests are given for determination of purity, although a few are rather hypercritical, as the substances attempted to be excluded thereby have not as yet been proved to be deleterious, nor has it been shown that anything has been gained by their exclusion, whereas those very substances may have therapeutic advantages to be recognised on further study.

Convallaria Majalis (lily of the valley) has now been added to the new United States Pharmacopoeia of 1890, and the committee of revision has adopted the rhizome and roots as the parts of the plant to be employed. In some quarters the flowers are insisted upon, but abundant evidence is now at hand to prove that the new officinal requirement gives the better therapeutic results.

Coryl is the short name given to a mixture of ethyl and methyl chlorides.

It is reported from Antwerp, Belgium, that it has proved of much value as an anaesthetic in minor and dental surgery. It is stated as being liquid at 0° C. (32° F.), whereas methyl chloride boils at 27° C. (—80.5° F.) and ethyl chloride (hydrochloric ether) at about 10° C. (50° F.), thus not producing the degree of cold that the former does, but giving better results than the latter. This is the claimed advantage of the mixture. It has made little record for itself as yet.

Creolin, the brownish-black, syrupy liquid known for some years past as liquor antisepticus, and previously stated to be a coal-tar product, has now been reported by Dr. F. Raschig, through an advertising circular, as nothing more than a mixture of about one part of resin soap with two parts of crude carbolic acid of about 20 per cent. strength, although the manufacturers have claimed that it is free from carbolic acid. It now becomes a question of veracity between the two claimants, but surely its disinfecting action for the past two years at least reminds one very strongly of carbolic acid.

The comment made here two years ago holds good to-day, and the relative efficiency reported here last year of lysol, creolin, and carbolic acid is still maintained by the results reported during the year past.

It is still used to a considerable extent, and no doubt will continue to be used as long as such desirable results are reported and it is kept prominent before the profession by judicious advertising; but it is difficult to understand why either lysol or carbolic acid is not chosen in preference to a substance whose composition is kept secret and whose clinical results in relative efficiency are undoubtedly somewhere midway between the other two agents.

During recent epidemics of cholera in the various countries of the Old World, some good results are reported from its use, but its disagreeable taste is against it, and Dr. W. Nicati, of Marseilles, France, suggests the masking of this taste to some degree by an intimate mixture of it with the clay called kaolin (hydrated aluminum silicate), thus presenting the agent in the form of granules. The practitioners of the island of Java report giving as much as 5 grammes (77 grains) during the first few hours of an attack, and this mode of administration by the above mixture, Dr. Nicati claims, renders the agent bearable to the patient.

Creosotal is the short name adopted recently for a so called creosote carbonate—a German article patented some three years ago. It has been revived by Dr. J. Brissonet, professor at the School of Medicine, Tours, France, who has prepared it, apparently, by a process of his own, independent of the patent. The process is too technical to repeat here, but it will suffice to state that it is a combination of carbonic acid with beechwood creosote. It is an amber-coloured, oily liquid at ordinary temperatures, becoming more fluid upon warming. It is neutral in reaction, odourless, with the faint sweetish taste of creosote, insoluble in water, dilute alcohol, and glycerin, but very readily soluble in alcohol, ether, chloroform, and benzine. It is an inviting substitute for creosote in the treatment of tuberculosis as, although it is about one tenth weaker in efficiency, it produces no irritation, and is well borne by the stomach and apparently does not take away the appetite—the great drawback to creo-. sote. It is given in doses as high as 20 grammes (about 5¼ drachms) daily. It splits up in the digestive track into its component parts, and creosote is found in the urine shortly after.

We know practically nothing of it in this country as yet, but should it be obtainable here, it surely should be tried wherever creosote may be expected to produce beneficial results but has failed.

Creosote is now thus spelled according to the most approved etymology of the new United States Pharmacopoeia of 1890. The previous spelling has been creasote.

A great mass of conflicting testimony has been presented during the past year in the way of results obtained from the use of this agent in the treatment of tuberculosis and tubercular affections. The profession on both continents has expressed itself pretty freely, but without enabling one to draw any definite conclusions as to the efficiency of the remedy. There appear to be careful observers and men of prominence arrayed on each side. However, good hygienic surroundings and proper attention to the diet are prominently gaining ground as the most effective treatment, whereas as many as 25 per cent. of the cases treated in some localities lose their appetite after taking creosote, and thus give poor results, on account of faulty dietary requirements to maintain what little strength may be left to the patient.

In the treatment of pertussis, tubercular pleurisy, tubercular manifestations of the larynx, and tubercular affections generally, aside from tuberculosis pulmonalis, better results are more frequently reported, but apparently there is anything but a favourable outlook for these distressing sufferers in the use of creosote.

Cresols are still used as disinfectants, but their disadvantages are such

23

that they apparently will continue to retard their usefulness. The so called "cresol-saponate" is now recommended by German practitioners, but it at once calls forth criticism in introducing an ingredient which renders its use still more disadvantageous. It is prepared by mixing crude carbolic acid with melted soft soap in equal proportions, to form finally a homogeneous mass which is soluble in water. Thus is increased the objectionable quality inherent in all the compounds of cresol, of rendering slippery the surgeon's hands and instruments.

Dermatol (bismuth subgallate) continues to receive attention in surgery, but less is heard of its previously boasted claims as an efficient substitute for iodoform. It is now being studied more on its own account, and found to be of service in many cases where iodoform was formerly used and complained of on account of its objectionable odour. Nothing like a complete substitution for the latter is, however, now claimed among conservative surgeons.

The reported success last year of Davidsohn in the treatment of otorrhoea is now followed by the report of 80 cases of acute and chronic purulent otitis, externa and media, by Dr. S. A. Chaniavsky. He washed the ear out with a 3 per cent. solution of boric acid, dried it with absorbent cotton, and applied a piece of the cotton covered with the dermatol powder well into the meatus. In all his cases the pus was dried up and rendered innocuous, but especially in the cases accompanied with acute otorrhoea were the results most satisfactory. Within three days, in otitis externa, the discharge markedly decreased, and a permanent result was reached sooner than with iodoform, tannic acid, calomel, boric acid, bismuth subnitrate, and the other usual agents. In otitis media, with perforation of the drum, however, the progress was somewhat slower.

Good results are reported by Matthews, H. Isaac, and others in the treatment of ulcers generally, and of burns, erosions, excoriations, and fissures, and although a local dermatitis may at times have been set up by the application, ultimate successful results were obtained, and without apparent loss of time by such a local complication.

Dr. G. Wicke, of Heinrichsthal, Prussia, reports marked analgesic effects when applied to parts rendered painful from the cauterising effect of silver nitrate. He noticed, by accident, in an exuberant ulcer of the arm, so treated for the purpose of reducing the profuse exudation, that great relief from the intense pain was remarked by the patient. This result led Dr. Wicke to try the same application on other cases, and with like good results.

The good effects previously reported in the treatment of diarrhoea are still further confirmed by the report of a case of severe diarrhoea, by Dr. John W. Martin, at the Sheffield Medico-Chirurgical Society of England. The case was that of a woman, age thirty-one, whose movements were involuntary and her condition alarming. The various astringents had failed, when about 2 gramme (30 grain) doses of dermatol were given every four hours, causing the diarrhoea to cease in twenty-four hours, and in two days the customary daily evacuations were again established.

Recently the great democratic principle recognised in this country of freedom has been rudely violated in the case of this article by the success of a foreign firm in obtaining a patent on even the process of manufacturing bismuth subgallate as well as on the trade name of Dermatol, and lends additional force to a recently expressed conclusion that the patent office had run mad, and now-a-days acts entirely without system, principle, justice, or the ordinary care and protection of home interests and the people at large. Is it not about time to call a halt and institute a course of discipline among the shiftless officials at Washington?

Diaphtherin (oxy-chin-aseptol), the new antiseptic and astringent of last year, has found a place of no little efficiency in the treatment of affections of the nose and throat. Dr. Albert Spengler reports very satisfactory results with a 1 per cent. solution in two persistent cases of empyema of the antrum of Highmore in which alumnol was unsuccessful. He found diaphtherin applicable in most affections of the nasal cavities, and especially in ozaena. Disagreeable effects were not noticed, and he concludes that after more experience diaphtherin will rank high in rhinological practice.

Dr. Rohrer, of Zürich, Switzerland, reports its beneficial use in fifty-seven cases of affections of the nose and ear, and predicts a future for it in this branch of practice, if not in general surgery.

Dr. Brandt, of Berlin, Germany, reports marked advantages in its use about the mouth and teeth. Its odour is so slight, and its freedom from irritation so pronounced, that patients are not at all averse to its use, giving great relief from foetid discharges of all degrees.

Diuretin (sodio-theobromine salicylate) still holds a place among the useful agents for producing diuresis in certain cases. The profession is now getting to acknowledge that it is not a specific, but has its decided beneficial effects in selected cases. Several foreign observers have made specially close study of this agent during the past year; and whereas they generally agree on some of the main points of its action, they differ somewhat on others.

Dr. R. del Valle y Aldabalde reports his unsuccessful clinical results in ascites due to hepatic cirrhosis, causing diarrhoea and anorexia. In cases due to renal origin it did cause a moderate diuresis; but in one case, pains in the head and loins, vomiting and diarrhoea were so pronounced that it could be continued no longer. In cases of cardiac dropsy, especially where calomel and digitalis had failed, however, reported results are very gratifying; and if the use of this agent had eventually to be limited to this one class of cases, it would thereby establish its claim to a place in the list of well recognised therapeutic agents.

Whether this agent owes its diuretic effect to action upon the renal epithelium or upon the circulation, still seems to be a mooted question among prominent observers.

Emphasis is still laid on the adaptability to the treatment of adults rather than children.

Genersich reports his experience in sixteen cases of dropsy due to various causes, but gives the following guarded summary:

"1. It increases the flow of urine in some cases of cardiac dropsy, but is uncertain in oedematous conditions due to other causes.

"2. It acts when digitalis, strophanthus, and calomel fail.

"3. It is not sufficiently reliable as a substitute for calomel.

"4. It only affects the heart slightly.

"5. Its disadvantages are in the price, unpleasant taste, derangement of the digestion, and in the headache, pyrexia, ecchymoses, and other dangerous symptoms occasionally produced, which require caution."

Massalongo and Silvestri report their results from quite an extended and careful series of experiments,—in cases of aortic incompetence, with oedema of the legs and diminished flow of urine; in oedema and ascites from mitral incompetence; in cases of combined valvular lesions and atheromatous condition of the arteries; in some forms of nephritis, and finally, in pleurisy with effusion and cirrhosis of the liver with ascites. In all these cases careful estimations were made of the amount of urine daily, of the pulse-rate and respiration, and in some cases, of the temperature. These observers confirm the above statement in regard to its best effects being noticed in renal, and especially cardiac, dropsy, and little effect in hepatic dropsy. They find that it never exhibited unpleasant consequences nor cumulative action when given in ordinary doses. However, in the earlier stages of cardiac trouble, it is much inferior to digitalis, strophanthus, convallaria, and like drugs. It is apparently only when oedema and anasarca are present that its effects are most pronounced. It acts best in mitral disease, next in aortic trouble, and least when diffuse atheroma of the peripheral vessels complicates these other conditions. The very best effects are obtained in acute nephritis and somewhat less marked in chronic cases.

Dr. Pawinski, of Warsaw, Russia, reports with great care eleven cases out of a series which include those of mitral insufficiency, accompanied with stenosis, aortic insufficiency, fatty degeneration, myocarditis, and parenchymatous nephritis. His observations were made with caffein and digitalis as well as the theobromine salt. His conclusions are, in general, the ones given above, with the addition of his directions in regard to the use of caffein and digitalis. He advises the use of these latter agents when diuretin has been given for about a week without a noticeable diuretic effect being produced, and in the choice between diuretin and caffein establishes the routine practice of giving caffein in adynamic cases, and diuretin in those showing evident irritability.

From this country, the report of Dr. James B. Herrick, of Chicago, Ill., is one of the most careful and complete. He read a paper on "Diuretin" before the Pathological Section of the Chicago Academy of Sciences, on February 9, last, in which he gave a detailed account of four cases of his own and four of Dr. A. E. Halstead. His conclusions are, in general, those before noted, but he sees fit to preface them with the following expressions: "While the exact pathological conditions that call for its exhibition cannot as yet be specifically stated, and disappointing failures will therefore attend its misapplied use in many cases where too much will be hoped for, yet a study and comparison of the results of the various observers who have employed this remedy in the past three years yield facts from which certain conclusions can be drawn." The article is well worth reading.[1]

Dulcin (para-phenetol carbamide), the synthetic sweetening compound discovered as far back as 1883 by Berlinerblau, and its practical use abandoned on account of its costliness, has now been brought forward again, as the process has been so cheapened that hopes are entertained of its practical application.

Its chemical composition and mode of preparation are too complex to be of interest here, but it may be stated simply that it is closely related to urea.

Professor DuBois-Raymond has experimented, through Kossel, upon its physiological action upon rabbits and dogs, and finds that it is comparatively free from objections. It apparently did not interfere with the appetite, or alter any of the healthy conditions of the animals. The dose was 2 grammes (31 grains) daily, which is found to be equivalent to 400 grammes (about 13 ounces) of cane sugar. This was continued for months without noticeable injury.

Dr. Ewald was then tempted to try it on human subjects, with very gratifying results.

Thoms and Stahl recently brought the subject up again, in confirmation of the above results, at a meeting of the Pharmaceutical society of Berlin, Germany, where they described the compound and its action more minutely than before. It forms colourless needle-like crystals, soluble in 800 parts of cold, 50 parts of boiling, water, and in 25 parts of 90 per cent. alcohol. It apparently takes very large doses—greatly above any ordinarily required quantity—to produce undesirable effects and inconvenience; but even then such effects are only temporary.

Its great insolubility is, no doubt, its chief disadvantage, but hopes are entertained of overcoming this defect. It is apparently more agreeable to patients than the other sweetening substitutes for sugar, and the diabetic, to whom it should be a desideratum, does not show the same dislike developed after a time when using levulose, saccharin, and the like.

Epidermin—the artificial skin for wounds and scratches—spoken of here last year, has been heard little of during the past year, and this may be due to the fact that it has not supplied the supposed want previously expressed for it. Surely nothing has been shown in its favour as a substitute for the efficient United States Pharmacopoeia collodium film.

Ether may be only alluded to again here in alphabetical order for the purpose of calling attention to the wise step taken by the recent revisers of the United States Pharmacopoeia in ceasing to recognise, in the new edition of 1890, the two different qualities previously known as ether (of about 74 per cent. of ethyl oxide) and stronger ether (of about 94 per cent. of ethyl oxide), for surely the stronger *only* should be used for anaesthesia, and there is little doubt that as a general solvent it is much superior—thus showing little practical use for any other than the higher grade article.

The standard for the now only officinal article, "Ether," has been raised to about 90 per cent. of ethyl oxide, and good tests have been furnished for verifying any product which may be offered, thus making it inexcusable for any physician or pharmacist to use an inferior quality.

Ethyl Bromide (hydrobromic ether) has increased in use during the past year, and many are the appeals, from those meeting with success, for its more extended use. All are very wisely particular to mention the selected class of cases on which to use it, and even give a list of the class of cases to be avoided, and thus warrant its legitimate use. As previously stated here, there is very little doubt but that the results when they are successful are surely very satisfactory, and many have continued its use now to their one, two, and four hundred cases without any unfortunate occurrence, but by far the largest and longest users are the continental practitioners, who are proverbially reckless in the way of taking the life of their patients in their own hands, and undoubtedly comparatively few of the unfortunate cases are heard of. They, in general, treat all patients as cases, and if they can make a correct diagnosis and have the always longed for post-mortem examination to verify it, they are perfectly happy and exult over their results, apparently oblivious many times to the fact that they lost the patient; but as it was a good case, and everything came out as desired—except death—they are thoroughly satisfied. This practice does not do at all for this country, where humanitarian ideas are uppermost and the desire to prolong the life of the patient is the starting-point for treatment—the correct diagnosis then being an additional achievement to be sought for, and, of course, the means by which correct treatment was attained and posterity benefited.

All who are most enthusiastic in its behalf miss the main point against its use, in not considering its inherent property of instability. There has been no one yet who has settled the question of the minimum amount of decomposition which may be accepted as safe. There are so many extraneous conditions which promote decomposition, that we do not know whether it is not practically going on all the time, and as it is so easy for a hurried or careless attendant to use a defective article, it makes the risks constantly present. With the other anaesthetics there are premonitory or accompanying signs in administration which simply annoy the patient and serve to warn the administrator, but rarely produce dangerous results except from gross carelessness.

Ethyl Chloride (monochlor-ethane) has been used with great success during the past year, both in the old country and this, but a word of warning comes from Dr. H. Radcliffe Crocker, of Harley street, London, W., England, in using the bulbs of Dr. Bengué, of Paris, as he found the inhalation of the vapour not altogether free from danger. He writes,— "Having occasion to scarify a small patch of lupus erythematosus on the nose of a young lady, I thought it a favourable opportunity to try a chloride of ethyl tube. The spot was frozen well enough, but the patient turned pale, slightly livid, and stopped breathing, looking very like a person under nitrous oxide gas. As I took away the ethyl at once, she recovered in a few seconds, but I should certainly not use it again to any part of the face where it was possible that the vapour could be inhaled. Chloride of methyl applied by means of a tampon is far safer and easier, but care must be taken not to over-freeze the skin, or a dermatitis may be set up."

Dentists are the most general users, but it has met with much favour in minor surgery. Drs. S. Ehrmann, of Vienna, E. Gaus, of Carlsbad, Austria, and others, have been very successful in operating on buboes, small tumors, and the nodules of lupus, also in very obstinate cases of neuralgia, lumbago, migraine and scrotal pruritus, with not more than one, two, or three applications. In three patients, Dr. Gaus believes he has cut short an approaching attack of gout, and looks forward to further success in this line. The methyl chloride produces a far greater degree of cold, and therefore the ethyl chloride is preferable in many cases. Dr. Gaus advises holding the bulb at a distance of 30 centimetres (about 12 inches) from the part, others state 15 to 20 centimetres (6 to 8 inches), as the degree of cold is then about sufficient for the necessary anaesthesia, and too low a temperature is not reached, thus avoiding any chance of inflammation, sloughing, or gangrene intervening.

Dr. Largeau reported recently at the French surgical congress the clinical results of an operation of double ovariotomy on a patient with heart disease, in which no general anaesthetic was used, but ethyl chloride as a local anaesthetic only. He previously operated in like manner on an adherent ovarian cyst and in an abdominal hysterectomy—all being successful and "perfectly justifiable and practicable when a patient is subject to cardiac or renal disease."

In our own country, Dr. C. L. Gibson, of New York city, gives results of his experience in some twenty-five cases of minor surgery, in an interesting article.[1] His cases were "chiefly cellulitis of the fingers, abscesses of the jaw, buboes, sinuses, boils, and carbuncles.

"Most of the cases were relieved by a single incision, and in such the anaesthesia was most satisfactory. Where more extensive procedures were demanded—where deeper structures were divided—for efficient curetting, etc., the agent was seldom efficient.

"Its action in certain cases, however, was ideal. In felons, for instance, the single rapid incision was generally effected absolutely without pain. Every one that is called upon to incise felons knows how excruciating the pain is. The patient winces at the slightest touch; the introduction of cocaine solutions subcutaneously is almost a cruelty, as intense pain results, both from the needle-pricks and from increase of the tension in the indurated tissues. Moreover, the cocaine often proves powerless to overcome the aggravated conditions.

"No attempts to use ethyl chloride were made in procedures requiring more than a few seconds' time, nor where careful dissection was needed, as the agent so changes the character of the tissues. It can, however,

[1] N. Y. Med. Jour., vol. 58, p. 351.

be employed to great advantage in removing small sections of tumors for microscopical examinations.

"It will occasionally be found useful to combine the action of the new agent with that of cocaine.

"The ethyl chloride will be found of considerable value in dermatological practice, especially for thorough scarification and application of the actual cautery."

Ethylene Bromide, the new sedative spoken of here last year as being introduced to avoid the undesirable symptoms often noticed from the effects of the alkaline bromides, has not been heard of much more during this year than last, except to record the undesirable results of the 87 per cent. of bromine in its composition so easily set free. It may be of service to repeat here the caution of last year, that care should be taken in prescribing not to confuse this with ethyl bromide (hydrobromic ether), as the difference in name is very slight when either pronounced or written. Fatal cases continue to be reported from this confusion of title.

Eucalypteol is a new antiseptic obtained by M. Anthoine by the treatment of eucalyptus oil with hydrochloride acid, producing chemically eucalyptene bichloride in colourless, scaly crystals with an odour resembling camphor, and almost without taste, as it is so insoluble that a taste does not develop until held on the tongue for some time, when a slight bitterness is manifested.

Dr. Lafage, of Neuilly, France, has undertaken some therapeutic examinations and finds that it is far superior to eucalyptus oil, eucalyptol, and other preparations of the eucalyptus leaves, being non-toxic and much more reliable in composition and uniformity of action. It is practically insoluble in water and in glycerin, but it is readily soluble in ether, chloroform, and alcohol, although it is decomposed by the latter.

Its antiseptic property is so pronounced that an exceedingly small quantity only is necessary to check the ordinary putrefactive changes, but it apparently does not retard the digestive ferments.

When given to animals, it is eliminated by the lungs, in the faeces, and in the urine. One hundred and fifty clinical cases were treated with gratifying results. In cases of phthisis it relieved the coughing and other distressing symptoms; in diarrhoea it cured some severe cases, and in typhoid fever it has worked well. The dose for adults in capsules is from 1 to 1.5 grammes (about 15 to 24 grains) in twenty-four hours, divided so as to come between meals; for children, from 250 to 750 milligrammes (about 4 to 12 grains) according to age.

It is still too new in this country to have been reported on.

Eucalyptol is not new by any means, but it is now destined to become more prominent from the fact that the new United States Pharmacopoeia of 1890 recognises it for the first time. It may be well then to recall here at this time, that it is the principal ingredient in eucalyptus oil, being that fraction which distils off between 175° C. (347° F.) and 177.2° C. (351° F.) from the volatile oil obtained from the fresh leaves of eucalyptus globulus and other species, and manufactured most largely in

Australia and neighbouring colonies. The oil is made there in as large quantities as 300 kilogrammes (over 600 pounds) a week.

As the old original recommendation for using the oil in intermittent fever has been pretty much abandoned, so the use of eucalyptol has been little applied in that direction. Eucalyptol being less irritating to the alimentary tract, it is practically substituted for the oil in all cases where the latter has been applicable; as a most active antiseptic in remarkably small quantities; as a general rubefacient; as an effective agent in lung and bronchial affections introduced by the spray and inhalation, and internally and locally with very good results in cases of diphtheria.

Eugénol Acetamide, the new local anaesthetic of last year, has been little heard of during the past year as far as published reports go, but this does not necessarily imply that it has not found a practical application, for the dentists were the ones to whom it was chiefly interesting, and their literature and writings do not reach as general a circulation among medical men as the other branches of surgical science; therefore their results may readily escape the general professional reader.

Euphorin (phenyl-urethane), the anilin product used as an antipyretic, has met with increasing usefulness during the past year, in a great variety of conditions, due to its non-toxic effects and rapidity of action. Dr. G. Cao has given us a summary of results up to the present time, by collecting together the observations made by Professor Giacosa, F. Adler, and R. Lépine, and Drs. L. Sansoni, L. M. Bossi, C. Curtis, G. Peroni, R. Bovero, Oliva Belfanti, Stillé, and himself, in the following recommendations for its use:

"1. It is a more efficient antifermentative and parasiticide than carbolic acid.

"2. It is more rapid and stronger in action as an antithermic than antipyrin.

"3. It is an energetic neuralgesic and analgesic in habitual hemicrania, in supraorbital neuralgia, sciatica and intercostal neuralgia, in syphilitic pains of the limbs and orchitis.

"4. It is superior in some cases to the salicylates in acute and chronic rheumatism.

"5. It is an efficient substitute for iodoform in major and minor surgical operations, being less poisonous and fully as antiseptic.

"6. It gives successful results as a disinfectant and cicatrising agent in bed sores, scalds, and other wounds.

"7. It acts well as an anodyne and healing agent in various forms of herpes.

"8. It is efficient in aphthous stomatitis.

"9. It is far preferable to iodoform, iodol, aristol, salicylic acid, resorcin, or chloral in the treatment of venereal ulcers.

"10. It is especially useful in tinea, trichophyton, favus, and various other parasitic skin affections."

Europhen (iso-butyl-ortho-cresol iodide)—the iodoform substitute, containing 27.6 per cent. of iodine which no doubt is the most effective element—aside from its use in minor surgery, still continues to be found invaluable in all venereal affections and particularly in soft chancres. Professor O. Petersen, of St. Petersburg, Russia, Eichoff of Elberfeld, Prussia, Sichel, Lowenstein, Kopp, and others in Germany, as well as elsewhere, are very decided in their marked preference for this agent over iodoform. Kopp reports his gratifying results in nineteen typical cases of soft chancre in which he used powdered boric acid mixed with the europhen for economical reasons, though when given alone, noticed no unpleasant effects. Healing occurred in all in from four to ten days. Nine cases of buboes were also thus treated, with healing in from fourteen to thirty-two days.

Dr. Julius Goldschmidt, being impressed with the noticeable fact that the tubercular form of leprosy manifests itself locally for years without spreading or becoming general, varied the routine practice generally adopted, of treating the affection locally only and not in conjunction with internal treatment, by using it in both ways simultaneously in five cases, for periods of eight to fifteen months. The results surprised him, as a marked diminution in the swelling was noticeable in four weeks' time, and in fifteen months the eyelids were normal and the affected spots entirely cured. The most marked case of improvement was one that had been under observation for many years with progressive tendencies, and Dr. Goldschmidt remarks that during his twenty-five years of experience with these cases no such result had ever before been reached.

Christmann recently reports his practical results in the treatment of tuberculosis. He employed europhen by three different methods,—by directly applying the agent to the culture of the tubercle bacillus; in an open test-tube suspended in a hermetically sealed glass containing the culture; as a concentrated emulsion in olive oil. Guinea-pigs alone were experimented on. His plan of operation was very carefully considered, and carried out with much pains. Owing to some negative results obtained when he used the emulsion, he noticed that the evolution of iodine was necessary to kill the bacillus, as it did not take place in these cases except when water was added to the emulsion, causing the decomposition.

His comparisons with iodoform used in the same way as the above, showed him that it was slower than europhen in its bacillicide effect, except when the iodoform was used in an emulsion, which result he attributes to some special action of that agent.

Dr. Eichoff emphasises the caution to be taken of not using europhen in conjunction with or after the use of corrosive sublimate, as mercuric iodide is formed, causing annoying irritation.

Finally, the great advantages of this agent over iodoform still continue to be prominent, and these are a lack of detrimental effects from any absorption that may take place, in the much more agreeable saffron or cresol-like odour, and the far better adherent property to the moist surfaces to which it may be applied. The chief requirement to be emphasised for its effective working is the necessity of applying it to secreting or otherwise moist surfaces. Its best effects by far are obtained in its external use only.

Exalgin (methyl-acetanilid), the analgesic, still shows its potency, and need for care in administration, by having cases of poisoning recorded against it. This, however, should not be a reason for anything like an abandonment of its use, but simply to treat it like all other well known potent agents, with care, and to prohibit its popular use (abuse). Too much emphasis cannot be laid on this latter point.

This agent finds its evident field of usefulness in neuralgic pains of a functional nature.

Dr. Edward G. Younger, M. R. C. P., of Mecklenburgh square, London, W. C., England, gives his interesting results of nine cases showing its marked analgesic effects. He found that one or two doses of the drug almost invariably procured immediate relief. He was unexpectedly successful in greatly relieving one epileptic patient, which now leads him to make further observations in the treatment of epilepsy, and report later. He states that he has never seen any bad results from its use, but he has never prescribed more than 130 milligrammes (2 grains) every four hours. In general he found 65 milligramme (1 grain) doses, repeated several times a day, to be sufficient for his results.[1]

Formalin is a patented article recently experimented with and brought forward by German investigators, particularly by Dr. J. Stahl, as an efficient general disinfectant. It is simply a 40 per cent. aqueous solution of formaldehyde. It is reported as being non-toxic and specially recommended for sterilising purposes. For sterilising bandages, for instance, a cartridge-like bolus of kaolin, impregnated with formalin, and known by the name of formalith, is introduced into a suitable tight receptacle with the bandages or dressings, whereby a permanent sterilising effect is accomplished, due to the spontaneous emission from the porous mass.

Formalin has a tannic-like effect upon the skin, producing a leathery condition, which passes on to the condition of a localised necrosis, without suppuration, leaving the surface with the appearance of a newly healed superficial wound.

This interesting property can readily be turned to good use by the surgeon, and unless there are objections to this agent not now apparent, we shall surely hear more from it.

Clinical reports have not been recorded as yet in this country.

Formanilid is a complex compound which has been known for some years, but has been recently brought into prominence by several physicians at a meeting of the Royal Medical Society at Buda-Pesth, Austria. It is a chemical compound of anilin and formic acid, and bears the same relation to anilin that acetanilid does. It occurs in elongated, flat, four-sided prismatic crystals, quite soluble in water, but much more so in alcohol. Its taste and action upon the tongue resemble cocaine, and although the biting or tingling sensation noticed at first is possibly more intense, and the numbness following much more persistent than cocaine, still the local anaesthesia is somewhat inferior.

[1] London Lancet, vol. 1, 1898, p. 785.

Drs. A. Bökal, Kossa, Meisels, J. Preisach, F. Tanszk, and M. Neumann all related at that society meeting their therapeutic results as showing a combination of desirable properties. It apparently combines the properties of an analgesic, anaesthetic, antipyretic, antineuralgic, and haemostatic. No such dangerous symptoms seem to follow its use as at times occur with acetanilid. Doses of from 250 to 500 milligrammes (about 4 to 8 grains) in twenty-four hours gave excellent results in neuralgic headaches, lumbago, and allied affections. The fever in rheumatism and typhoid was markedly abated almost immediately (in some cases as quickly as five minutes), and relief lasted from three to fourteen hours. A 3 per cent. solution, injected subcutaneously or directly into the urethra, produced decided anaesthesia and paresis of the bladder. Its haemostatic effect was well proved by dusting it on bleeding wounds, where the effect was immediate. Cyanosis at times was produced, but anything like collapse was not seen. In affections of the air passages pain is almost immediately relieved by insufflations (with equal quantity of starch), or gargles, and local operations are then undertaken with satisfaction. Dr. Meisels opened two large abscesses without pain by the subcutaneous injection of only 1 cc. (16 minims) of a 3 per cent. solution.

Verification of these satisfactory results from other sources will be awaited with interest.

Gallacetophenon (tri-oxy-aceto-phenon), a derivative of pyrogallol and commercially known as a dye-stuff under the name of "alizarine—yellow C," alluded to here last year as being of some promise to the dermatologists, according to the favourable reports then presented, has made little progress during the past year. Practically nothing has been written in its favour, and it may be almost considered as retired.

Even Dr. Hermann Goldenberg, of New York city, who last year pointed out its advantages, now states that he has not used it very freely of late, as he finds other agents give better results and are not so dear. He calls attention to the fact that the price is against its more general use. He cites one of his cases of psoriasis, in which a 10 per cent. ointment produced quite an intense irritation, which disappeared in a few days on discontinuing its use. His results began to be varied and lacked uniformity, and he immediately suspected adulteration. A number of his professional friends tried it as well, and although they obtained some good results they had their failures with it. His impression is that if pure it will be found to work as well, if not better, than pyrogallic acid (pyrogallol) in psoriasis, but not as well as chrysarobin. It undoubtedly has a great advantage over some of the other agents in not staining the linen.

Gallanol is the name given the compound formed by the action of the gallic acid in tannin when presented under certain conditions to anilin. It is described as occurring in colourless crystals, with a bitter taste, soluble in alcohol, chloroform, and boiling water, but sparingly in cold water, and possessing marked astringent properties. It is chiefly used externally in skin affections. It surpasses chrysophanic acid and pyrogallol as being far less irritating, and without poisonous properties.

At the last annual meeting of the French Society of Dermatology and Syphilography, Drs. Cazeneuve and Etienne Rollet, of Lyons, described its marked advantages in psoriasis and eczema when applied in the form of a 10 per cent. solution or ointment (which may be increased, if called for, to 25 per cent.), or suspended in chloroform. It rapidly allays itching, and thus gives much relief to the patient from the beginning of the treatment.

Gallobromol (di-bromo-gallic acid) is a recently introduced neurotic prepared by Dr. Grimaux by substituting for two hydrogen atoms in gallic acid two atoms of bromine. It occurs in colourless, needle-like crystals, freely soluble in alcohol, ether, and boiling water, but much less so in cold water.

Dr. R. Lépine, of Lyons, France, has employed it for more than two months in his practice with gratifying results, giving as large a dose as 15.5 grammes (4 drachms) without any inconvenience being noticed. It apparently does not produce the depressing effects noticed with potassium bromide, but in his few cases of epilepsy, although the attacks were arrested, his impression is that it is inferior to the latter. In chronic chorea, however, it showed decided improvement.

It is too early to predict in any way for this agent, especially as practically nothing is known of it as yet outside of France.

Glycozone is the compound produced when one volume of chemically pure glycerine is acted upon by fifteen volumes of ozone under certain conditions of temperature and pressure. It rapidly absorbs moisture, and therefore must be kept tightly sealed. It is largely used in intestinal affections, as reported by Dr. Cyrus Edson, of New York city, in gastric ulcer, catarrh of the stomach, and dyspepsia. It acts more slowly, but fully as efficiently, as hydrogen dioxide. It has met with many favourable results.

Gold Chloride, both alone and in conjunction with sodium in the "cure" of inebriety, has been rapidly on the decrease, due to an increasing number of exposures of its fallacies. The promoters of this system attempted to establish branches in England and elsewhere, but received little sympathy from either the medical profession or the laity.

The "institutes" still exist in scattered places in this country, but they are losing ground very rapidly, and one of the chief means of hastening this rational end is by such exposures as furnished in a paper written by Dr. B. D. Evans, of Morris Plains, N. J., on "Keeleyism and Keeley Methods, with Some Statistics,"[1] in which he closes as follows: "After careful examination into 'Keeleyism,' actuated by a desire to learn something of its merits and statistics from a source other than Keeley organs, paid Keeley lecturers, and newspapers subsidised by Keeley gold, I have been led to the following conclusions:

"1. That it is, as Dr. Keeley says, 'A system'—a system of charlatanism of large proportions.

"2. That the system is carried into effect in a purely mechanical way, and that the 'institute physicians' are little less than local commercial agents, knowing nothing of the 'cure' which they handle and administer.

"3. That the statistics published by the 'Keeley people' cannot be relied upon in the slightest, inasmuch as secrecy is their motto, whenever and wherever it pays in gold.

"4. That their so called 'cure' contains dangerous and poisonous drugs, calculated, by the indiscriminate manner in which they are administered, to produce insanity and other serious psychoses.

"5. That the remedy has an intoxicating and exhilarating effect, and that many of the finely written testimonials are written while the patients are under this influence.

"6. That secrecy is maintained purely for the purpose of enhancing the commercial value of the commodity, and not because a valuable discovery has been made—speculating upon the fact that with the masses *omne ignotum pro magnifico* holds good.

"7. That many ministers and prominent gentlemen who have spoken publicly in behalf of Keeley remedies and methods were actuated to do so by a desire to welcome any agency that would alleviate the evils of alcoholism, and not by any knowledge of the real merits of the 'cure' or the nature of the results that follow its use.

"8. That any physician who allows himself to indorse the Keeley cure, either in words or by advising a patient to take it, not only commits an act unprofessional, but forfeits his right to the respect of his professional brethren."

The whole article is interesting and worth reading.

Guaiacol, the beech-wood tar product containing a maximum of 90 per cent. of creosote, still claims marked attention. The literature of the year is quite voluminous, and much diversity of opinion is expressed. Naturally the largest number of reports are made on its use in pulmonary tuberculosis, but it has been used in an increasing number of cases of typhoid fever. The carbonate of guaiacol, as stated before, is the salt rightly chosen to give the best results. Dr. F. Hölscher, of Mülheim, Prussia, calls especial attention to this treatment. He gave it in 1 gramme (15.4 grains) doses night and morning in sixty cases, all of which recovered. He does not believe the carbonate is an antipyretic, but simply an antiseptic in these cases, the fever being reduced indirectly only. Other observers have verified these results, and urge further trials.

As a true antipyretic, however, Dr. S. Sciolla, of Genoa, Italy, claims very striking results when he applies it externally to the skin of the extremities, back, and abdomen. It is free from caustic action, is rapidly absorbed, and reduction of temperature is marked. He tried creosote in similar cases, but had to abandon it on account of its caustic effects.

Many continental practitioners have followed Dr. Sciolla, and have abundantly verified his results.

The almost universal testimony for the year from internal and hypodermic administration in pulmonary tuberculosis is very disappointing, and the most conservative observers finally conclude that little or no benefit is derived in advanced cases, and nothing very encouraging can be looked for in incipient or early cases. They reluctantly fall back, for the most part, on the conclusion that good hygienic environment, wholesome food, attention to person and habits, and desirable climate are of far more value than any medicaments yet discovered.

Some of the disappointing results may have arisen from the poor quality of much of the commercial guaiacol offered, as the recent investigations of Profs. A. Béhal, E. Choay, Liebreich, and Dr. H. Thoms have shown that it rarely contains more than 50 per cent. of the pure compound. It has been customary to describe it as a liquid, but it has now been produced synthetically as a colourless solid compound, which crystallises readily in the prismatic form. It has a sweet and decidedly astringent taste, but does not attack the mucous membrane.

Its use will no doubt continue until some other agent is forthcoming which will give even a glimmer of hope for better results.

Haemogallol and *Haemol*, the oxydised products of the haemoglobin of the blood alluded to here last year, have received further attention from Drs. A. Grünfeld and Lange on the continent, and from Drs. Wm. Henry Porter and Paton in this country. They have continued to obtain gratifying results in many cases of anaemia which had resisted other treatment. The fact of these agents lacking any disagreeable taste, and of their harmlessness to the teeth, at once gives them prominence in practice.

Aside from the above, there are no other reports of note except that the price has been reduced somewhat, which will be an incentive to give them further trial.

Helenin, the white acicular crystals obtained from the root of inula helenium (elecampane root), alluded to last year as being used in the treatment of tuberculosis and as an antiseptic, has been practically unheard of during the past year, possibly on account of its continued costliness. It may have been used successfully in the localities mentioned last year, but no reports have been made of it.

Hydrastinin, the oxidation product of hydrastin (one of the alkaloids found in the root of hydrastis Canadensis) and alluded to here last year as being reported on as a haemostatic in gynaecological practice, has been little heard of during the year, possibly on account of its recognised uncertainty. of action.

Hydrogen Dioxide (peroxide of hydrogen) has steadily advanced in usefulness during the past year. A larger number of physicians now recognise its marked advantages, where they hesitated to make use of it before. The comment made here last year holds good to-day, but with more emphasis, however, as the results there stated have been still further verified.

Dr. Cyrus Edson, of New York city, has recently urged a more universal use of it in the treatment of contagious diseases, as previously recommended by Dr. Elmer Lee, of Chicago, Ill. This is not a new application, but considerable experience has now been attained, and therefore Drs. Lee and Edson rightly urge more attention to it.

The new United States Pharmacopoeia of 1890 has wisely introduced a 10 volume or 3 per cent. solution, with a detailed process for preparing it, under the head of Aqua Hydrogenii Dioxidi.

Hypnal (mono-chloral-antipyrin) has not been reported upon during the past or previous year to any marked extent (the last comment made here was in 1891). Whether this is because of its universally accepted usefulness, or, on the other hand, due to its abandonment as a hypnotic, is not apparent.

Dr. Filehne, however, continues to find it of sufficient importance to retain it, although it is not uniformly favourable in its action. He points out that its hypnotic action is not due to the chloral alone, for the proportion of chloral present (about 45 per cent.) is just as active in this combination, where the effective dose is about that of chloral alone; and not only much better results are at times obtained, but much less prostration is produced. Its tastelessness, ready solubility of 1 : 10 in water, and rapid effects, give it attractive advantages. It will, however, sometimes fail. Dr. Filehne reports, out of 124 observations on patients, no action was noticed in 27, and slight effect in 20. In the minor forms of excitement in the insane, in the early stages of delirium tremens, and in chorea good results were obtained. Simple insomnia appears to yield to its action, and sleeplessness caused by pain is often overcome.

Ichthyol (ammonium ichthyol-sulphonate) has received marked attention during the past year, particularly from the Germans, and the reports of successes have been very numerous, although not uniformly so.

The gynaecologists have probably been the largest users of it, next to the dermatologists. The reports on its use in endometritis have been conflicting. Dr. N. P. Mariantchik used it in 19 cases with much disappointment, whereas E. Curatolo obtained excellent results. This is not the only instance, by any means, of opposite conclusions, and the explanation for these opposing views is still to be made.

Jadassohn, with others, reports much success in treating gonorrhoea in both men and women. Thirty-seven cases of female patients gave excellent results with a solution of from 1 to under 10 per cent. He applied it both to the cervix and endometrium with great benefit. The best results were obtained in the early acute stage. Freudenberg recommends it in the form of suppositories in prostitis. Out of his 30 to 40 cases— mostly subacute or chronic—during the past two years, only two failed to obtain relief. Two or three suppositories were used daily, and any irritation noticed was avoided at the time of the next application by reducing the proportion of ichthyol.

The marked success obtained by Dr. H. W. Freund, of Strasburg, Germany, with this agent in the treatment of fissured nipples, led Dr. A. von der Willigen, of Rotterdam, Holland, to employ it in fissure of the anus. One female patient, who had tried all the forms of treatment except the surgical one, was reported cured in one week by painting the part with pure ichthyol; another patient only required ten days to restore him to the normal condition, while a third healed up in two weeks, after receiving no relief from a surgical operation. There were no relapses in any of his cases.

Dr. L. Herz, of Pilsen, Austria, reports good results in most inflammations of the throat, in which he used a 2 or 3 per cent. solution in the form of a gargle. The so called follicular tonsilitis, however, was the only affection which did not respond favourably. Cases of very marked inflammation, in which the tonsils and soft palate were so swollen that the mouth could scarcely be opened, were relieved in twenty-four hours by the pain disappearing and the swelling subsiding.

The two great disadvantages of this agent, its disagreeable odour and tendency to soil the linen, are still persistent and without remedy.

Iodoform has had its usual varied uses during the past year, and apparently has lost little ground in professional estimation. Its suggested use in tuberculous joints, especially the knee, has met with some good results in the hands of a few, but others think it dangerous to pack a mass of such toxic material into a cavity of that kind, and even when there they maintain that it does not show uniformly beneficial results. The dentists also are not now united on their previous practice of packing a tooth cavity with it. Its injection, however, in goitre, in the form of a solution of one part to seven each of ether and olive oil, as Kapper has done, has been followed by gratifying results; and, again, the introduction into the peritonaeal cavity in abdominal operations by dusting the powder on the surrounding tissues, as Frederick Treves, of London, England, has done, gives a fresh impetus to that field of application.

Sir Joseph Lister has recently been instrumental in calling attention to the antiseptic property of this agent. This property has not been acknowledged heretofore, but, on the contrary, has been refuted. Now Sir Joseph Lister, Behring, and others call attention to this advanced theory of its action, that its purpose is to destroy, by chemical changes set up, the products of the bacterial action, rather than, as heretofore claimed, to destroy the bacteria themselves.

Many have reported on the decided irritation set up when iodoform is applied locally to raw surfaces, and thus have been driven to the use of some of its rivals.

Its extremely disagreeable, penetrating, and persistent odour is still against it, and deodourisers continue to be recommended from every quarter. It will not be necessary to repeat the various expedients to mask its odour mentioned here on a previous occasion, but they are all being resorted to in suitable cases. Still two others may be mentioned—the addition of ¼ per cent. of carbolic acid and 1 per cent. of essence of peppermint; and Dr. E. Cavazzani's recommendation of the following powder, without disagreeable odour, as a dressing:

Iodoform..55 parts.
Salicylic acid..20   "
Bismuth subnitrate..............................20   "
Camphor 5   '
24

It should be constantly borne in mind that the characteristic odour of iodoform is inherent to it, and we might just as rationally expect to remove the sweetening property of sugar and still expect to retain the usefulness of that necessary article, as to remove the odour of iodoform and retain its identity. We can adopt all manner of expedients to mask this objectionable quality, but we may rest assured that the iodoform is still there as long as we hold its combining elements together, and as soon as we split these up we no longer have this useful agent.

Iodol (tetra-iodo-pyrrol) is still a very close rival to iodoform, and is used in almost every place where the latter is applicable. As its identity has not been referred to here before, it may be well to just allude to its production and form at this time for the sake of ready reference. It is obtained by treating pyrrol (a coal-tar product) with a solution of iodine in iodide of potassium, usually known as iodo-iodide of potassium. As it is seen in the market it occurs in very long minute delicate prismatic crystals of a yellowish tint, sparingly soluble in water, but readily in alcohol. When even slight decomposition is going on, the crystals take on a brown tinge, due to the free iodine. Its odour is very slight (practically odourless when pure), and, unlike iodoform, possesses no toxic properties when undecomposed. It contains about 89 per cent. of iodine.

Dr. H. Chatellier, of Paris, France, has recently recommended it in the treatment of eczema of the ear. In moist confluent eczema of the pinna, extending within the auditory canal, he insufflates the powder into the canal and surrounding parts after thoroughly cleansing the surfaces. In dry external eczema he applies it in the form of a lanolin ointment. The inflammation disappears completely, as a rule, in two weeks, but irrigation is kept up for a short time afterwards to complete the treatment.

To remedy the at times dangerous defect in this agent, of gradually liberating its constituent iodine after long keeping, E. Konteschweller mixed caffein with iodol in stoichiometrical proportions in a solution of alcohol to produce a permanent light gray crystalline combination, without odour or taste and practically insoluble in most solvents—containing 25.4 per cent. of caffein and 74.6 per cent. of iodol.

Clinical reports on this caffein-iodol have not made their appearance as yet, either in this country or abroad.

Iodopyrin (iod-antipyrin), the chemical combination óf iodine and antipyrin recommended as an efficient antipyretic, and alluded to here last year in a very unpromising way, has not taken any prominence whatever in its line of supposed usefulness, and its theoretical applicability in certain cases has not been fulfilled.

Iodozone, the name given to a solution of iodine in ozone, and alluded to here last year, has not made its appearance in any of the current medical literature of the year, and may be considered as being of so little value as to pass unnoticed by the majority.

Izal is the trade name given by an enterprising English firm to a very recent "non-poisonous" antiseptic, and consisting of an emulsion containing 30 per cent. of a new oil produced by a patent process employed in the manufacture of a special form of coke. It appears to belong to a series analogous to the terpenes, with characteristics between those of the paraffins and the benzins. No phenol proper can be detected in the emulsion. The London *Lancet*[1] thus reports on a sample submitted to it for examination: "Its antiseptic power appears to be considerably greater than that of carbolic acid, whilst it is practically non-poisonous. At any rate, it exerts nothing like the poisonous action of carbolic acid, and, according to Dr. Klein, is without injurious effect upon the economy, unless taken in unreasonably large quantities. Dr. Klein has conducted a large number of experiments with this substance, with the view of ascertaining its value as a disinfectant and germicide. Some twenty-five species of microbes were experimented with, and the results were highly satisfactory, and such as to compare most favourably with similar experiments with well known members of the disinfectant group. The preparation submitted to us for examination consisted of a milky emulsion, doubtless produced from the oil referred to, which was markedly alkaline to test paper, and from which a mixture of oily bodies separated on the addition of acid and on warming. The oils so separated occupied about half the original volume of the liquid." . . . . . It "mixes well with water, has an agreeable smell, leaves no objectionable greasy stain, and is entitled to rank amongst the foremost disinfectant and antiseptic preparations which are at the present time available."

Mr. Wm. Bruce Clarke, F. R. C. S., of Harley street, London, W., England, gives an interesting account of his experience with it in the treatment of wounds.[2] His conclusions are as follows: "From a consideration of Dr. Klein's experimental researches in connection with the substance, and from my own practical experience of it, I have no hesitation in saying that the antiseptic in question seems likely to prove more efficacious practically than any at present known. It will be obvious to any one who peruses critically the account of the cases in which I have employed it, that in many of the instances referred to it was put to a very severe test, and that by its aid some excellent results were obtained. At the same time, it is equally clear that its behaviour under all circumstances must be submitted to the test of a more lengthy experience before one can be in a position to predict that exact place which it is destined to take amongst the antiseptic fluids of the future. One thing, however, is certain, viz., that the surgeon will rejoice to hear that at last an antiseptic has been found which is easy to use, does not irritate his own hands or his patient's skin, and is at the same time by far the most powerful with which he is yet acquainted."

It has not yet made its appearance in this country.

Jambul (jamun), the seeds and bark of the Eugenia Jambolana, has still a very varied history of successes and failures in the treatment of diabetes.

Dr. Vix now comes forward with his report of successes in the use of preparations of the bark. He describes two severe cases out of twelve,

---

[1] Vol. 2, 1898, page 86.
[2] London Lancet, vol. 2, 1898, page 18.

in which 7 per cent. and 8 per cent. of glucose were excreted without marked polyuria, in which he brought the urine back to normal, and kept it there for two years, when the patient died from other causes. He emphasises the need of general treatment in conjunction with the use of this agent, and feels confident that jambul is of the greatest value, as its action may always be relied on, and with no unpleasant symptoms appearing, as far as his cases are concerned. He advises it to be given with or after meals, in water or wine sweetened with a small quantity of saccharin.

Dr. V. E. Lawrence, of Halstead, Kansas, has met with favourable results after abandoning all the usual remedies.[1]

Kresin is the trade name given to a very recent antiseptic and disinfectant brought out by German chemists. It is described as being a simple mixture of 25 per cent. of cresol and 25 per cent. of cres-oxyl acetate in water, of a brown colour, and retaining the odour of the cresol in it. It is readily diluted with water in all proportions, making a clear solution. Some of its claims to attention are that it is relatively less poisonous, causes less irritation, and is efficient in smaller quantities than carbolic acid.

Little has been heard of it as yet, except through the manufacturers and their agents.

Losophan (tri-iodo-meta-cresol) is a new antiseptic produced by the action of iodine upon *m*-oxytolic acid, according to a complex reaction of little moment here. It is described as occurring in colourless needle-like crystals, containing about 80 per cent. of iodine. When dissolved in as weak an alcohol as 50 per cent. it readily decomposes, but in a 75 per cent. alcohol it remains practically permanent.

It appeals especially to the dermatologists. Dr. Edmund Saalfeld, of Berlin, Germany, gives his experience with it, as being of considerable value in animal and vegetable parasitic affections of the skin. Out of 16 cases of tinea tonsurans of the face and body, 13 were cured, and the remaining 3 much improved. Out of 3 cases affecting the scalp, 1 was cured and the other 2 much improved. In all these cases he used a 1 to 2 per cent. alcoholic solution. In cases of pityriasis versicolor he used petrolatum ointment of the same strength with success. In cases of pediculi capitis and pubis a 1 per cent. solution was found to be most serviceable. The ordinary treatment for scabies proved more efficacious than with this agent. In some cases of prurigo, chronic eczema with infiltration, sycosis vulgaris, acne vulgaris, and rosacea it was found to be efficient. In cases of psoriasis and primary syphilitic affections it gave no satisfaction. In acute inflammatory conditions of the skin it causes annoying irritation, and therefore is contra-indicated.

More extended trials are necessary before establishing its general usefulness.

Lysol has had an extended use during the past year. Nothing astonishing, however, can be reported in its favour, but it has evidently come to stay.

[1] Medical News, vol. 62, page 46.

The conclusions of Cadéac and Guinard, mentioned here last year, may be taken as conservative for the present time as well:

"It is superior as a microbicide to carbolic acid, creolin, cresyl, and other analogous coal-tar products.

"It has not, however, any advantages over the antiseptics of established reputation.

"It is only really efficacious when used in solutions which may be irritating or caustic.

"Although not destined to play a great part in surgery, it may often be useful in the prophylaxis and arrest of epidemics.

"It is likely to be particularly serviceable in the disinfection of premises, privies, ships, and stables.

"It is readily soluble, reasonably active, and very cheap."

Methacetin (para-oxy-methyl-acetanilid) has been of little prominence since last alluded to here a year ago. It was announced then by its promoters with great confidence that it would supersede its analogue phenacetin, but little evidence is now present that anything has been accomplished in that direction. It may die a natural death.

Menthol (peppermint camphor) has now been introduced into the new United States Pharmacopoeia of 1890, as an agent of sufficient value to merit the increased attention it will receive.

In milder facial neuralgias and rheumatic pains the relief continues to be quite evident, although at times it does not last long. This was an early criticism, alluded to here two years ago, and still continues to be noticed.

It seems to be of marked value in most all cases of pruritus, from whatever cause.

Dr. James McNaught, M. R. C. S., of Waterfoot, near Manchester, England, has met with considerable success in injecting guaiacol and menthol within the larynx for the treatment of foetid conditions of the sputa.

Dr. A. L. Benedict has introduced the vapour of menthol into the stomach through a tube, by means of an aspirator, directly against the mucous membrane of that organ, in cases of atony or catarrh. His results were gratifying.

Dr. R. Blondell again recalls his observations of its marked antiemetic property. He has seen nausea and gastric spasm stopped by the action of menthol at such a point that ipecac even loses its power of producing emesis.

Dr. Moriz Weil has confirmed the results of many well known observers before him, in successfully using this agent to check persistent vomiting after all the usual remedies had failed. He employed either Gottschalk's formula (menthol 1 part, alcohol 20 parts, distilled water 150 parts), or Weiss's formula (menthol 1 part, alcohol 20 parts, syrup 30 parts), making a better solution than the former, or finally his own (10 drops of a 20 per cent. solution in olive oil dropped on powdered sugar). His dose averaged 65 milligrammes (1 grain).

Methyl salicylate (synthetic oil of wintergreen) is mentioned here simply to call attention to the fact that it has now been introduced into the new United States Pharmacopoeia of 1890.

Methylene blue (tetra-methyl-thionine chloride), the anilin derivative, is still in dispute as to its efficiency in the affections for which it has been recommended. Much conflicting testimony is on record from the discussion which has taken place in and out of medical societies during the year past, leaving the matter still in doubt in the minds of conservative observers.

First, in the treatment of malaria, Neumann relates three cases treated with this agent with fair success, but he is not assured that he has reached the proper dose as yet. He has found that about 300 to 450 milligrammes (5 to 7 grains) per day for eight or nine successive days gives satisfactory results.

During a discussion in the Berlin Medical Society, on January 25 last, Prof. Senator stated that in his experience both methylene blue and quinine fail in patients who bring back malarial fever when returning from Africa. Dr. Kohlstock, however, maintained that this fever was a marsh fever, entirely distinct from malarial fever. Dr. Strassman then further made the statement that he had given this agent to puerperal women without the least benefit. He called especial attention to its disadvantage of colouring everything blue that it came in contact with. The amnionic fluid was so coloured, and even the urine of the child remained blue for at least four days after birth. These were not necessarily contra-indications, but simply decided disadvantages, and unless its superiority over other agents was definitely manifested these would militate against it.

At the next meeting of the same society, on February 1, Dr. Paul Guttmann called attention to the fact, that so many had reported failures with this agent that he would suggest the probability of impurity in the article used. He could not explain otherwise how its action varied so in different types of malaria. He insisted that its administration should be continued for at least four weeks, in capsules of about 100 milligrammes (1½ grains) each, five times a day. In confirmation of the successful use by many observers now on record, he cited the experience of Prof. S. Parenski and Dr. S. Blatteis, of Cracow, Austrian Galicia, whose 35 cases of malarial fever, with 33 recoveries, stand as proof. These observers administered the agent sometimes by the mouth in the powder form, and at other times in solution hypodermically by means of a Pravaz syringe.

Dr. Moncorvo also has met with success in the use of this agent in this affection, and calls attention to its special adaptation to children in being tasteless, and therefore easier to give them than quinine.

Dr. Ferreira, of Rio Janeiro, Brazil, has likewise met with great success in the same way. He treated 40 children affected with malaria, and concludes as follows:

"1. It is especially satisfactory in cases which have resisted other methods of treatment.

"2. It is useful both in the intermittent and remittent varieties when not very severe.

"3. It does not produce the vomiting, diarrhoea, nor headache, often occurring with quinine.

"4. It rapidly causes diminution in the size of the liver and spleen, and appears to have a distinct action on the micro-organisms of malaria and its products.

"5. It causes a definite reduction of temperature, but not so marked as with antipyrin.

"6. It may be safely administered to very young children, and should be continued for some days after the disappearance of all manifestations of the malarial poison.

"7. It should be more largely used in this class of cases than is the custom at present."

Dr. A. Kasem-Beck reports his favourable results in 30 cases of malarial fever, but only used this agent either when quinine disagreed with the patient or other remedies failed. He also treated 14 cases of diphtheria with a watery solution of 1 to 9 with marked success, which he attributed to both the local and general effects. Three to four milligrammes (1-20 to 1-16 of a grain) of pilocarpin were given to assist in the separation of the membranes. All his cases progressed to recovery.

In this country, Dr. A. Rose, of New York city, has met with success in its use in diphtheria, after losing cases by other treatment. Even in "simple non-diphtheric ulceration of the throat, patients would, after one or two applications of the solution, express themselves with great delight as being cured." He concludes by adding that, for theoretical reasons, he will try this agent in whooping-cough when an opportunity presents itself.[1]

Netschajeff, of Moscow, Russia, has used this agent in acute nephritis, in order to prevent the growth of the streptococcus assumed to be present there. He treated 15 cases, without any noticeable unpleasant effects, and in 3 of his cases the rapidity of recovery was remarkable. He concludes that it would be erroneous to assign the improvement to a diuretic action of the agent, since in other conditions it shows no diuretic action, but the beneficial effect must be attributed to the restoration of the renal function by a specific action of this agent, rendering the tissues unsuitable for the streptococci to lodge.

Lastly, A. d'Ambrosio, of Naples, Italy, ventures to give some encouragement in the treatment of cancer by means of this agent. He relates the remarkable case of a woman under treatment with this agent, whose enlarged breast had shrunk to the normal size in four months, and the axillary glands responded in like manner. He is convinced that the treatment certainly prolonged the life of the patient more than a year, and although unfavourable conditions existed afterwards, due to a developed pleurisy, he confidently looked for a complete cure.

Many will be rather skeptical of this conclusion, but the Italian is hopeful.

[1] N. Y. Med. Record, vol. 44, p. 267.

Microcidin (sodium naphtholate) has practically retired from the field since last alluded to here two years ago, for although it has been in use as an antiseptic agent during this period, so many other agents give such satisfaction that it hardly finds a place for itself.

Dr. V. Cozzolini, of Naples, Italy, very recently ventures to give it credit for excellent results in the treatment of acute and chronic suppurations of the ear, and of all forms of rhinitis, ozaena, and tonsilitis. He used either a weak solution, or an ointment with vaseline as an excipient, and incorporated with cocaine hydrochlorate. It seems odd that he does not recognise *a priori* that any of the benefit may come from the cocaine.

Monochlorphenol has spread little further than Italy—its original source of introduction—since last alluded to here. They may still have it under investigation at home, but nothing of any importance has drifted into the medical literature of the past year.

Myrrholin is the very unnecessary name given to the simple solution of equal parts of myrrh and oil, which has been used very successfully as a vehicle for creosote by Dr. Kahn, of Würzburg, Bavaria, Germany, in laryngeal and pulmonary tuberculosis. He observes that the creosote is much better borne by patients when given in this way. He is as yet undecided whether the myrrh assists the creosote in the remedial action or not, for he finds a simple cerate of myrrh very useful in eczema of the nostrils and in both simple and foetid atrophic rhinitis, but in doses of 300 milligrammes (about 4 grains) of creosote and 200 milligrammes (about 3 grains) of this excipient, thoroughly mixed and given in capsules, he has met with gratifying results.

Naphthalin (naphthalene) has been in steady use during the past year. Its efficiency has been recognised by the revisers of the new United States Pharmacopoeia of 1890 by now introducing it there.

Many patients object to its decided odour, which is even nauseating to some sensitive stomachs. Various means have been suggested to mask this objectionable feature, such as oil of bergamot, camphor, and the like, which seem to blend their odours to such a degree that it becomes much more bearable. Dieterich, of Antwerp, Belgium, offers a formula which he claims to be efficient:

Naphthalin...............................	3,000	parts.
Camphor.................................	1,000	"
Coumarin (the chief constituent of Tonka bean)	2	"
Oil of orange flowers.......................	1	"
Nitrobenzol..............................	10	"

Naphthol (naphthyl alcohol) has been brought into greater prominence at this time by being now recognised by the new United States Pharmacopoeia of 1890, under the head of naphthol (*B* naphthol).

Reports of its beneficial action as an antiseptic, as first recommended, are increasing in number, and its field has broadened out on this line to a considerable extent. The most prominent and interesting contribution on the action of this agent during the year is an article by Dr. D. D. Stewart, of Philadelphia, Penn., on "The Prevention and Treatment of Cholera by the Naphthols," [1] including a bacteriological report by Dr. George M. Sternberg, U. S. A. It was found that both the *a* and *B* form had just about the same power of preventing the growth or destroying the vitality of the cholera spirillum, and both are recommended in the treatment of the early stage of the disease.

Although, as before alluded to here, the *a* form is less poisonous, more soluble, and more efficient, it still proves to be somewhat more irritating, and therefore the *B* form is preferred as a prophylactic, particularly as it is less disagreeable in taste.

Mons. Dubois, of Amiens, France, reports a case of its successful use as a vermifuge after all others had failed. The case was a sixteen-year-old girl who had been suffering from vomiting for many months, resulting in a diagnosis of worms as the cause. The vomiting was so persistent and prolonged that the girl was greatly emaciated. He prescribed about 250 milligrammes (4 grains) of naphthol three times a day. In a few days she passed thirty-four round worms, the vomiting ceased, and recovery was rapidly completed.

Dr. Jules Reboul, of Marseilles, France, continues to obtain the good results reported here last year with naphthol camphor (camphorated naphthol), for he now reports seven new successful cases of tubercular adenitis, particularly a case of multiple enlargement of the cervical glands, in which the treatment was continued for nearly one year.

Dr. Nélaton reports to the Paris Chirurgical Society three of his own cases of enlarged cervical glands of both sides of the neck from the submaxillary region to the clavicle, and producing considerable deformity all of which was reduced to the normal in eight months by the use of this agent. In the discussion brought out by Dr. Nélaton's results, many prominent observers differed considerably from his conclusions, going even so far as to emphasise the fact that it is not rare for tubercular glands to diminish in size and even to return to normal, without treatment.

At a subsequent meeting of the same society, Dr. Nélaton called attention to the liability of an intoxication occurring in some cases, as mentioned by Dr. Calot, of Berck-sur-Mer, France, where the injection of a large dose might be followed by very serious manifestations and possibly fatal results. Others corroborated this liability, but Professor Verneuil was rather inclined to believe that this should not be attributed to this agent but rather to the condition of the kidneys.

Orexin (phenyl-dihydro-quin-azoline) has not advanced much in the estimation of observers during the past year, and it still remains difficult to determine accurately the extent to which the appetite is promoted by any single agent when so much has to be taken into account. The hydrochlorate of orexin has heretofore been the form most used, but now Paal has found that the base orexin itself is preferable, in the way

[1] Amer. Jour. Med. Sciences, vol. 105, p. 388.

of being less disagreeable in taste, to say the least; and Dr. R. Frommel and Professor Penzoldt both find that it acts fully as well. Dr. Frommel relates his experience in cases of loss of appetite after serious operations. He used it in four cases of young pregnant women suffering with uncontrollable vomiting. All were relieved within two weeks.

Professor Penzoldt, whose results have been alluded to here for the past two years, still has a leaning towards the hydrochlorate, and has now published his results of 273 additional cases. One hundred and forty-three were successful, and 130 were either total failures or doubtful in benefit. He admits that the subjects were not well chosen, but considers his results are relatively satisfactory. Should failure result after using it as long as five or ten days, he advises its suspension for a week, after which success often attends its subsequent use.

Ouabain, the glucoside obtained by extraction from the root and wood of the Ouabaïo, growing in Africa and used there as an arrow poison, has been little heard of during the past year, either in pertussis or as a local anaesthetic. The two observers alluded to here last year have apparently not reported further on their continued results, whether good or bad, and we know practically nothing as to its standing at the present time.

Paraldehyde has now been introduced into the new United States Pharmacopoeia of 1890, and thus is recognised as a product of sufficient merit to warrant more extended trials, in spite of its disappointing results at times. It is there described as a " polymeric form of ethylic aldehyde."

Many expedients have been adopted to disguise its two objectionable features of taste and odour, and now almost every physician and pharmacist has his own effective excipients.

Another disagreeable feature has recently been noticed as being among the possibilities, to say the least, and that is *a habit*. Dr. F. A. Elkins, of Scotland, reports an interesting and instructive case of his in the Edinburgh asylum—a man 65 years old who had suffered for seven years from insomnia and had begun taking paraldehyde two and a half years ago. The habit was not long in being acquired, and at the time of his admission to the asylum he had taken nearly 500 grammes (16 ounces) a week, which even then hardly satisfied him in the way of producing sleep, as he could obtain but little more than a half hour. Upon entering the asylum he looked anxious, anaemic, greatly emaciated, tremulous, restless, and with unsteady gait. His breath had the odour of paraldehyde and his heart acted feebly, irregularly, and intermittently. After being under strict observation for a few days, his mental symptoms became more pronounced, and he had visual and aural hallucinations as well as unpleasant delusions. For the first three nights paraldehyde was continued, and in about one week sulphonal was substituted with apparently good results. Dr. Elkins very naturally calls attention to the similarity to *delirium tremens*, for the aldehyde element is in both alcohol and paraldehyde. The only points of dissimilarity are the extreme emaciation, the heart effects, and the abnormally large appetite noticed with paraldehyde. The man was discharged well in three months.

Mr. Wm. Mackie, of Elgin, N. B., was led to try this agent in the spasm of idiopathic asthma, from the noticeable fact of its free elimination by the breath, and he administered it in about 12 cases with uniformly successful results. It rapidly relieved the distressing spasm and promoted sleep. Many of these cases had tried all the well known agents with less relief than with this one. This was usually given in about 2 cc. (30 minim) doses, every hour or half hour, until relief was obtained. In none of his cases were more than three doses required, and frequently only one. In a thirteen-year-old boy with a history of asthma "from his birth" a dose of about 1.25 cc. (20 minims) was found to have a "miraculous" effect.

Following up the idea of looking to the functional disturbances which may be produced by the administration of some of the newer hypnotics, and which began by a series of experiments in 1891 on the gastric disturbances, Dr. John Gordon, of Aberdeen, Scotland, made some interesting observations on the influence on pancreatic digestion. Paraldehyde was one of the hypnotics chosen for observation, and no attempt was made to study more than the action which the pancreatic fluid has upon starch, of converting it into maltose and dextrin. His conclusions were as follows: "That paraldehyde in weak solutions had a distinctly retarding influence of four to eight minutes; and that when five minims were added to 60 cc. of mucilage of starch, retardation was complete in presence of 0.75 cc. of pancreatic solution."

Pental (tri-methyl-ethylene) has steadily progressed in usefulness during the past year. Conflicting reports are at times published, but the success of this anaesthetic is now pretty general, especially in the hands of the dental surgeons, where the minor operations offer the most favourable field for its use.

Among those who rather discountenance its use, Dr. David Cerna, of Texas, stands out most prominently during the past year. He read a paper before his state medical association last May, on "The Actions and Uses of Pental," in which he carried on a special series of experiments exclusively on dogs, and he apparently conducted them with much care and with considerable thoroughness. He made careful notes on the circulation and respiration, giving sphygmographic tracings, and finally summed up the meagre clinical history from other sources than his own. He does not agree with previous reports as to its pleasant after-effects or its suitability to general anaesthesia. He believes a noticeable after-effect to be excitement, and that it not only cannot be considered safe, but is decidedly inferior to ether and chloroform.

Fortunately for its own progress into usefulness, if it really has the advantages claimed for it, Dr. Cerna is in the minority.

Dr. P. F. Féodoroff has used it in 117 minor operations, including teeth extraction, opening abscesses, amputations about the hands and fingers, and the like, on patients of all ages, from fourteen up to fifty-six. The duration of anaesthesia was always short, varying well within the limits of from a half minute to fifteen minutes. In cases of incomplete narcosis, tactile sensation at times appeared to be present, though analgesia was complete. Complete anaesthesia of the cornea could not be uniformly obtained, and muscular relaxation could not be accomplished even when the narcosis was very pronounced. As a whole, it can be stated that no excitement whatever was noticed. In the way of unpleasant after-effects, only occasional weakness in the limbs, tremor, headache, giddiness, and uncalled-for laughter or weeping were observed, but these all disappeared of their own accord in about five minutes at the outside.

Dr. C. G. Velez also has used this agent in 106 of the same class of cases, with very gratifying results. His experience completely corroborates that of Dr. Féodoroff, and he emphasises the fact that patients take this anaesthetic repeatedly without the least repugnance. He cautions all concerning its inflammability.

Some observers have claimed that this agent produces albuminuria, but from experiments recently tried for minor operations of the human jaw and teeth, and on dogs and rabbits, Dr. Bauchwitz has found neither sugar nor albumin in 18 cases out of 20 of his series—the two exceptions being in menstruating women. His conclusion is that by reason of its satisfactory after-effects, its harmlessness, and its certainty of action, he considers it the best anaesthetic for short operations.

Prof. L. Holländer, whose cases had amounted to 400 at this time last year, reports that he has now had as many as 1,200 on whom he has successfully used pental, and fully corroborates Dr. Bauchwitz.

Pharmacopaeia, U. S., of 1890, was issued on August 19, 1893, and proved to be the best production any country has ever published. It has been issued well in advance of the date of its official recognition, in order to allow all those who should be intrinsically interested in it to become familiar with its contents. The Committee of Revision have set the date for its official recognition as January 1, 1894.

It is sincerely hoped that all physicians and pharmacists will take an increased interest in its authoritative contents and lend their influence to its more complete recognition by attempting to make far more use of its well tried remedies than has been the tendency. There is little doubt whatever in the fact that suitable remedies will be found there for the great majority of man's ills, and thus render comparatively unnecessary the vast multitude of new and little tried agents.

Phenacetin (para-acet-phenetidin) has been confined pretty strictly during the past year to a somewhat restricted use in influenza, and as an analgesic in all forms of pain, with remarkable success. Its fatalities do not apparently increase, but on the other hand its favourable reception in the profession is much on the increase.

Its alleged ill effects, together with antipyrin and acetanilid, created so much professional attention a year ago that the British Medical Association was induced by one of its members to instruct its Therapeutic Committee to investigate the whole subject and report. The report is as follows:

"During the past year the committee has conducted an inquiry into the frequency and importance of the ill effects alleged to attend the use of phenazone (antipyrin), acetanilid (antifebrin), and phenacetin, as anti-pyretic and analgesic agents.

"In carrying out the inquiry, the committee have had the coöperation of the secretaries of twenty-seven branches of the Association, and, in the case of the South Wales and Monmouthshire branch, of a local Therapeutic Committee. This latter has been formed, with Dr. D. R. Paterson as honourary secretary, to assist the central committee in conducting inquiries of this kind.

"The inquiry, which was addressed to those likely to possess the necessary experience in the use of drugs, has recently been concluded, and its results tabulated and analysed. Two hundred and twenty reports in all have been received.

"It would appear from these reports, that both the frequency and importance of these ill effects have been considerably exaggerated. The predominant opinion is, that with due care, especially as regards the initial dosage, ill effects, other than those connected with idiosyncrasy, are extremely infrequent, of little or no importance, and are not of such a character as to limit in any material way the usefulness of the drugs. This conclusion does not so fully apply to antifebrin, the action of which has been frequently followed by ill effects. In the case of antifebrin the dosage employed has in the majority of cases been too large.

"Wm. Hunter, *Hon. Secretary.*"

Phenocoll (amido-para-acet-phenetidin) is still in use by itself, but the most favoured forms at present are the hydrochlorate and the salicylate (now under the assumed name of salocoll). Reports of its use continue to be somewhat conflicting, but so much has been accomplished with it that one is strongly inclined to attribute any lack of success either to idiosyncrasy of the patient or error in the choice of a remedy whose promoters never expected it to furnish satisfaction in such cases.

In "A Preliminary Communication concerning the Antiseptic Value of Phenocoll Hydrochloride,"[1] Dr. Carl Beck, of New York city, gives an interesting study of the comparative value of acetanilid, phenacetin, and phenocoll, by applying them to wounds, open sores, etc., in the form of powder, 5 per cent. aqueous solution, 10 and 15 per cent. alcoholic solutions, 10 and 20 per cent. gauze, and 10 and 20 per cent. vaseline and lanolin ointment. Acetanilid caused no irritation, and is classed with boric acid. Phenacetin produced no bad effects and appeared to be more powerful, thus ranking between boric acid and iodol. Phenocoll, however, greatly surpassed both, and in the form of the hydrochloride was fully as efficient as iodoform, and more potent. It excels iodoform as being without odour, readily soluble, without irritating effects, non-toxic—therefore enabling it to spread over large surfaces in considerable quantities, and not contra-indicated in kidney affections.

It has had quite an extended use during the past year in malarial conditions. Italian observers appear to have given special attention to it. Following up Prof. Peter Albertone's successful results alluded to here

[1] New York Med. Jour., vol. 57, p. 488.

last year, Dr. V. Cervello, of Palermo, Sicily, reports his 18 cases of quotidian, tertian, and erratic forms treated by this agent, with 15 cures and only 3 failures—the latter being his earlier cases and of especial obstinacy.   The dose should be from about 1.3 to 1.6 grammes (20 to 25 grains), given twice or three times every two hours, so timed that the last dose should come about two hours before the beginning of a chill.   This course is continued, not only until the attacks disappear entirely, but for some little time after.   Dr. Cervello concludes that "we have in it a veritable substitute for quinine."

Dr. Giovanni Cucco also reports almost as great a success as Dr. Cervello in 84 cases, of which 52 were cured, 21 doubtful, 4 without effect, and 7 were too recent to report upon conclusively.

Probably the most conservative summary of the experience with this agent in malarial conditions at this time, is given by Dr. v. Dall'Olio. He summarises about as follows:

"1. It does not appear to have potent antipyretic properties as regards fever in general, but it is at least as effective as quinine in the malarial state.

"2. It does not cause ringing in the ears, cutaneous eruptions, or other toxic symptoms, as quinine is apt to do.   .

"3. It succeeds in a certain number of cases in which quinine absolutely fails.

"4. Its taste is not difficult to mask, and thus is of marked value in the treatment of children."

Phenolid, the 50 per cent. mixture of acetanilid and sodium bicarbonate alluded to here last year, has been practically unheard of during the past year.   It has no doubt passed into oblivion.

Pheno-Salyl has been little heard of during the past year.   Being little more than a mixture of carbolic, salicylic, and lactic acids, it has attracted very meagre attention.   Since alluding to it last year, the published formula is now found to be somewhat more extended by the addition of eucalyptol in small quantity along with the menthol, and then the whole mixed with four times its volume of glycerin.

Dulerly reports using it with success in various uterine affections, in gonorrhoea, and as a wash for rectal sores, for its antiseptic effects.

Picrol (di-iodo-resorcin-mono-sulphonic acid) is the name given a new antiseptic containing 52 per cent. of iodine, described by MM. Darzens and Dubois as being of great potency.

It is prepared by adding, with constant stirring, an alcoholic solution of iodine and iodic acid to resorcin-mono-sulphonic acid.   The latter is produced by treatment of resorcin with concentrated sulphuric acid, by a detailed process not of moment here.

The potassium salt is the one most minutely described, as being in the form of colourless and odourless crystals with an extremely bitter taste. It is not considered poisonous, although too reckless use is not without danger.   It is readily soluble in water and most of the ordinary solvents.

Nothing has been heard of it clinically as yet.

Piperazin (di-ethylene-di-amine) has increased in use considerably during the past year, and has been employed strictly in the same class of cases as for the past two years, with particular attention given to cases of gout. The explanation of its beneficial action has been, up to this time, that it dissolves the uric acid of the gouty diathesis; but this has recently been questioned.

There has been some discussion on the erroneous statements claimed to have been made in several recent text-books on the identity of piperazin, as made by the process of W. Majert and A. Schmidt, and the di-ethylene-di-amine produced by A. W. von Hoffman and by Ladenburg. The latter article is claimed by Majert and Schmidt to be an impure piperazin. To those who may be interested in the chemistry of the subject, the report of the paper by Majert and Schmidt, as read at a meeting of the London Chemical Society on February 2 last, and reported in the London *Chemical News*,[1] will be worth reading.

The most thorough paper on the use of this agent, recently published in this country, is that of Dr. D. D. Stewart, of Philadelphia, Penn., on "Piperazin in the Treatment of Stone in the Kidney—Report of Cases." A detailed account is given of three cases of uro-lithiasis, with stone in the kidney, treated with this agent, on the whole, with satisfactory results.

From across the Atlantic, Wittzack reports his experience of the changes occurring in the urine after administration, as seen in six patients, with different forms of the uric acid diathesis—one with advanced rheumatic arthritis, accompanied with gout, and the remaining five affected with gravel, although two of these appealed for relief from catarrh of the bladder. All the cases proved successful, and furnished him a good basis for his theory, based on his chemical investigations, that this agent does not really possess any solvent power in this connection, but rather possesses the property of collecting together the uric acid throughout the system, of combining with it, and thus being excreted by the kidneys.

He calls special attention to the fact that this agent is quite hydroscopic, in some cases containing as much as 50 per cent. of water, and thus allowance must be made when administering.

Dr. Biesenthal's communication at the meeting of the Berlin Medical Society, on July 12 last, on the artificial production of gout in animals, by the administration of potassium chromate, attracted considerable attention. The results were obtained under Professor Virchow's direction at the Pathological Institute, and some of the animals killed after this was accomplished were shown at the meeting. Such artificially gouty animals were claimed to have been cured by the administration of piperazin.

At the following meeting of the same society, on July 19, Dr. Mendelsohn declined to admit that the gout produced by Dr. Biesenthal was at all related to true gout, and he does not believe that Dr. Biesenthal's artificial condition can be cured by piperazin. He agrees with Wittzack above, that it has no solvent power whatever on uric acid, and, therefore, no beneficial results should be looked for either in uric acid diathesis or

[1]Vol. 67, p. 108.

renal calculus. Professor Virchow replied to Dr. Mendelsohn that he had been verifying Dr. Biesenthal's observations for the past few months, and finds that in fact the artificial gout is identical with the form in man, but, on the other hand, agrees with Dr. Mendelsohn that piperazin has no influence at all on the gouty diathesis.

Dr. Röhrig believes that this article is anything but a harmless agent, as he has noticed albuminuria produced by it, but as he mentioned he had used the picric-acid test to determine its presence, Dr. Biesenthal questions his conclusions. The picrate formed by the use of this test is mistaken for albumen.

According to Dr. Biesenthal's investigations, he accounts for the control of subsequent deposition of the acid crystals as being due to the dissolved urates preventing further formation.

Dr. T. Hewson Bradford, of Philadelphia, Penn., calls attention to the liability of this agent to cause urticaria, as he unexpectedly noticed it in a case of his about a year ago. The case progressed to final recovery, but this interposed complication caused him to report his case as a warning to others.

Pyoktanin (methyl-violet), the anilin dye, is still battling away to hold its own in professional estimation. Nothing definite can be reported as yet one way or the other, as the profession appears to be still divided.

Dr. E. J. Doering, of Chicago, Ill., read a paper before his local medical society, in March last, on "Pyoktanin in Diphtheria," in which he relates his experience in five cases of true diphtheria. The youngest patient was two years old and the oldest thirteen. All recovered; but as he used iron and stimulants internally, careful feeding, constant spraying of the throat with hydrogen dioxide solution, inhalation of steam by slaking lime, and using steam atomisers in conjunction with the applications of pyoktanin, it is surely a very reasonable question as to how much of the success may be attributed to the accompanying proceedings, and he himself observes that he did not place entire reliance on the pyoktanin. In conclusion, he expresses his belief that in this agent *we have a most valuable aid in the treatment of diphtheria* and infectious diseases of the throat, and earnestly requests all who have not yet tried it to give it an early trial.

In otology, several observers have reported upon it. Dr. Rohrer, of Zurich, Switzerland, obtained rapid and successful results in superficial and deep-seated inflammations about the ear.

Dr. Nathan S. Roberts, of New York city, gives some brief notes of four out of a number of cases under his care, and concludes "that it is of much less value than the standard remedies now in use, but is worth thinking of when these fail. It has the disadvantage of highly colouring the skin or clothing, and is, therefore, an awkward remedy for home use."[1]

Dr. Felix Baron von Oefele, in Bad Neuenahr, Germany, has used it quite freely in subcutaneous injections for malignant growths, producing rapid reduction of carcinomatous and sarcomatous tissue.

[1] N. Y. Med. Record, vol. 43, p. 110.

Dr. von Schlen, of Hanover, Prussia, reports the cure of rodent ulcer in a man of seventy, after the use of resorcin had failed. At the time he had made his report, the spot was simply designated by a faintly coloured stain with a slightly elevated border.

Dr. Julius Goldschmidt has found upon trial that this agent is useless in lepra tuberosa.

Dr. M. Heimann reports a case of ptyalism in which the discharge was quite offensive, and apparently came from a greatly congested alveolus of the upper jaw. He applied various agents, but without success, except with potassium iodide. This, however, only gave temporary benefit. He then resorted to a 1-10th per cent. solution of pyoktanin. In three weeks the applications were discontinued and a cure was established.

Pyrogallol (pyrogallic acid) is too well known to need any comment here, but it now has been advanced into greater prominence by being introduced into the new United States Pharmacopoeia of 1890.

It may, however, be of interest to some to recall at this time P. Cazeneuve's process for preparing it. He mixes one part of gallic acid with two parts of anilin, which soon solidifies. Then he heats this up to 120° C. (248° F.), until carbonic acid gas is no longer given off, and allows it to cool, when the long needle-like crystals of anilin pyrogallate form. These are treated with either benzol or toluol, which dissolves the anilin, leaving the pure pyrogallic acid, whose melting point is 132° C. (269.6° F.).

Quinine Chlorhydro-Sulphate is a new salt, claimed to be of great therapeutic value by its promoters, MM. Grimaux and Laborde, of France. Its mode of preparation is not yet published, but two of its advantages over the simple sulphate are pointed out. It will dissolve in its own weight of water, thus fitting it for hypodermic use. It contains for the same weight the same quantity of quinine as the sulphate, and therefore the doses are equivalent.

Little, of course, is given concerning clinical experience with it, as it has not been known long enough.

Resopyrin, the compound of resorcin and antipyrin, has been very little heard of during the past year, and may, no doubt, be practically considered as permanently laid aside.

Resorcin (resorcinol), one of the phenol derivatives, by its steady and successful progress into usefulness well merits the place given it, by being introduced into the new United States Pharmacopoeia of 1890.

It continues to be used with considerable success in the same class of cases as reported on last year—gastritis, gastric ulcers, diphtheria and affections of the larynx generally, pertussis, and others.

About the only original application during the year is that of Dr. Unna and some of his pupils, who applied it successfully to the face to promote peeling of the skin in the treatment of acne rosacea. A paste of 50 per cent. resorcin and zinc oxide is applied to the affected part several times a day. In three or four days the skin becomes like parchment, and the application must be stopped at once, for the cracking of

25

the skin, which will begin at that stage, must be avoided. A dressing of gelatin, glycerin, zinc oxide, and hot water is then applied, covered with cotton wool. In a few days the dressing will come off, bringing the skin with it. Some dangerous and unfavourable results have followed this practice, but they are few. The patient, of course, is confined to the house on account of his appearance, and the urine at times is coloured black; but these objections are very trivial when the number of satisfactory results are taken into account. Freckles and other superficial spots may be removed by the same treatment.

Retinol (resinol), obtained by distillation of Burgundy pitch, is still pretty generally used as a useful solvent for many medicinal agents, to which it lends efficiency by virtue of its own antiseptic property.

Salacetol (salicyl-acetol) is a new synthetic compound introduced by P. Fritsch as a substitute, like salophen, for salol, by elimination of the objectionable carbolic-acid element and introducing another to better its general effects. It is obtained by the decomposition of sodium salicylate with mono-chlor-acetone while heat is applied. It appears either in fine needle-like crystals or scales, according to the solvent used for purification, and has a slightly bitter taste. It is only sparingly soluble in cold water, but freely in hot alcohol and other ordinary solvents.

Dr. Bourget, of Lausanne, Switzerland, has made good use of this agent in incipient diarrhoea and choleriform affections, in doses of 2 to 3 grammes (about 30 to 45 grains) introduced into 30 grammes (about 1 ounce) of castor oil early in the morning, before eating, and, if required, may be repeated for two or three days. A child of one year old may take 500 milligrammes (about 8 grains) a day with good effect and no inconvenience.

It has been found efficient also in genito-urinary affections, sub-acute rheumatism, and gout.

It is rather too early as yet to hear more definite reports.

Salicylamide, the substitute recommended for salicylic acid, has not made its appearance in print during the past year, and may be considered as having been retired.

Salipyrin (antipyrin salicylate) has now been attainable in this country since December last,—after the conflicting proprietary interests had been adjusted, so that now the difficulty alluded to here last year, of obtaining this agent, has been removed. Notwithstanding this incentive to more general use, nothing has been reported to show that far better results cannot be obtained from the administration of the two component ingredients in proportions varying with the circumstances of each case, rather than being compelled to give the proportions offered in the compound.

Salocoll is the trade name given to phenocoll salicylate, which is claimed to have the advantage over the hydrochlorate of being less soluble, and, therefore, less liable to produce the bad accompanying and after-effects of the latter. Very gratifying results are claimed for it in influenza.

Salol (phenyl salicylate) has now been added to the new United States

Pharmacopoeia of 1890, and although some conflicting opinions are still given, yet, on the whole, it is found to be a very valuable agent in many of the numerous affections in which it has been tried. The literature for the past year is very voluminous, and naturally cannot be alluded to here in a detailed way. Some few of the prominent results may, however, be referred to.

In cholera epidemics, Dr. M. Volkovitch, of Warsaw, Russia, believes this to be an excellent remedy, but it must be given in considerably larger doses than are usually administered in such cases.

Dr. Patrick Hehir, F. R. C. S. E., health officer of Chadarghat, Deccan, India, after employing it in sixty-eight cases in an epidemic, reports that it " is of no more value in the treatment of cholera than the many vaunted specifics that have preceded it, and the probability is, that in the epidemic under reference, better results would have been obtained under treatment based on general principles. In point of fact, the cases not brought under the salol treatment indicate this. Like all other drugs which have been recommended as possible specifics in the treatment of cholera, salol has failed to justify one's expectations from it, and I think it must be relegated, like its predecessors, to the limbo of oblivion, as far as its special usefulness in cholera is concerned."[1]

Dr. F. Reiche also reports, that although salol was the routine practice early in the Hamburg epidemic of 1892, it was found to be very decidedly useless later, when given either internally or by injection in ethereal solution.

Finally, Dr. Girode exhibited at the meeting of the Biological Society of Paris, on May 20 last, two masses of salol as found in the stomach of a woman who had died of cholera. She had taken at intervals of three hours six doses of 500 milligrammes (about 8 grains) each. On the following day it was discontinued, on account of the vomiting following each dose. There is little doubt but that some was vomited after swallowing it; but on post-mortem examination, in less than three hours after death, two lumps were felt about the middle of the great curvature of the stomach, which were found to be the lumps exhibited. Each lump lay in a small pouch moulded to it. At those points the stomach wall was thinned and congested. Dr. Girode raised the question of the propriety of giving salol in a disease in which the mechanism of digestion is so disordered.

In diabetes mellitus, Dr. A. Nicolaier, of Göttingen, Prussia, obtained results which varied considerably. In some cases it showed no action at all, but in others more or less favourable results were noted. It apparently is contra-indicated in cases suffering from albuminuria and nephritis.

As an intestinal antiseptic, it has shown little better results. Dr. V. D. Posajyni used it in forty-nine cases of typhoid fever; three of the cases died, from lung complications principally; relapse took place once; intestinal haemorrhage twice; about 25 per cent. did not appear to be

---

[1] London Practitioner, vol. 49, p. 329.

affected favourably, and the remaining 75 per cent. were markedly benefited by checking the intestinal fermentation.

Dr. E. Mansel Sympson, who made good use of this agent in chronic
cystitis last year, now reports on its use as an intestinal antiseptic.
This field of usefulness appears to be the chosen one for this agent.

In dyspepsia he has obtained very gratifying results. In infantile
diarrhoea the good results reported before have now been repeated by
Dr. Sympson.

In typhoid fever he has used salol, not so much for the purpose of
counteracting the specific microbe or ptomaine, but for cleansing the
whole intestinal tract, and thus reducing the irritation of Peyer's patches.
It was also found to prevent the excessive formation of gas in the intestines.

As an antiseptic in surgery, Dr. Reynier reported to the Chirurgical
Society of Paris, on July 12th last, that salol, either alone or combined
with iodoform, produced excellent results in the disinfection of ragged
cavities, in tubercular abscesses, in deep sinuses, and in large bony
cavities.

At the following meeting of the same society, on July 21st, he confirmed his former commendation of this agent as an antiseptic, by speaking of its decided value in cases where one desires to procure asepsis in
the urinary passages. He believes that, even if given internally, it will
sterilise the urine unless the pus be large in amount, but its administration must be continued for some time. The lack of this latter precaution, he thinks, may account for some of the failures already reported.

Dr. G. N. Grivtzoff, of Sebastopol, Russia, has obtained particularly
good results in acute and subacute cases of gonorrhoea by internal administration. Urethral injections should also be used in conjunction
with the internal use in cases of very long standing.

Dock has used it successfully in the treatment of pleurisy.

Dr. G. Grossi has obtained very gratifying results through hypodermic
injections in pulmonary tuberculosis. He reports on eleven cases, ten
of which were greatly benefited; the other case was apparently too far
advanced to hope for much.

Salophen (acetyl-para-amido-salol), or salol in which the carbolic-acid
element, with all its accompanying poisonous properties, has been substituted by an allied, but comparatively harmless and far more useful,
element, has gained steadily during the past year in professional estimation. Its use has been pretty generally confined to the class of cases in
which it produces its best results, namely, cephalalgias, neuralgias, and
migraine, although rheumatic affections have received marked attention,
but not with as uniformly favourable results.

Caminer has used it in 1-gramme (15.4 grains) doses in all the above
affections with much satisfaction. He finds that if it is used early in
cases of migraine it aborts the attacks, but does not influence their
frequency.

Hitschmann gives his experience principally in acute rheumatism,
where it appeared to him to be a specific. He obtained good results in

one case where other salicylates had failed, and in one where they could not be tolerated. Its analgesic effects were also good in his hands, but the sweating produced varied somewhat in amount, and upon evaporation from the skin showed evidences to him of salophen crystals being eliminated by that channel as well as by the previously observed outlets of the urine and faeces. Although it has been definitely stated that it splits up before absorption, still Hitschmann and others believe some enters the circulation undecomposed, and thus appears on the skin. He also alludes to the appearance of sodium salicylate, acetanild, and phenacetin crystals in a like way.

Dr. H. A. Hare, of Philadelphia, Penn., believes that we have in this agent a very valuable remedy in rheumatism—four favourable cases which he reports had not responded to the ordinary treatment, and included sciatic neuralgia with myalgia, rheumatic neuralgia affecting the brachial plexus, and neuralgia of various parts accompanied with headache, and rheumatic middle ear disease. He, however, very wisely cautions too great an enthusiasm, as there are many instances in which cessation of all treatment, or the use of comparatively mild agents, has produced equally favourable results.

Dr. E. Koch finds great satisfaction with this agent in rheumatism and neuralgias. The more recent the attack, the quicker and more certain the action; but in chronic cases, and in arthritis deformans, its best results are obtained by alternating it with other remedies.

He finds its antiseptic action only trifling, and its chief field to be that of nervous affections of various forms; neuralgia, sciatica, pleurodynia, neuritis, cephalalgia, hemicrania, and other painful affections.

Gerhardt concludes, after an experience with sixteen consecutive cases, that it is particularly indicated when gastric sensitiveness is present, when other remedies fail, or when the use of salicin and the other like agents are objected to on account of the disagreeable taste, as in the case of children.

Lütze has made some experiments, directed chiefly towards the unpleasant after-effects of this agent, in comparison with its rivals. He treated seventeen cases of various rheumatic muscular pains, without any disagreeable symptoms or interference with the appetite; twenty cases of headaches of various origin, with only three cases showing no improvement. In several neuralgic cases it proved as efficient as other modern agents, and in acute rheumatism as good results were obtained as with salicylic acid. The only symptom ever complained of was profuse sweating.

He emphatically denies the excretion of salophen by the skin, as claimed by some observers.

Dr. Karl Osswald confirms the above favourable results in most particulars, and, finally, Dr. D. B. Hardenbergh, of New York city, reports on its use in ten cases of acute rheumatism, as occurring in the wards of Bellevue hospital, all of which were cured in less than ten days on an average.

Saprol, the so called "Disinfection Oil," has not been reported upon

during the past year, and although theoretically its disinfectant properties were very manifest, still no notice has been forthcoming as to its
practical working.

Solutol, the new disinfectant alluded to here last year, has been practically unheard of during the year past, and, if still in use, is not of sufficient importance to be reported upon by any one.

Solveol is in almost the same position as solutol. It, however, has the
advantages over the latter of being far less caustic, of being superior to
carbolic acid in antiseptic properties, and of not possessing the greasi-
ness of creolin and lysol. It therefore claims more attention, and has
received it from Dr. F. Hueppe, in his published comparisons between it
and lysol.

Somnal, the liquid hypnotic compound made by the union of chloral,
alcohol, and urethane, continues to show good results in selected cases
of insomnia, such as those occurring during convalescence from acute
diseases, but has little effect when the insomnia is due to acute inflammation.

Dr. E. Marandon de Montyel, of Paris, chief medical officer of the
lunatic asylums of the department of the Seine, has tried its effects in
various forms of insanity, and concludes that it is injurious in acute
mania and general paralysis, but is of great value in cases of melancholia, where it promotes sleep and produces a soothing effect to the
mental condition by removing the depression and gloomy forebodings.
He finds it contra-indicated when the digestion is out of order.

Sozal, the antiseptic allied to carbolic acid, and alluded to here last
year, has been practically unheard of during the year past, and may
surely be considered as having been retired for lack of applicability.

Sozo-Iodol (di-iodo-para-phenyl-sulphonic acid), the antiseptic substitute for iodoform, is still in use to about the same extent as last year,
not having apparently gained much in favour, if it has done as much as
hold its own. The sodium salt of this acid compound has been quite
freely used in pertussis during the last year. Dr. Paul Guttman reports
having treated thirty cases with insufflations of about 200 milligrammes
(3 grains) into each nostril once a day. Six of the cases were children;
two were discharged cured in eight days, and in the remaining four the
frequency and violence of the attacks were greatly diminished in from
three to six days. The remaining twenty-four cases showed favourable
results in general.

Dräer claims to have proved, in direct contradiction to Dr. F. Hueppe's
results, that preparations of this agent, and particularly the free acid
and the mercury salt, possess marked disinfectant properties upon the
growth of cholera bacilli, and that they completely prevent their growth
if the agent is used sufficiently strong and contact is sufficiently prolonged.

Spermin (testicle juice) is still warmly advocated by Brown-Séquard,
as he has now reached the large number of 100,000 injections, according
to his own report, with a gratifying proportion of successful cases. Few
conservative observers, however, have sufficient faith, even in its theoret-

ical promises, to carry on any systematic study, and have left the field pretty clear for the originator's own manoeuvres.

Dr. A. W. Poehl, however, believes that he has recently proven that spermin possesses a catalytic action in relation to general oxidation, and· an "intra-organic oxidation" of leucomaines in particular, and, therefore, has published his investigation of its effect on cholera microbes. He apparently has satisfied himself, if no one else, that this agent checks the formation of the ptomaines.

Steresol is the name adopted for an antiseptic varnish to be used in diphtheria and some skin affections, and introduced therapeutically by Professor Berlioz, of Grenoble, France.

Dr. Blanc gives the formula for it as,—

Gum Lac	5 grammes (80 grains).
Gum Benzoin	5 "	(80 ").
Balsam Tolu	5 "	(80 ").
Cryst. Carbolic Acid	1.5 "	(24 ").
Alcohol sufficient to dissolve.		

Another formula, from another source, is

Purified Gum Lac	270 grammes (9¼ ounces).
Purified Gum Benzoin	10 "	(150 grains).
Balsam Tolu	10 "	(150 ").
Cryst. Carbolic Acid	180 "	(6¼ ounces).
Oil of Cassia	6 "	(93 grains).
Saccharin	6 "	(93 ").
Alcohol sufficient to make up to 1 litre (about ¼ gallon).		

No clinical results have been reported as yet.

Strophanthus calls for little comment here. Its reputation is now well established in the profession, and it has its fitting position of an efficient alternate to digitalis in most cases, aside from effects peculiar to itself.

It has now been admitted to the United States Pharmacopoeia of 1890, by which it receives authoritative standing.

Recently its original introducer, Dr. T. R. Frazer, read a communication to the Royal Society of Edinburgh, Scotland, carefully reviewing its complete history, which may be found in full, by those interested, in the Transactions of that Society.

Sulphaminol (thio-oxy-di-phenyl-amine), the antiseptic introduced to replace iodoform, on account of its lack of odour, has not been in general úse during the past year, and the verdict of the Polish practitioner, Wojtaszek, alluded to here last year, that it "is devoid of any physiological action," still holds good at this time.

Sulphonal (di-ethyl-sulphon-di-methyl-methane) still receives well-merited attention from the profession, both for its good results, disappointing results, and toxic effects. Its abuse is still common, and the greatly-to-be-deplored practice of the laity, using it promiscuously, continues unabated. Self-medication is surely increasing, and thoughtless or apathetic physicians are much to blame for the spread of this habit.

The most rational use and study of this potent agent, as well as that of most other hypnotics, are obtained in insane asylums, where these drugs have been of such inestimable value. For a more correct and just opinion of their true worth, the medical reports of such institutions should be consulted.

Mr. Wm. J. Smith, M. B., of London, England, has made quite a careful study of "The Chemico-Physiology of Sulphonal,"[1] as a continuation of previous experiments, and concludes that it seems to split up in the system, in an indirect way, so as to yield ethyl-sulphonic acid, and that this is eliminated in the urine unaltered.

Dr. John Gordon, of Aberdeen, Scotland, draws the following conclusion upon its action on pancreatic digestion, obtained from his experiments made in connection with some other of the recent hypnotics: "From the results of numerous experiments, the smallest quantities delayed the pancreatic digestion the most—that is, from three to five minutes,—while the stronger solutions had no appreciable effect."

Toxic effects continue to be reported all too frequently, and if it were not for the very evident advantage of the drug, when used with care and under medical supervision, it would stand a very fair chance of being either excluded from practice or restricted by legislative authority. Quite an array of observers have published their warnings, but only a very few can be enumerated here. Dr. R. Lépine, of Lyons, France, again brings before the profession his experience of the therapeutic effects of sulphonal, but this time treats of its poisoning properties,[2] in which he considers the cases of serious poisoning only where, in the large proportion, death follows; but he calls especial attention to the fact that prolonged use may produce minor toxic effects which merit attention, viz., "Noises in the ears, headache, vertigo, weakness, and incapacity for mental or physical work. The patient may next pass into a condition of drowsiness or stupour, or he may suffer from difficulty of speech," etc. Ptosis, oedema of the eyelids, and, in certain cases, cyanosis may occur as signs. These are "some of the signs and symptoms of *sulphonalism*, which resembles morphinism so far as the suspension of the administration is followed by vertigo, motor disturbances, general weakness, digestive troubles, etc. The difficulty experienced by the physician, in ascertaining whether the symptoms observed are produced by the remedy or the disease, is accordingly very much increased.

"The fact cannot be too strongly insisted upon that drugs are not harmless substances, and that, although they are often useful, they are also sometimes injurious, especially when their administration is prolonged. A special class of disease is associated with the toxic action of drugs, and this class is constantly receiving new additions every year, in proportion as new remedies—which are sometimes somewhat carelessly used—are introduced into medical practice."

C. Fuerst, in speaking of its toxicity, emphasises the fact that recovery rapidly follows if the whole alimentary track be thoroughly purged;

[1] London Practitioner, vol. 49, p. 413.
[2] The Medical Week, vol. 1, p. 26.

for just as long as it is kept free, and the kidneys act efficiently and normally, the drug may be considered harmless.

Dr. Kast suggests, as a remedy against cumulative action and consequent poisoning effects, to interrupt its administration from time to time, so as to secure elimination. Anorexia, vomiting, or pains in the stomach may be regarded as indications for immediate discontinuance.

Gonzales realises that the effects of sulphonal upon man are not as satisfactory as the experiments on animals gave us reason to expect, and, therefore, he attempts to reinforce its action by giving it with morphine hydrochlorate. The sleep of sulphonal, according to his observations, is neither very sound nor of sufficient length, and to supply these deficiencies he added morphine hydrochlorate to it, and undertook some interesting experiments on frogs and rabbits with the mixture, and finds that it is perfectly successful as far as these two animals go. The sleep appears to be a physiological sleep and lasts from seven to ten hours, is not followed in the least by disagreeable sequelae, and the heart and respiration perform their functions normally. He concludes by recommending this mixture as an efficient and safe hypnotic, without depressing action on the heart, and of great benefit, even, in insomnia due to neuralgia and nervous excitement. The proportion of the two drugs may very naturally be varied to suit individual cases, but the one used in these experiments on dogs was 40 milligrammes ($\frac{2}{3}$ of a grain) of the sulphonal to 8 milligrammes ($\frac{1}{8}$ of a grain) of morphine hydrochlorate.

An English practitioner recently asked the profession at large, through the medical journals, whether continued use of this agent had been noticed to produce a complete cessation of the catamenia. His question is apparently yet unanswered. He had under his care an unmarried woman, for whom he had prescribed 1.3 grammes (20 grains) of sulphonal fifteen months before an existing attack of influenza. Unknown to him, the patient had continued the use of the drug in that dose *every single night* since. She appealed to him now for amenorrhoea and for no other symptom. She looked, and actually was, perfectly well, and no suspicion of anaemia was noticeable.

Terebene and *Turpin Hydrate*, the former produced by the action of strong sulphuric acid on oil of turpentine, and the latter by the action of nitric acid and alcohol on oil of turpentine, need no comment here. They are pretty well recognised by the profession, and have now been admitted to the new United States Pharmacopoeia of 1890.

Teucrin is the name given to the extract of the European perennial plant, teucrium scordium (water germander or woodsage). Although this extract has been known for some years, and at one time received some attention as a tonic on account of its bitter, pungent taste, it fell out of use until, at a meeting of the Vienna Medical Club on February 1 last, Professor von Mosetig-Moorhof related his experience with it for the past five years in the local treatment of tuberculosis.

The details of the preparation of this extract are not of special interest, but the finished product is a dark brown liquid of the consistency of honey, acid in reaction, with a garlic odour, bitter taste, and containing a considerable portion of calcium sulphide and other sulphur salts. After sterilisation it is used hypodermically, and shows general as well as local effects.

Successful results are reported with it in cold abscesses. Professor von Mosetig-Moorhof has noted in these cases a rapid change into the acute condition, the skin becoming red, local temperature raised, and the indolent condition becoming painful. Two or three days after, the abscess is opened up, and healing rapidly takes place. In ulcerative adenitis, caseous glands, recent carcinomatous growths, lupus, and actinomycosis very satisfactory effects were produced.

The above uses of this resurrected extract need further confirmation before much more can be reported in its favour.

Thilanin (sulphuretted lanolin) has not received much favourable report during the past year.

Dr. Saalfeld, of Berlin, speaks well of it in some cases of eczema and superficial inflammations, as he claims it has the advantage of not irritating; but Dr. G. H. Fox, of New York city, does not agree with him at all. From his careful study of twelve cases of eczema, representing various conditions of the skin, he is convinced that the agent possesses no advantages whatever over other commonly employed remedies. It is decidedly objectionable in private practice on account of its colour and odour, and in dispensary service on account of its greater cost. Out of some seventeen other cases he states, if some were taken alone, they might serve as a justifiable basis for a strong recommendation, while others would as strongly condemn it; but taking all together, they apparently prove that it is of some value under certain conditions only.

Foreign observers will have to give this agent a little more attention in order to substantiate their previous claims.

Thiol, the German artificial ichthyol, has received most attention from the gynaecologists and dermatologists during the past year, although it has been put to some other uses. Good results have pretty generally been obtained, and nearly every one remarks on the marked advantages over the natural ichthyol, for the same reasons as pointed out here last year.

Thiophene, the iodoform substitute, obtained from all commercial benzenes (from coal-tar), has not been heard of in this country during the past year, and only one prominent observer from abroad, Dr. O. Zuckerkandl, of Vienna, has favoured the profession with his experience in the use of the di-iodide, which was the form Dr. Augustus Hock spoke so well of last year.

Nothing apparently has been added to the advantages alluded to here last year, but simply its agreeable odour, non-toxic and non-irritating properties have been verified and emphasised. It has even been of service in cases where iodoform produced eczema.

Thiosinamine (allyl-sulpho-carbamide) is not a new compound, but has recently been brought forward by Dr. Hans von Hebra, of Vienna, Austria, as being of service in the treatment of lupus, based on his experiments carried on for about two years.

It comes in the form of colourless prismatic crystals, soluble in water, alcohol, and ether; but as it is readily decomposed by water, alcoholic solutions are used. It has a mustard-like odour and bitter taste. The crystals are obtained by heating together and boiling down to concentration,—

Essential Oil of Mustard............................. 2 parts.
Absolute Alcohol.................................... 1   "
Strong Ammonia Water............................ 7   "

Dr. von Hebra made his preliminary report before the last International Dermatological Congress, where he reported using a 15 to 20 per cent. alcoholic solution hypodermically injected, usually in the back between the shoulder blades. He found not only lupus much benefited, but cicatricial tissue generally was softened and rendered pliable, glandular swellings, except those from syphilis, diminished, and exudations absorbed. No general systemic disturbance was produced.

Dr. Latzko reported to the Imperio-Royal Medical Society, of Vienna, at its meeting on January 27 last, his experience with this agent in forty cases, including large tumors of the uterine appendages, slight perimetritis and salpingitis, uterine displacements, and other gynaecological cases. He observed its peculiarly beneficial action on the cicatricial tissue, and its great benefit in restoring retroflexions to the normal position and reducing the size of enlarged growths.

Dr. A. Hanc, of Vienna, reports having used it hypodermically in two cases of urethral stricture, with what at first appeared to be very gratifying results, the effect being produced very rapidly, enabling the patients to micturate without pain and to discard the catheter. Improvement appeared to progress upon further injections, four injections being given to each. One of the cases continued to retain his improved condition, but the other relapsed. Dr. Hanc therefore concludes that such injections are of transient duration only, and naturally does not put much faith in its use.

Further experience is surely necessary before it can be recommended very strongly.

Thymacetin (oxy-ethyl-acet-amido-thymol), the new agent reported last year to be an analgesic, has now been carefully studied by Dr. E. Marandon de Montyel, who finds that it is without effect either as an analgesic or hypnotic, and what few effects it does have (which are peculiar to itself) are not sought after, so that one might rightly conclude that little use will be found for this agent.

Thymol (propyl-meta-cresol), being now officinal in most of the prominent National Pharmacopoeias, calls for little comment here, but for those who may be interested in its use as an anthelmintic, a few references to such use during the past year may save some one a little time in looking up the literature.

Dr. Prospero Sonsino, of Pisa, Italy, asserts, as the result of his experience, that it is an effective agent generally against anchylostoma (a very common worm in Egypt, lodging itself in the small intestine). For ascarides he finds it no better than santonin. For tapeworm it is useless.[1]

Dr. F. M. Sandwith, of Cairo, Egypt, confirms the general results of Dr. Sonsino, and relates some of his own details.[2]

Surgeon-Lieutenant-Colonel Edward Lawrie, of Hyderabad, Deccan, India, believes that thymol will kill the filariae as found in the blood of cases in which it is supposed to have caused chyluria.[3]

Dr. Patrick Manson, M. R. C. P., of London, England, relates an interesting case of filariae in the blood, directly from India, which he treated with thymol, and as he could not obtain the favourable results of Dr. Lawrie, urges the latter to multiply his experiments down there on the spot where such cases are of frequent occurrence.[4]

Mr. Charles Williams, of Norwich, England, relates two cases of filariae, similarly treated to the above, and with the same results as Dr. Manson.[5]

Tolypyrin is the trivial name given to a new synthetic antipyretic, similar to antipyrin, in that one hydrogen atom of the phenyl radicle in antipyrin is replaced by a methyl radicle. It would be natural, then, to expect that it would resemble antipyrin in its action, as it actually does. Professor Liebreich points out its relation to antipyrin as being the same as that of chloralose and chloralamide to chloral.

It was first produced in the establishment of J. D. Riedel, of Berlin, by Dr. H. Thoms, and occurs in colourless crystals, quite soluble in water, with a very bitter taste.

Dr. Paul Guttmann, of Berlin, has been one of the chief investigators of its action, finding its effects in pyrexia very marked. His general conclusion is, that it is quite equal to antipyrin in the degree of its effects as an antipyretic, antirheumatic, antineuralgic, as 4 grammes (about 62 grains) accomplishes the same effect as 6 grammes (about 93 grains) of antipyrin, and, therefore, in consideration of its lower price, it is to be preferred to antipyrin.

No other investigator has yet reported further than this, so that the year to come may show something of value.

Tolysal (tolypyrin salicylate) is another new antipyretic from the firm of J. D. Riedel, of Berlin, formed by the combination of tolypyrin with salicylic acid, in like manner to antipyrin and salicylic acid to form salipyrin. It occurs in fine, delicately pink crystals, sparingly soluble in water, but readily in alcohol, and with a bitter taste.

Dr. Arthur Hennig, of Königsberg, Prussia, is about the only one who has given any definite report on the use of this agent, and he gives some results which are very remarkable, both as to rapidity and certainty of action in the treatment of acute rheumatism of the joints. He also finds it to be of decided value as an analgesic, antipyretic, and antiseptic, with no cumulative effects. It does not produce ringing in the ears, digestive disturbances, sweating, rigours, collapse, or cyanosis.

[1] London Lancet, vol. 2, 1892, p. 1156.
[2] London Lancet, vol. 2, 1892, p. 1357.
[3] London Lancet, vol. 2, 1892, p. 1247.
[4] London Lancet, vol. 1, 1893, p. 387.
[5] London Lancet, vol. 1, 1893, p. 1466.

Further observations will now be in order for the coming year, and it is to be hoped that the above statements may be confirmed.

Trional and *Tetronal*, the two hypnotics closely allied to sulphonal, both in composition and action, have become very prominent during the past year, and justly so from the great number of favourable reports now on record. There is little to add to what was stated here last year, as the remarks then made hold good now, except, as stated above, accumulative testimony is already quite voluminous, being almost without exception in their favour, and surpassing sulphonal in many ways. Some few reports, particularly from New York city, give trional second place to sulphonal, but practically all observers agree as to its being a very efficient hypnotic.

The only present drawback to their more general use in this country is the fact that their producers have patented them, thus making them less accessible, and, as rightly pointed out by Dr. Wm. C. Krauss, of Buffalo, N. Y., in an article on the use of trional,[1] "thus making its scientific, humane importance secondary to the commercial."

Tropacocaine (benzoyl pseudo-tropeine), sometimes called tropsin for short, has received increased attention during the past year, chiefly owing to the marked notice called to it by an American practitioner, Dr. Arthur P. Chadbourne, of Boston, Mass., in an interesting and concise paper read before the Section on Pharmacology and Therapeutics of the British Medical Association, at its meeting in Nottingham, England, in 1892.[2] His results were based on extended investigations with the synthetic article in the Berlin university, assisted by two of its professors.

It occurs with cocaine and other bases in the small Java coca leaves, and somewhat in other species. Giesel first isolated it the year previous. Liebermann, who then studied it thoroughly, succeeded in making it synthetically. The base itself is insoluble in water, and, therefore, like cocaine, the hydrochlorate is almost universally used. The base itself occurs in the form of colourless plate-like crystals of fatty lustre.

Dr. Otto Seifert experimented with a 5 per cent. solution as an anaesthetic in laryngeal and nasal surgery, and found it necessary to increase the strength to 10 per cent. to obtain the same anaesthetic effect that cocaine produces. This strength then was apt to produce irritation, and "intense haemorrhage" occurs, requiring special precautions to check it.

Dr. George Ferdinands, C. M., of Aberdeen, Scotland, has followed up Dr. Chadbourne's results with those of his own, and presents a paper on the "Clinical Observations on Tropacocaine in Ophthalmic Practice,"[3] and concludes as follows:

"1. Tropacocaine is more reliable and deeper in its action than cocaine, and the anaesthesia it produces lasts a little longer. Unlike cocaine, it anaesthetises inflamed tissue—at least more deeply than does that salt. There is complete absence of the haze over the cornea which

[1] N. Y. Med. Jour., vol. 57, p. 443.
[2] Brit. Med. Jour., vol. 2, 1892, p. 402.
[3] Brit. Med. Jour., vol. 1, 1893, p. 1318.

is so characteristic of cocaine anaesthesia. This was specially appreciated when needling. The strength of the solution depends on the requirement. For general use 2 or 3 per cent. is sufficient, and a 5 per cent. solution may be used with safety when anaesthesia of the deepseated parts is required.

"2. Solutions of tropacocaine made with distilled water keep well and retain their strength for months. One solution (3 per cent.), prepared in January last, although now a little cloudy, has not lost its activity. So far no fungus has been noticed growing in the solutions.

"3. With the exception of the one case mentioned in which the 10 per cent. solution was used, tropacocaine gave rise to no disagreeable symptoms. It practically has no mydriatic action; neither is it haemostatic. But it certainly did not give rise to 'intense haemorrhage,' as was the experience of Seifert. ·

"I am inclined to think that cocaine will eventually be replaced by tropacocaine, when its advantages are fully understood. Even if it were only for its antiseptic properties, the new anaesthetic should be given the preference. The price is not prohibitive, and increased demand will place it within the reach of all."

Dr. Hugenschmidt, a dentist in Paris, France, confirms the above results, as far as they are related to his specialty, as he has performed such dental operations as perforation of the alveoli, removal of sequestra, and teeth extraction—all without pain.

More will surely be heard of this very promising agent.

Tuberculin (parataloid) is now receiving quiet attention from conservative observers who, although many of them get diverse results, are studying this agent rationally and beneficially, because the whole subject is now devoid of the excitement of novelty and of greatly over-estimated results.

The present condition of the whole subject is well put in an article on "The Effects of Koch's Tuberculin Combined with Surgical Measures in the Treatment of Lupus," by Mr. Malcolm Morris, F. R. C. S.,[1] and may be aptly quoted here: "The exaggerated hopes to which the premature announcement of the discovery of a remedy for tuberculosis by Professor Koch gave rise, were followed by so great a reaction that there is now a danger of the real therapeutic virtue of the remedy being lost sight of in the disappointment caused by its failure as a specific. It cannot be denied that disappointment seemed at first to be fully justified by the fact that after Koch's method had been applied in strict accordance with his own directions, the last state of the patient was in too many cases worse than the first. It appears to me, however, that in absolutely condemning tuberculin as useless, or worse than useless, we do not take sufficiently into account the generally unsatisfactory nature of the results of other methods of treatment in cases of tuberculous disease, and notably in cases of lupus."

This about speaks the sentiments of many observers at the present time, and the literature is now becoming voluminous in reporting the varied field in which this agent is being used. Diverse opinions still largely exist, and it must needs be, but so much individual testimony is being accumulated that when collected in the future something of its true value may confidently be expected, either in the way of proving this present agent of service, or developing modifications which will outrank the original. This is not an extravagant prognostication, for it is the almost universal rule that much more is learned from failures than from successes, and such knowledge often gives greater and more far-reaching results. Therefore, the "greatest ill to mankind" may not receive its death-blow by means of this agent, as was promised, but the temporarily discarded agent may still find its appropriate place in the list of efficient remedies.

Tuberculocidin (alexin), modified tuberculin, has received little attention during the past year. Dr. Langermann reports on its use in four cases of pulmonary tuberculosis, with varied results.

He admits that it does not cause either serious constitutional effects, as tuberculin does, or irritation at the point of inoculation; but as to its curative action, he has great doubts.

This probably is the verdict of the profession at this time.

Tumenol, the compound closely allied to ichthyol, and whose name is derived from the bituminous matter from which it is obtained, continues to be of great service to the dermatologists, to whose practice it is pretty generally confined. The solid form is readily softened by heat and incorporated into ointments and salves.

Dr. G. H. Fox, of New York city, finds that it immediately allays the itching, and does not have the irritating qualities of the tar ointments, but is otherwise fully as efficient in acute and chronic infiltrated eczema.

Urethane (ethyl carbamate) has not yet completely recovered from the excessive crowding to the front of its vigourous rival hypnotics. It, however, is very steadily in use, and will in time be fully appreciated for its mild, moderate, and safe action, which is so well suited to so many cases of insomnia not due to pain. It is such a safe and effective hypnotic to give children, that it should receive decidedly more attention than it now does.

Weights and Measures by the decimal (metric) system have received an increased impetus during the past year.

On January 1, last, the government of Nicaragua adopted the metric system, and later in the same month a deputation representing the "New Decimal Association" (spoken of here last year), the chambers of commerce and trades unions, as well as various scientific societies, were received, according to agreement, by Sir William Harcourt, British chancellor of the exchequer, to urge the government to adopt the decimal and metric system of weights, measures, and coinage, or to appoint a committee of inquiry into the whole subject. Not much encouragement was given this representative deputation, as the reply was made that the proposed change seemed insurmountable for the present, as the English people were very slow to change, and they would have to be educated up to it. Such a movement showed very conclusively, however, that the subject was gaining ground rapidly, the people *were* becoming educated up to it, and all that was needed was steady perseverance and long waiting. From what is known of the English in habits and temperament, it may be predicted they will probably be the very last to make the change, when they will practically be compelled to it for commercial reasons alone.

At the World's Auxiliary Congress of Engineers, held in Chicago, Ill., on August 1, last, Mr. T. C. Mendenhall, superintendent of standard weights and measures at Washington, D. C., read a paper on the "Fundamental Units of Measure," in which he stated that his bureau would in future regard the international prototypes, metre and kilogramme, as fundamental standards, and the yard and pound would be considered as fractions of them. This is equivalent to an official notification that this government has formally adopted the metre as the standard of measurement.

This surely is a long step forward in the introduction of the system in this country; moreover, the progress of the system has been still further advanced by the convention for the seventh decennial revision of the United States Pharmacopoeia, which declares the metric system official in their revised edition, taking effect on January 1, 1894.

THE OBSTETRICAL AND GYNAECOLOGICAL WORK OF THE ASSOCIATION DURING ITS FIRST DECADE.

By GEORGE TUCKER HARRISON, M. D., of New York County.

Read by title October 12, 1893.

The contributions to the science and art of obstetrics and gynaecology respectively, or gynaecology in the widest acceptation of the term, made during the comparatively short period of the existence of this Association, embrace a wide field, and are of very great value to all interested in the department of medicine to which they relate. It is exceedingly interesting, as showing the rapid progress of medical knowledge, to note that pathological, aetiological, and therapeutical views advocated in 1884 must be modified considerably in 1893 to be in harmony with more recent investigations. To the student of the history of medicine, the material found in the Transactions is invaluable for obvious reasons.

The first paper coming under the above category, read at the first meeting in 1884, was from the pen of Dr. Wm. H. Robb, of Montgomery county, and is entitled "The Management of Criminal Abortion." This paper is well written, and shows evidence of large experience and skill. The author will find few, however, nowadays to follow his recommendation to use tents introduced into the cervix to control haemorrhage.

Dr. T. G. Thomas next delivered an address on obstetrics and gynaecology to a large and appreciative audience. The address, it need hardly be said, was written in his usual felicitous style, and had for its matter many of the most important questions pertaining to this branch of medicine. The views maintained by the learned author as to the therapeutic

26

value of the electric current in ectopic gestation are not, however, in harmony with modern opinion, nor has the author's estimate of the value of laparo-elytrotomy stood the test of time.

The paper of Dr. Darwin Colvin, of Wayne county, on "Venesection in the Convulsions of Pregnant and Parturient Women," presents a number of interesting histories which seem to illustrate the value of venesection. It is a valuable contribution to the subject.

Dr. Nathan Bozeman, of New York county, read a paper on "Extra-Uterine Pregnancy, with an account of two cases and their treatment," going into its history to a considerable degree. No subject has received more illumination than this theme during the last few years, and, as a consequence, the therapeutical views advocated by Dr. Bozeman are not in accordance with present attainments. In a case of tubal pregnancy, instead of using electricity, gynaecologists are now agreed that the extirpation of the sac is indicated.

An interesting "Case of Ovarian Cystoma, with operation," complicated by fatty degeneration of the heart, was reported by Dr. T. M. Lloyd, of Kings county, and read by title.

Dr. Frank W. Ross, of Chemung county, reported a case of rupture of the uterus in which the entire uterine contents escaped unruptured into the abdominal cavity. The author very properly draws attention to the great importance of the study of this accident, in order that the practitioner may be prepared to cope with its difficulties. We now know the circumstances under which a rupture is likely to occur, and the importance of prophylaxis.

The subject of the protection of the perinaeum was discussed carefully in a paper by Dr. Jacob Hartmann, of New York county. This paper was read by title.

"The Curette, its Place and its Power in Uterine Therapeutics," was the title of a paper read by myself. Since that time the field of usefulness of this instrument has been enlarged, and its use has been recommended in peri-uterine inflammations, in association with drainage, by Polk, Pryor, and others.

Dr. Wm. T. Lusk, of New York county, presented a very valuable paper on " The Mauagement of Breech Cases in which both extremities are reflected upward parallel to the body of the child."

Dr. T. H. Manley, of New York county, read a paper on " Women as Midwives," well worthy of careful perusal.

At the second annual meeting, the first paper on a gynae-cological subject was read by Dr. R. H. Sabin, of Albany county, and was entitled " Rupture of the Vagina, through Douglas's *cul-de-sac*, at the first coitus."

Dr. Ely Van de Warker, of Onondaga county, read a paper on the " Medico-Legal Bearing of Pelvic Injuries in Women," a timely and interesting theme.

What a host of memories come trooping up at mention of the name of Dr. Isaac E. Taylor, of New York county ! The paper contributed by him was entitled " Recto-Labial and Vulvar Fistulae." It was characterised by his usual accu-racy of observation and thoroughness of research. Long will abide with us delightful recollections of his noble pres-ence, his charming manners, his lofty integrity, and unselfish devotion to the best interests of the medical profession.

"Remarks on Peri-Uterine Haematoma" was the title of a paper I had the honour to read at this meeting.

"Pelvic Haematocele: Its Diagnosis and Treatment," was a paper from the pen of Dr. Wm. Wotkyns Seymour, of Rens-selaer county, read by title. The value of the paper is im-paired from the failure of the learned author to discriminate between effusion of blood into the connective-tissue of the broad ligaments and neighbouring parts (haematoma), or into a closed part of the peritonaeal cavity (haematocele), or into the free abdominal cavity (intra-peritonaeal haemorrhage).

A paper on "Two Peculiar Conditions of the Mammary Glands," was contributed by Dr. Simeon Tucker Clark, of Niagara county.

Dr. Thomas H. Allen, of New York county, furnished a

valuable paper on the "Removal of the Uterus for Cancerous Disease."

At the third annual meeting, Dr. John G. Orton, of Broome county, in a short paper, called attention to "Peculiarities 'in a Case of Ovariotomy."

The subject of "Eclampsia" was chosen as the obstetrical theme for discussion. Dr. Wm. T. Lusk opened the discussion in a carefully prepared paper, in which he called attention to the divergent views in regard to aetiology and treatment. The questions he propounded were answered by Drs. Tyson of Philadelphia, Isaac E. Taylor, T. Gaillard Thomas, George T. Harrison, Darwin Colvin, James R. MacGregor, and G. Alder Blumer. The general discussion was participated in by Drs. Hovey, Didama, E. R. Squibb, T. M. Lloyd, J. P. Garrish, E. D. Ferguson, and E. M. Moore. The widest divergence of views developed during the discussion related to the therapeutical value of venesection.

At the fourth annual meeting, the President, Dr. Isaac E. Taylor, devoted the chief part of his address to a consideration of the subject, "Lupus of the Cervix Uteri and Female Genitalia." The illustrations add very much to the value of this contribution.

"Placenta Praevia" was the subject of discussion in the field of obstetrics. The introductory remarks were by the author. The questions propounded were answered by Drs. C. C. Frederick, Isaac E. Taylor, Darwin Colvin, S. B. Wylie McLeod, T. Gaillard Thomas, W. T. Lusk, Rollin L. Banta, John Shrady, John G. Orton, and Wm. H. Robb. In this discussion Dr. Isaac E. Taylor entered at length into an account of his views with reference to the behaviour of the cervix during pregnancy. He showed conclusively the justness of his claims to priority of discovery in regard to the maintenance of the entire cervix up to the time of labour. This discovery is well fitted to illustrate, in a conspicuous manner, the accurate powers of observation and sagacity of Dr. Taylor.

"Two Cases of Epithelioma of the Labium Majus: Operation and Recovery," was the title of a paper furnished by Dr. Thomas H. Manley, of New York county, well worthy of perusal.

At the fifth annual meeting, the first paper on a gynaecological subject was a short one by Dr. E. J. Chapin Minard, of Kings county, under the title, "Does the Menstrual Flow Originate in the Tubes? The Act of Menstruation Viewed from an Inverted Uterus." The observation is an exceedingly interesting one.

Dr. Isaac E. Taylor furnished a most interesting paper on "Inversion of the Uterus after Somatic Death." According to his theory the mechanism is, that the cervix is unfolded first, then the body, and the fundus last. The inversion is therefore, according to him, from below upward, instead of from above downward. In the discussion Dr. Leale expressed the opinion that Dr. Taylor had presented a theme of great medico-legal importance.

The address in obstetric medicine was delivered by the writer.

The subject of "Puerperal Septicaemia" had been selected for discussion at this meeting, and was introduced by Dr. Carlton C. Frederick, of Erie county, in a paper showing extensive knowledge and large experience. He propounded a number of questions, the solution of which engaged the efforts of Drs. Biggs, Ferguson, McLeod, Carroll, Ross, Shrady, Robb, Grauer, Lusk, and Banta. Undoubtedly, on the whole, the student of medicine will find a great deal of value here, associated with some antiquated doctrines which seem strangely out of harmony with present views.

Dr. Leighton, of Kings county, narrated an interesting case of "Parturition in a Room Infected with Rubeola, and the Consequences."

At the sixth annual meeting, the President, Dr. Wm. T. Lusk, in his annual address narrated a case of tubal pregnancy in which rupture occurred, and for which he performed laparotomy and extirpated the sac. Recovery followed. He discussed the question of aetiology, diagnosis

and treatment as related to ectopic gestation in his usual lucid
manner. Drs. William Goodell of Philadelphia, Henry O.
Marcy of Massachusetts, Janvrin, and Risch participated in
the general discussion that followed.

Dr. George E. Fell, of Erie county, reported a case of partial inversion of the uterus, with his method of treatment
by uterine irrigation. Dr. Marcy discussed it. Dr. Fell also
read a paper on " The Latero-Dorsal Position in Gynaecic
Irrigation."

The late Dr. Charles S. Wood reported "A Case of Laparotomy for Ruptured Pyosalpinx. Error in Diagnosis: Recovery." The case is very important, as demonstrating the
difficulty of making the differential diagnosis between pyosalpinx and appendicitis.

Dr. Henry D. Ingraham, of Erie county, contributed a
paper on " The Treatment of Uterine Fibroids by Electricity." The author has stated his views with a spirit of judicial fairness, and an evident desire to arrive at the truth.

" The Use and Abuse of Forceps in Obstetrics " was the
theme discussed by Dr. J. P. Garrish, of New York county,
in a paper read by title only.

Dr. Wm. H. Robb, of Montgomery county, read a paper
on " Pelvic Cellulitis in Women," in which he maintains the
pathological importance of this morbid condition. It is a
most excellent contribution to this subject. Drs. Henry O.
Marcy, E. M. Moore, E. D. Ferguson, and John Cronyn participated in the general discussion.

At the seventh annual meeting, Dr. A. Palmer Dudley, of
New York county, described "A New Method of Surgical
Treatment for Certain Forms of Retro-Displacement of the
Uterus, with Adhesions." According to this method, an
oval surface is denuded on the anterior wall of the uterus;
then each round ligament is brought up, and a portion of the
peritonaeal covering upon the inner side of it denuded to
correspond with that upon the uterus. The denuded surfaces are brought together by continuous catgut sutures. In
this way the round ligaments are shortened, as will be readily

perceived. The future must determine the value of this operative procedure.

Dr. S. B. Wylie McLeod, of New York county, propounded a number of questions relating to the management of labour and the puerperal state; also one in regard to the influence of a more advanced obstetric science on the biological and social condition of the race. Those selected to discuss these questions were Drs. Ira B. Read, Wm. McCollom, Joseph Wm. Steckler of New Jersey, George Tucker Harrison, T. J. McGillicuddy, Wm. H. Robb, Alfred L. Carroll, A. Palmer Dudley, and E. D. Ferguson. In this discussion one of the speakers advocated the use of hot uterine irrigations after delivery, and antiseptic vaginal injections for a week or more following. It is needless to say that such recommendations are fraught with danger to the patient, and are uncalled for except where infectious germs have gained access into the genital tract.

Dr. C. C. Frederick, of Erie county, delivered the address on obstetrics, and ably discussed many of the burning questions of the day.

Dr. Charles S. Allen, of Rensselaer county, reported at length "A Case of Scarlet Fever in the Puerperium, Complicated with Cerebral Haemorrhage, Convulsions, and Hemiplegia, with remarks,"—a very interesting case.

Dr. Darwin Colvin, of Wayne county, read a paper entitled "Abortion, What of the Placenta after the Second Stage." He argued in behalf of active intervention. The paper was discussed by Drs. Carroll, Ferguson, McLeod, and Jewett.

At the eighth annual meeting, Dr. E. T. Rulison, of Montgomery county, read a paper on "The Use of Chloroform in Labour." He argued with force and ability in favour of a wider application of this therapeutic agent. Dr. Ogden C. Ludlow, in the discussion, coincided in his views. Dr. M. W. Townsend, of Genesee county, was opposed to its general employment. Drs. Murray and Douglas also participated.

Dr. Alfred L. Carroll, of New York county, introduced the discussion on "Acute Diffuse Peritonitis" in a masterly manner.

To the writer was assigned the task of discussing "Acute Diffuse Peritonitis as it Occurs in Gynaecological Practice."

Dr. W. D. Granger, of Westchester county, read a paper on the "Causes of Insanity Peculiar to Women." He shows conclusively that alienists have exaggerated the influences of causes peculiar to women in producing types of mental disease.

Dr. A. Palmer Dudley, of New York county, delivered "An Address on Gynaecology: Some of the Accidents which have Attended the Progress of Gynaecology during the Past Ten Years." He showed in clear terms the great advance made in surgical gynaecology in modern times.

Dr. George E. Fell, of Erie county, reported two cases of interest, one "A Case of Puerperal Eclampsia at Seventh Month. Induced Labour: Recovery;" the second, "A Case of Embolism of a Branch of the Pulmonary Artery following Childbirth. Oxygen Inhalations: Recovery."

Dr. John A. Wyeth, of New York county, read a timely paper on "Carcinoma Mammae: What may we Expect after Operative Treatment? How may the Ratio of Mortality be Diminished?" He argued correctly on the importance of early diagnosis, and immediate and wide removal of the organ in the very commencement of invasion.

At the ninth annual meeting, the first paper relating to gynaecology was read by Dr. Henry D. Ingraham, of Erie county, with "Ectopic Pregnancy" as his subject. The object of the paper was particularly to call the attention of the general practitioner to the earlier symptoms of ectopic gestation. Drs. E. M. Moore and Janvrin discussed it. Dr. Janvrin referred to the fact that he had been one of the earliest in the field to recommend surgical intervention in cases in which the symptoms pointed to this abnormal form of pregnancy. Dr. Janvrin brought before the attention of the Association "The Palliative Treatment of such Cases of Cancer of the Uterus and its Adnexa as are Not Amenable to Radical Operative Measures." The subject was treated in a careful and skilful manner.

Dr. Douglas Ayres, of Montgomery county, narrated "A Case of Puerperal Eclampsia at the Seventh Month, with a few Thoughts from Practical Experience as to Treatment." He regards chloral hydrate as one of the most important therapeutic agents at our command. He is also an advocate for venesection in the case of women of full habit, with suffused face and full, slow pulse, showing much arterial tension. Dr. Delphey, in the discussion, also advocated the use of venesection. It seems to me that the constant resort to the use of the lancet in the treatment of puerperal eclampsia is greatly to be deprecated. Venesection depreciates the quality of the blood, and therefore the eclamptic seizure is not an indication for its employment. The recurrence of such attacks also is much more certainly prevented by the use of narcotics.

Dr. H. S. Williams, of New York county, discussed "The Question of Maternal Impressions," in a learned and philosophical manner, in a paper read by title. His views, it may be remarked, are not in accordance with those of the best modern obstetricians.

"Mitral Stenosis in Pregnancy" formed the title of a paper by Dr. Zera J. Lusk, of Wyoming county, which is an important contribution to the subject. It was discussed by Drs. Ross, Cronyn, Higgins, and Armstrong, with the result of bringing out a number of valuable suggestions available in practice.

Dr. Ogden C. Ludlow, of New York county, presented an excellent paper on "The Use of Electricity in Midwifery."

"Abdominal Hysterectomy for Myoma" was illustrated by an instructive case in a paper read by Dr. Frederick A. Baldwin, of New York county. The case shows how much may be accomplished in shock following operations by persistent efforts to sustain the heart. Drs. Ingraham, Cronyn, Ross, and Truax participated in the discussion.

Dr. T. J. McGillicuddy, of New York county, argued at length upon the advantages of pelvic version as compared with podatic version. His facts and arguments are worthy of careful study.   Drs. Ludlow and O'Brien took part in the discussion.

It will thus be seen from this review that many of the most important questions pertaining to gynaecology and obstetrics have been brought to discussion before this Association, and it is certainly within the bounds of moderation to assert that this field of medicine has thereby been greatly enriched.

PENETRATING WOUND OF ANTERIOR FOSSA THROUGH ORBITAL PLATE OF FRONTAL BONE—RECOVERY.

By Z. J. LUSK, M. D., of Wyoming County.

Read by title October 12, 1893.

On July 11, when Mrs. H. and her mother were out driving, the horse became unmanageable and ran furiously up the street. In turning toward a yard he dashed diagonally across a board sidewalk; the carriage was partly overturned, the cover catching upon the top of a lamp-post. Mrs. H. was thrown violently against the post, driving a piece of gas-pipe, with a blunt end five eighths of an inch in diameter, into the forehead to a depth of three and one half inches. Her swaying body remained suspended in this position until removed by two strong men, one lifting the body, while the other pressed her head off the tube. The accident occurred about 1:30 p. m., on the day of the meeting of the Wyoming County Medical Association, and several physicians, myself among the number, were eye-witnesses.

She was carried to a house near by, and I was invited to take charge of the case. She was unconscious; pulse 50 and irregular; respiration 14, laboured and irregular. There was a ragged scalp wound, beginning at a point over the left parietal foramen, extending forward and downward to the glabella or smooth surface between the superciliary ridges, thence extending outward along the upper border of the left superciliary ridge to the external angular process, forming a triangular flap of the scalp, which was torn from its attachments and turned down, covering the left ear.

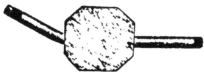

Fig. 1. Section of Lamp-post.

Another laceration began at the glabella, extended downward one half inch below the inner angle of the orbit, thence outward, along the upper margin of the malar bone, to a point on a perpendicular line with the external angular process and two and one half inches below it, forming a quadrangular flap, which was turned down, covering the left side of the face. This flap contained, along its upper margin, the eye-brow, and farther down the contents of the orbit. The eye-ball was uninjured except being completely separated from its attachments. The bones uniting to form the orbital floor were as completely removed as though it had been the work of the most skilful hand. Beginning at the external angular process, thence along the border of the supra-orbital ridge, to a point mid-way between the supra-orbital notch and attachment of the corrugator supercilii muscle, thence downward to the lachrymal groove, thence along the lower border of orbit, there was not within this boundary the slightest evidence of ossiffic deposit. There was also a fracture of the nasal eminence of the frontal bone, extending one and one half inches to the right of the left supra-orbital notch, the inferior fragment being elevated one eighth of an inch, caused by pressure against the gas-pipe. It was impossible to force the fragments back in line, and a perceptible elevation remains. The gas-pipe must have entered near the external angular process, and torn through the tissues until the force became expended against the unyielding frontal eminence. Very likely the tube was not driven to its full extent until thus arrested, although in clearing the wound of débris so as to make sure of the removal of all spiculae of bone, quite a sweep could be made with the finger with very little resistance.

Haemorrhage was quite profuse, but was controlled by cold compresses of sublimated water. I gave early a hypodermic injection of ¼ gr. sulphate of morphine. The parts

were thoroughly washed with hot sublimated water, 1 : 2000.
At the point of deepest penetration, which was about three
and one half inches, I used a 1 : 3000 solution in the cavity,
the patient lying on her back; by turning slightly the face
downward, the water ran out.   After making the parts as
thoroughly aseptic as possible, I introduced several strands
of aseptic silk in the deepest perforation, and united the
flaps by interrupted sutures.   The external dressing consisted of iodoform and boracic acid, and I covered the whole
with sublimated gauze and absorbent cotton.

I saw her several times during the afternoon.   She rested
quietly, occasionally sighing; saw her at 9 p. m., and found
her pulse 50, respiration 14, temperature 98°.   Soon after

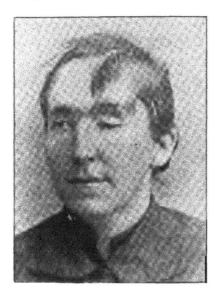

leaving her, and while visiting a patient across the
street, I was hurriedly summoned.   T h e   gentlem a n
who came for me said she
was dying in a fit.   I
learned that she had had
a convulsion soon after I
left her, which was so violent that they were unable
to hold her on the couch,
from which she had not
been removed since the
operation.   She was now
breathing irregularly; pulse .
36, respiration 12.   Fearing

Fig. 2.   Present Condition.

the trouble was due to
blood-pressure on the base of the brain, and that the drainage had become choked, there having been very little discharge, I had her replaced upon the couch, enlarged the
opening, giving more free drainage, moved the strands of
drainage silk, and turned her nearly over face downward.
Following this, blood flowed freely with several small clots;
her breathing became better, the circulation improved, and

the dyspnoea and cyanosis disappeared. When I left her at 10:30 p. m., her respiration was more natural than at any time since the accident; pulse 60, respiration 16. At 3 a. m. she had slight convulsive twitches, the respiration became again embarrassed, drainage had become choked again by a coagulum. I turned her on her face, moved the drainage silk, and introduced a grooved director two and one half inches, broke up the coagulum, when several large clots of blood escaped, followed by quite free haemorrhage, so much so that I was obliged to cover the head with an ice-bag, which controlled the bleeding; pulse and respiration became more regular, and continued so through the day.

July 13. She rested quietly through the night, had taken one half glass of milk every three hours. She was semi-conscious; speech monotonous and slow. Temperature 98¼°, pulse 60, respiration 16. When asked if in pain, she answered no. Had up to this time passed urine involuntarily; bowels moved freely in response to enema. She continued quiet through the day.

July 14, 10 a. m. Had rested well during the night, no muscular twitching; pulse 62, respiration 16, temperature 98¾°. Showed more signs of consciousness.

July 16, 11 a. m. Had a good night. I removed dressings. No inflammation or redness, scalp wound healing nicely, very little discharge. Removed drainage silk, and washed out cavity with a weak sublimated solution; dusted boracic acid over the wounded surfaces and covered with sublimated gauze.

July 17, 18, and 19. Patient continued to improve, and on the 20th, dressings being loose, I removed them. The scalp wound being thoroughly cicatrised, indeed the wound thoroughly healed externally, except over the inner canthus, I removed the stitches Subsequent dressings consisted in dusting the wounded surface with boracic acid and covering with sublimated absorbent cotton. From this time the patient continued to improve without interruption, and on Tuesday, August 8, four weeks from the date of injury, was able to sit up and be about. On Saturday, August 12, she was able to ride three miles to her home in a carriage.

In looking up the literature of injuries of this kind, I can find no parallel to this case. Gun-shot wounds through the orbital and frontal region are nearly always fatal. In this case the injury was caused by being impaled on a blunt tube five eighths of an inch in diameter and four inches long, the tube entering at the external angular process, and tearing everything before it until arrested by the nasal eminence, which was fractured one and one half inches to the right of the left supra-orbital foramen. The tube was driven through the orbital plate of the frontal bone and into the anterior fossa, three and one half inches, making an opening sufficiently large to admit the index finger, the head striking the tube with sufficient force to bend it to an angle of thirty degrees. The body swaying upon this bent tube, increased the injuries to the cranial viscera. The following blood-vessels and nerves were completely divided, viz.:

At the apex of the optic foramen the *optic nerve* and the *ophthalmic arteries*. External to the optic foramen, at the back part of the outer wall of the orbit, is the oblique sphenoidal fissure which transmits the ophthalmic division of the trifacial nerve and the nerves to the muscles of the eyeball, together with the *ophthalmic vein* and some sympathetic filaments from the carotid plexus. The ophthalmic is a large vein which connects the frontal vein at the lower angle of the orbit with the cavernous sinus. From the foregoing will be seen the importance of the vessels and nerves divided, especially the *ophthalmic vein*, which bears such intimate relations to the cavernous sinus   The dura mater sustained a slight rupture, nearly admitting the end of finger, but too deep to suture.

Mrs. H. is able to be about the house, visited me at my office a few days ago, and was able to walk to the photographer's to have her picture taken. Her sense of smell is slightly perverted, and hearing in the left ear nearly abolished. She cannot hear a watch tick two inches from the ear, and complains of peculiar noises.   Aside from these, she considers herself perfectly well.

I have reported this case, believing it of interest (1) because of the shocking manner in which the injuries were received; (2) because of the enormous extent of injured surface, nearly one half of the scalp and the integument of the left side of the forehead and face being torn from their attachment, with extensive injury to cranial viscera, together with a compound comminuted fracture of the frontal bone; (3) the rapidity with which complete repair took place under antiseptic treatment.   There was at no time a drop of pus, the entire wound healing in about four weeks.

In the photographs are seen the cicatrix of the triangular flap, part of which is concealed by the growth of hair since the injury, the cicatrix of the quadrangular flap, and the points of entrance and deepest penetration of the gas pipe.

MEMOIR OF WILLIAM R. BALLOU, M. D.

By WILLIAM T. WHITE, M. D., of New York County.

. WILLIAM RICE BALLOU, son of John W. and Mary H. (Smith) Ballou, was born in Bath, Me., July 27, 1864. He died at Thomasville, Ga., March 9, 1893, from phthisis pulmonalis. His early education was obtained in the public schools of Bath. He first attended lectures at the Medical school of Maine, and afterwards at the Bellevue Hospital Medical college, where he graduated in the spring of 1886. A few months later he passed his examination and took a degree from the former school. After serving the usual term of eighteen months in Bellevue hospital, he commenced practice in New York city. He soon had a class in the Bellevue dispensary, where he worked diligently until the spring of 1892, when on account of failing health he was obliged to give up work and go South, in the hope of regaining his health. He thought that he contracted phthisis from dispensary patients. As a " quiz-master " he was quite popular. In 1890 he wrote a compend on " Equine Anatomy and Physiology," which was published by P. Blackinston, Son & Co., Philadelphia. For three years he was professor of equine anatomy in the New York College of Veterinary Surgeons. He was an excellent teacher, and deservedly popular with the faculty and the students. He was a member of the Episcopal church. In April, 1889, he married Miss Louisa Morse Bridges, who, with one son three years old, survives him.

MEMOIR OF ALFRED LUDLOW CARROLL, M. D.

By JOHN W. S. GOULEY, M. D., of New York County.

Another founder of the New York State Medical Association, and faithful friend of the people, is gone forever; this once bright light of science is extinguished; his fertile mind is at rest, his pure soul is at peace, his suffering is ended! ALFRED LUDLOW CARROLL, the learned physician and eminent sanitarian, is no more, but his good works will long survive the death of his body, and his name will be placed high on the roll of honour. His loss is deeply mourned by all lovers of truth, justice, wisdom, and industry, which he typified in the highest degree. His illness was of many months' duration, and he bore its pain with the unfailing courage, patience, fortitude, and heroism which had characterised his whole life.

Alfred Ludlow Carroll was born in the city of New York on the 4th day of August, 1833, and died on the 30th of October, 1893. He was the grandson of Anthony Carroll, who was a great-grandson of Long Anthony Carroll, the eldest son of Daniel Carroll, of Litterluna, King's county, Ireland. The Carrolls and Ludlows began to intermarry three generations before that of Alfred Ludlow Carroll, whose father and mother were first cousins. Alfred's father, Anthony Carroll, born in New York city, was a lawyer of distinction, an accomplished classical scholar, and an earnest student of English literature and of archaeology. Among the objects of interest left by him to his son is a valuable numismatic collection.

His mother, Frances Ludlow, was a woman of superior attainments and of excellent literary taste. Her husband dying young, she devoted her life to her son's education, which she rendered very liberal. Never was youthful mind more receptive of instruction than his, or more quick in acquiring the knowledge which made him what he became. His mental soil was peculiarly adapted to those rudiments of wisdom which so soon took firm root, grew luxuriantly, and bore precious fruit, which ripened in good time to be gathered and used with masterly art; for both parents had bequeathed to him their strong characteristics of heart and mind. He was a good Latin scholar, and had a fair knowledge of Greek. His English was of the finest polish. He spoke and wrote French with uncommon accuracy, and understood German. He learned the higher mathematics, physics, and chemistry, and was conversant with several branches of zoölogy and botany, all of which were of the greatest value to him in his subsequent labours in state medicine.

He began the study of his profession at the age of eighteen as a private pupil of the late Dr. Valentine Mott, attended three winter courses of lectures, and was graduated Doctor in Medicine at the Medical Department of the University of New York in the year 1855. For eight years after graduation he enjoyed special advantages as an assistant to Dr. Mott in private and public practice. In later years circumstances changed his early bent for surgery, and he turned his attention to general medicine. His medical essays bear testimony to his vast acquirements in this department of science. The many physicians who sought his aid in consultation highly prized his opinions, which were never given until he had completed the most painstaking and thorough analytical investigation of each case, using all the modern instruments of precision that could assist him in arriving at a correct diagnosis. His wise and rational selection of therapeutic agents never failed to inspire the greatest confidence in his judgment.

While engaged in general practice he found time to cultivate his taste for literature and art. He always deplored

literary and medical brigandage, and, as editor of a medical
journal, laboured industriously to raise the standard of medical morals and of scientific essays.   He believed, with the
sage of old, that he who would gain a knowledge of men
and things must first understand the meaning of words.
His reviews of literary and scientific works are so many
pleas for thoroughness in research, accuracy in statement,
simplicity in diction, and good taste in composition.   These
and his other writings show acute discernment, profound
dialectics, and rare discrimination.   His dislike of shams and
of irrational methods is exhibited throughout his essays, both
medical and literary, in verse and in prose.   His keen sense
of the ridiculous is admirably depicted in many epigrams,
and in a profusion of sketches which are remindful of the
extraordinary delineations of the renowned John Leech.
The Carrollian sketches mirror the most glaring side of human
foibles, of the abuse of official station, of social obliquities,
of exaggeration in fashions, and of hygienic improprieties,
while they are never gross, and were never intended to be
offensive to the most delicate sensibilities of members of
refined society.   His dextrous hand was ever obedient to the
precise commands of his clear head, whether engaged in scientific labour or in home diversion—always able to illustrate
his ideas with a quickly but well made drawing, or a model
in wood.   In recreation, his intimate friends were often as
much astonished as they were amused by his suddenly exhibiting a sketch made while, apparently, he was paying
little attention to a discussion.   The sketch showed the
humorous features of the subject, and also the weak points
of the contestants.   This picture was sometimes the main
part he took in the debate, and was, perhaps, quite as forcible
a method of expression as any oral utterance that might have
been elicited by the disputants.   His artistic sense was irre-
pressible, and was always pictured in symbols appropriate to
each occasion.   His love of the good, the beautiful, and the
true was boundless.   In him the sacred fire of poetry ever
burned: it glowed through his verses and his musical essays,

through manifestations of his love of song, and through his admirable drawings, many of which were clothed in the richest colouring.

His numerous miscellaneous literary essays are scattered in various lay publications, and, if collected, would fill several large volumes.

One of his earliest medical contributions, if not the first, appeared in the *American Medical Monthly* for January, 1857. Afterward he wrote many papers and editorial articles for the *Medical Gazette*, the New York *Medical Journal*, the Journal of the American Medical Association, and other journals. From 1867 to 1871, inclusive, he edited the *Medical Gazette*, a publication full of spirit, wit, and wisdom. His weekly editorial articles were always instructive and entertaining, and often filled with humour and satire— notably one on the "Language of Science," in the *Medical Gazette*, Volume I, page 322. He ceased his official connection with the *Gazette* at the end of the current year of 1871, and established himself, for the practice of medicine, in New Brighton, Richmond county, Staten Island, where he remained until the year 1889; then, at the solicitation of friends, he returned to New York city.

The lively interest he took in the prosperity of the New York State Medical Association, from its beginning, is manifested not only by the annual contribution of an interesting and useful essay, but by the active part he took in the discussion of papers, and in the general conduct of the affairs of the organisation by the Council, of which he was one of the most efficient members, and in the formation of the Association's library, to which he contributed more than two hundred volumes. For three consecutive years he edited the Transactions of the Association, and performed this arduous task efficiently, promptly, and in admirable style. All of the literary and scientific labour he ever undertook was done with diligence, exactitude, and good taste. His introductory remarks to the discussions on typhoid fever (1887), on nosography (1888), and on acute diffuse peritonitis (1891),

27

were all master-pieces, resulting from long and extensive experience and due deliberation.

It is in sanitary science, however, that his genius found room for its greatest expansion. It is particularly in this department, all-important to the people, that he was able to apply so well the knowledge he had acquired, by untiring industry, in different branches of learning, both in medicine proper and in its allied sciences. What appears to be his first extended contribution to sanitation is published in the second volume of the *Medical Gazette*, July, 1869, and bears the title Hygiene in its Relations to Therapeusis. The following named editorial articles on public health appear in the *Medical Gazette*, beginning with,—

Volume II, 1868 and 1869:—Sewage. New York versus Brooklyn. The Health of Brooklyn. Hygiene. Earth Closets and Infection. Food for Infants. Civilisation and Nervous Diseases.

Volume III, 1869:—The Infection of Crime. Police Orders versus Disease. Hygiene and Hygrometry. Impure Croton Water.

Volume IV, 1869 and 1870:—A Hygienic Hint. Tobacco. "Hygienic Sociables." Heated Air and Evaporation of Water. Sanitary Legislation. Law and Lunacy. Relapsing Fever. The Sanitary Department of the new City Charter. Syphilisation. Bills of Mortality. New Board of Health.

Volume V, 1870:—Adulteration of Food. Control of Prostitution. Care of Abandoned Children. The Sanitarian Abroad. The Spread of Contagion. The St. Louis "Contagious Diseases Act." The Census. Yellow Fever and Quarantine.

Volume VI, 1870 and 1871:—Control of Prostitution. Physiological Effects of Alcohol. The Insanity Commission Bill. Treatment of the Insane. Vaccination. Wanted—A National Sanitary System.

Among his popular articles on hygiene are the well known Ollapod Papers, published serially in the *New York World* during the year 1873, and signed Doctor Ollapod. These articles, which if reprinted in duodecimo form would cover several hundred pages, are replete with the most useful information respecting the prevention of disease and the general care of the person, conveyed in the most pleasing style, and abounding in wit and humour. The Ollapod Papers attained great celebrity among the laity as well as among the profession, and were reproduced even in distant parts of this country and quoted largely in many journals.

In February, 1874, he delivered an address on The Philosophy of Health before the Alumni Association of the University Medical College of New York. This address, found in manuscript among his papers, like all of his other work, bears the stamp of deep thought, great erudition, and ripe scholarship, besides being very suggestive and original concerning questions of sanitation. His addresses on Public Health before the New York State Medical Association (1885) and the American Medical Association (1890) are of the same high character.

In 1880 he organised the Board of Health of Castleton township, Staten Island, and was its first president. His report for 1880 to the State Board of Health is a model of thoroughness in method and exactness in statement, whilst it shows his ability in the administration of health laws and his profound knowledge of all that concerns sanitation.

During his residence at New Brighton he gave some interesting and instructive free popular lectures on hygiene, notably one entitled "The House that Jack Built," with the quaint illustrations of the nursery book, but enlarged by himself and adapted to the purposes of the lecture, whose characteristic exordium is well worthy of reproduction. It begins as follows:

" There is an old nursery rhyme which tells of a way to be 'healthy and wealthy and wise.' I quote this, not as a believer in the supreme efficacy of early rising—which is one of the worst things that a man can do in a malarial region— but because it shows that even uncouth folk-lore, in its earliest teachings of infancy, puts health before all other worldly possessions. And, indeed, neither wealth nor wisdom can avail much, in the absence of health, to enjoy the one and to apply the other. But if 'early to bed and early to rise' be not the sole secret of salubrity, the one underlying principle of all sanitary science may be condensed into even shorter phrase, and summed up in the single word *cleanli-*

ness, which, from my present point of view, is not 'next to godliness,' but of fully equal importance. By 'cleanliness' I do not mean merely the removal of superficial and visible dirt, such as can be effected by ordinary ablutions of tariff-protected soap and water, but perfect purity and freedom from contamination; cleanliness of soil, air, water, food, as well as of body and of mind.

"Simple as is this end in view, the methods for its attainment involve infinite details, and their difficulties are increased by the aggregation of population in civilised communities, and by the perverted ingenuity with which civilised man endeavours to multiply his luxuries and to warp natural laws to suit his convenience. Primitive man, with many square miles of earth to his own share, 'the sky for a coverlet,' and immeasurable cubic space to breathe, was in little danger of 'filth-poisoning' from soil-pollution or close air;—but put his evoluted descendants in a settlement of twenty-five-foot lots; let them, aided and abetted by builders and plumbers, crowd themselves into houses with what they are pleased to term 'all the modern improvements,'—and they will probably soon succeed in sickening themselves and each other. Since the sanitation of the household is a prime factor, without which neither personal hygiene nor the best efforts of the public authorities can suffice to preserve health, I purpose briefly to examine not merely the house that Jack built at a time when fermenting malt was kept in a rat-infested cellar, but the sort of house that Jack ought to build nowadays; and, generally speaking, how Jack ought to live in it."

He then proceeds with the subject, which he treats in his wonted masterly style. His statements are forcible pen-pictures, and his manner is original, happy, and tinctured with a quaint satirical humour; but the composition is full of the most sagacious suggestions.

In 1884 he succeeded Dr. Elisha Harris as Secretary of the New York State Board of Health. This was the first opportunity he had to expand his genius; and what he accomplished during a brief tenure of office, though well told by Dr. Smith in another paragraph of this memoir, can be fully appreciated only after examination of his admirable annual reports published in octavo volumes. While on duty at the Capitol he delivered an acceptable course of lectures on hygiene at the Albany Medical College. In 1890 he gave, at the Mott Memorial hall, a course of twelve lectures on hygiene, and in 1891 a similar course at the New York College of Veterinary Surgeons. His quickly and well made black-board illustrations formed a remarkably interesting feature of these lectures.

Among his papers was found the manuscript of an unfinished work on public health, also a translation from the German of a work on hygiene—this last was, however, made by his mother, who was an excellent German scholar—and many letters showing that he was often consulted on intricate questions relating to health laws and general sanitation by health officers of cities in and out of the state of New York.

The highest eulogia of his personal character, of his literary and artistic accomplishments, of his ability as a physician, and of his sagacity as a sanitarian, have appeared in the public prints and medical journals throughout the land.

The following communications give evidence of the estimation in which he was held by prominent sanitarians at home and abroad:

Dr. Stephen Smith, of far-reaching repute as a surgeon and sanitarian, writes as follows respecting the acquirements of Dr. Carroll: "He became one of the leading contributors to the current literature in the department of preventive medicine. He had a mind trained to analytical studies in medicine and surgery; but it was not until the year 1870 that his attention was directed to problems relating to public health. At that period he was in close and friendly relations with Dr. Elisha Harris, then connected with the New York Board of Health, and subsequently with Sir John Simon, Medical Officer to the Privy Council of England. These eminent sanitarians were then actively engaged, officially, in developing, in their respective spheres, the new methods of sanitary administration. Dr. Carroll entered this unexplored field with the ardour of an enthusiast, and his writings soon began to attract attention. On the death of Dr. Harris, in 1884, the position of Secretary of the State Board of Health became vacant, and Dr. Carroll was selected to fill the vacancy. This selection was in accordance with the wishes of Dr. Harris. The office was one which, in many respects, he was eminently qualified to fill. He was very exact in all of his studies, and very methodical in all of his work. The business of the Board was conducted with the greatest promptness, new lines and methods of investigation were adopted, and order and system characterised every branch of the service. But Dr. Carroll's tenure of office was brief—far too brief for the interests of the public health of this state. He resigned his position quite unexpectedly to the Board and his friends, alleging that the influence of other officers at the Capitol interfered with the success of his work. Dr. Carroll's interest in sanitary science continued, and he wrote many valuable papers for different societies during his remaining years. In his death that science has lost an ardent student and a successful administrator of health laws."

Dr. Edward M. Moore, of Rochester, formerly President of the New York State Board of Health, entertained the highest opinion of Dr. Carroll's abilities as secretary and executive officer of the Health Department of the state. In a letter lately written, he warmly renewed his commendations, and said that he regarded Dr. Carroll as "one of the best, and probably the best, informed man on the subject of hygiene in the state," and that he had always greatly prized his advice on all important questions relating to public health.

Dr. Lewis A. Sayre, for many years city physician, writes: "I knew him well for nearly forty years, and always found him the same polished, finished gentleman in his deportment with every one he met—more refined and elegant in his manners than any other person that I have known in the profession. He had great classical and literary tastes, and was a most laborious student all his life. In all subjects relating to public health he was considered an authority, both at home and abroad. I know of but few writers in this country who have done so much for the public welfare in sanitary matters as Dr. Alfred Carroll, and I am glad to add my meed of praise to his worth as a man, and my admiration of him as a skilful and scientific physician."

The following letter from Dr. Thudicum, of London, is an additional tribute to Dr. Carroll's memory:

"LONDON, November 27, 1893.

"*Dear Sir:* I was very much grieved to receive from Sir John Simon your letter of November 11, conveying the sad news of the death of my friend, Dr. A. L. Carroll, of your city. Sir John, who is very feeble in consequence of long illness, has requested me to reply on his behalf also, and I do so with a heavy heart. Dr. Carroll was a man of rare scientific accomplishments, and fully imbued with the best modern developments of sanitary science. I travelled with him in Ireland and in the south of England for many days together, so that I had ample opportunity for judging of his ability and acquirements, and I congratulated your state of being provided with so able and successful a principal medical officer. I do not know many of his earlier publications, but his later ones, with which I am acquainted, are full of original observations, keen application of the most progressive science, and conclusions of the greatest practical value. I had formed a plan for a manual of public health, to be published on both sides of the Atlantic, but the greater scheme was never carried out, and only my small volume appeared, which pleased my friend so that he quoted several passages from it. That he should have died so early, when full of work, thought, and promise of his ripest results, is a great loss to the state of New York, and, as he gave an excellent example, to the United States in general. The profession, of which he was an ornament, has great reason to deplore his loss, and we, who had known and loved him here, will preserve to him an affectionate memory. . . .

"I remain, dear sir, ·

Yours very faithfully,

J. L. W. THUDICUM, M. D., F. R. C. P., Lond., etc."

The official positions occupied by Dr. Carroll are as follows:

Health Officer of Castleton, Staten Island.
Secretary of the New York State Board of Health.
Physician to the Smith Infirmary, Staten Island.
Consulting Physician and President of the Medical Board of the Nursery and Child's Hospital, Staten Island.
President of the Natural Science Association of Staten Island.
President of the Board of Trustees of the Mott Memorial Library.
Secretary of the Medical Journal and Library Association of New York.
· Secretary of the National Institute of Letters, Arts, and Sciences.
Editor of the *Medical Gazette.*
Corresponding Member of the Boston Gynaecological Society.
Member of the American Public Health Association.
Member of the American Medical Association.
Member of the British Medical Association.
Member of the Richmond County Medical Society.
Member of the New York County Medical Association.
Fellow of the New York State Medical Association.

In 1862, Dr. Carroll was married to Miss Lucy Johnson, who, with his two sons, survives him.

Dr. Carroll's bearing was noble, and his manners courteous, gentle, easy, and graceful. His frame was ample, his muscular development good, but the provision of adipose substance in his body was always scanty. His height was six feet. His head was large, the frontal part expansive. His nose was prominent, his eyes large and blue, and his hair and beard of a light brown hue. His mouth was large, his utterance clear. His language was precise and pure, and he was never at a loss for the right word, in conversation or in debate. His facial expression depicted thoughtfulness, high mental power, and inflexible resolution. He was charitable, kind in disposition, loving to his family, and affectionate and steadfast to his friends. His body was the casing of a noble soul, and of a mind of highest intellect. It may be said with truth, that he was a man of powerful mind, rare sagacity, great genius, and profound erudition. His brilliant career—as a man of letters, as a physician, as a sanitarian—is glorious to American literature, honourable to medicine, and consoling to the people.

For the information of those who may wish to know precisely the kind of work Dr. Carroll has performed in general medicine and sanitation, the following catalogue of a part of his essays is appended:

PAPERS ON GENERAL MEDICINE.

"Is Suspended Animation during Anaesthesia always Attributable to the Anaesthetic?" American Medical Monthly, January, 1857.

"Homoeopathic Tolerance and Allopathic Bigotry." A criticism of homoeopathic practices. American Medical Monthly, January, 1859.

"Improved Instruments for Physical Diagnosis." The Medical Gazette, May 23, 1868. Read before the New York Medical Journal Association, May 15, 1868.

"A Curious Case of Congenital Deformity." Exstrophy of the bladder, treated by plastic operation, April 13, 1858. The Medical Gazette, September 5, 1868.

"On Hydrophobia." Medical Gazette, Volume II, 1869.

"Two Cases of Aniline-Poisoning." Medical Times, March, 1873.

"A Case of Enteric Fever, apparently of Pythogenic Origin." Death on the twenty-seventh day, after a seemingly favourable course of the disease. London Practitioner, May, 1875.

"Clinical Notes on Some Common Disorders of the Nervous System." Medical Record, February 6, 1875. Delivered by request before the Richmond County Medical Society, December 2, 1874.

"Management of the Gouty Temperament." The American Practitioner, December, 1875. Read before the New York Medical Journal Association, November 19, 1875.

"Reflex Nervous Disorders from Dental Irritation." Dental Register, February, 1876. Read before the American Academy of Dental Surgery, October 19, 1875.

"The Clinical Use of the Sphygmograph." New York Medical Journal, September, 1877. Read before the Richmond County Medical Society, July 11, 1877.

"A Contribution to the Aetiology of Puerperal Infection." The Medical and Surgical Reporter, April 6, 1878.

"Congenital Absence of the Rectum." The Medical Record, December 13, 1879.

"Congenital Malformation of Tricuspid Valve; Lesions of all Four Valvular Orifices; Survival for Twenty Years, with Few Heart Symptoms during Life." Medical Record, 1879.

"Medical Fees." Medical Record, 1880.

"Abuse of Medical Charities, and Unprofessional Conduct of Clinical Examiners." Medical Record, 1880.

"Medical Registration Law." Medical Record, 1880.

"Chronic General Peritonitis." New York Medical Journal, 1881.

"Consultation with Irregulars." Medical Record, 1882.

"On the Duration of Contagiousness after Acute Infectious Diseases." Transactions of the New York State Medical Association, 1884.

"A Case of Meningeal Extravasation, with Remarks on the Localisation of the Superficial Lesions." Gaillard's Journal, July, 1886. Read before the New York State Medical Association, Fifth District Branch, March 23, 1886.

"Remarks on Leptomeningitis Infantum." Gaillard's Medical Journal, November, 1886. Read before the New York State Medical Association, Fifth District Branch, October 12, 1886.

"Recovery versus Cure." Transactions of the New York State Medical Association, 1886.

"Remarks Introductory to a Discussion on Typhoid Fever." Transactions of the New York State Medical Association, 1887.

"Sphygmographic Tracings." Read before the New York State Medical Association, Fifth District Branch, November 15, 1887. Gaillard's Medical Journal, December, 1887.

"Mineral Water Miracles." Gaillard's Medical Journal, January, 1888. Read before the New York County Medical Association, October 17, 1887.

"Perfected Obstetrics." Times and Register.

"Remarks Introductory to a Discussion on Nosography." Transactions of the New York State Medical Association, 1888.

"What is the Rate of Mortality from Malignant Neoplasmata, as Compared with Other Diseases?" Transactions of the New York State Medical Association, 1888.

"Remarks on the Mortality from Puerperal Diseases in the State of New York." Transactions of the New York State Medical Association, 1888.

"Remarks Introductory to a Discussion on Acute Diffuse Peritonitis." Transactions of the New York State Medical Association, 1891.

EDITORIAL ARTICLES ON GENERAL MEDICINE.

"Prurigo Secandi." The Journal of the American Medical Association, August 10, 1889.

"The Errors of Statistics." The Journal of the American Medical Association, August 31, 1889.

"State Examinations and Schools of Medicine." The Journal of the American Medical Association, November 16, 1889.

Many more editorial articles on general medicine were written by Dr. Carroll and published in various journals, and more than a hundred and fifty such articles from his able pen appeared in the *Medical Gazette* from 1867 to 1871, inclusive.

PAPERS ON HYGIENE AND PUBLIC HEALTH.

"Hygiene in its Relations to Therapeutics." The Medical Gazette, July 3, 1869. Read before the New York Medical Journal Association, June 25, 1869.

"Science and Alcohol." The Nation, July 20, 1871.

"The Question of Quarantine: The Nature and Prevention of Communicable Zymotic Diseases." The Medical Gazette, 1872. Read before the Medical Library and Journal Association of New York, January 5, 1872.

"Sewer Gases and their Effect upon Public Health." The New York World, February 2, 1873.

"Hygienic Philosophy." An oration delivered before the alumni of the Medical Department of the University of New York, at the seventh annual meeting, February 6, 1874. The New York World, February 7, 1874.

"Preventable Sickness." The Sanitarian, November, 1875.

"The Enemy in the Air." The Messenger of Staten Island, March 1, 1878.

"The Personal Factor in the Aetiology of Preventable Disease." Transactions of the American Medical Association, 1880.

"Filth Diseases in Rural Districts." Medical Record, 1883.

"The Proximate Cause of Malarial Disease." Report of the Board of Health of the State of New York, 1884.

"Sewage Disposal and Contamination of Water-Supply." The Medical Annals, 1884. Read before the Albany Institute, Albany, N. Y., October 7, 1884.

"An Address on State Medicine." Transactions of the New York State Medical Association, 1885.

"The Report of the State Board of Health on Beer." Medical News, 1886 (editorial).

"The Financial Aspect of Sanitation." Proceedings of the State Sanitary Convention, Philadelphia, May, 1886.

"Vital Statistics." The New York Times, July 9, 1889 (editorial).

"Bedside Hygiene in Typhoid Fever." The Journal of the American Medical Association, July 13, 1889 (editorial).

"The Registration of Vital Statistics." The New York Medical Journal, July, 1889 (editorial).

"Health Boards and Phthisis." The Journal of the American Medical Association, August 3, 1889 (editorial).

"Disposal of House-Refuse." The Journal of the American Medical Association, February 15, 1890.

"Address on State Medicine." The Journal of the American Medical Association, May 24, 1890.

"The Water-Supply of New York." The Evening Post, January 12, 1892.

"How Long Shall a Cholera-Infected Vessel be Detained at Quarantine?" The New York Medical Journal, September 24, 1892.

The thirty-six editorial articles of the *Medical Gazette*, on sanitary questions, named in the text of this memoir, added to the catalogue of papers on hygiene and public health, give a total of fifty-eight printed contributions to sanitary science made by Dr. Carroll, in addition to his elaborate reports as Secretary of the New York State Board of Health.

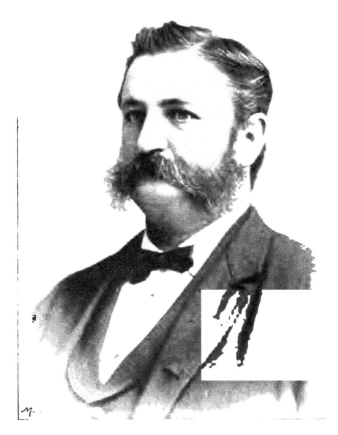

Simeon Tucker Clark

MEMOIR OF SIMEON TUCKER CLARK, M. D.

By W. Q. Huggins, M. D., of Niagara County.

Dr. Clark was born in Canton, Norfolk county, Mass., October 10, 1836. His parents were Rev. Nathan Sears Clark, and his wife, Laura Stevens Swift. The father was engaged in the ministry of the Methodist church, and no unimportant part of Dr. Clark's early education was undoubtedly the development in his youth of his ready understanding of human nature by the changing associations of his life under the itinerant system of his father's church. The father was a man of high character, mentally and morally, and the mother possessed marked poetic genius, and from her the son doubtless inherited his poetic nature.

In his youth Dr. Clark was given the best education within the reach of his parents, and he received the degree of M. D. from Berkshire Medical College in 1860, and the degree of A. M from Genesee College in 1866.

Before the completion of his medical studies, in 1857, he married Miss Ruth J. Mendell, and in 1861 Dr. and Mrs. Clark went to Lockport, making that city their permanent home. Here the doctor attained his high rank in his chosen profession, and during all this time he was blest in his domestic life by the loving ministrations of the wife of his youth, and the addition to his family of a daughter and a son,—Mrs. Ermina C. Bissell and Nathan M. Clark, who, with the fond mother, survive the ever affectionate and indulgent husband and father. He was the friend of all who would admit him to their hearts, and in the case of those with whom he was wholly congenial, this friendship ripened into a tender and sweet feeling of kinship. While all who knew him may say they have lost a friend, there are

many who feel bereft of a brother. Especially will he be
missed in Grace Episcopal church, of which he was a member, and in his Masonic associations, to which he was particularly devoted. He was Past Master of Red Jacket Lodge,
in the city of Lockport, and Grand Steward of the Grand
Lodge of the state.

In character, Dr. Clark was a remarkable man. He was a
noble type of the duality of the material and spiritual in
human nature. His strong physical and intellectual nature,
finely organised, and richly endowed with a susceptibility to
impressions of either a painful or a pleasurable character,
enabled him to enjoy all the blessings of material life with
the greatest satisfaction, while his spiritual sense was so pronounced as seemingly to put him in touch with the unseen
world in which are the real potencies of life and being.
This spirituality of his nature pervaded all his work. It led
him to study the sciences as a revelation giving him a knowledge of the Supreme Intelligence whose purposes are disclosed in the material world to whose analysis science is
devoted. It bound him with bonds of sympathy to the
afflicted who sought his professional services, and none knew
better than he how to sweeten the bitter cup of pain and
bereavement by kind words of encouragement or deeds of
personal aid. It brought him so close to his fellows that the
mystery of the human mind was almost like an open book to
him, and enabled him to attain his marked prominence as an
expert in mental alienation.

In fact, so dominated was he by this spirituality of his
nature, that he was not in accord with his times in the greed
for money-making, and never even marked out the line of
his professional work by the remuneration he might receive.
He was as faithful to the poorest of his patrons as to the
wealthiest, and always felt rewarded when he had saved a
life, however humble it might be. Still, his profession
brought him the comforts of life, and in his assiduous devotion to it he attained a merited high rank, both at home and
abroad. He was pension examiner for ten years. In 1876

he was chosen a permanent member of the New York State Medical Society. He was also a member of the American Association for the Advancement of Science, and his contributions to medical journals, especially upon mental alienation, received merited attention, both in this country and in England. , For the three years preceding his death, he had ably discharged the duties of Professor of Medical Jurisprudence in the Niagara university.

His sense of right was aroused in the unfortunate ethical controversy which divided the profession of this state in 1888-'84, and he early gave his earnest efforts in support of the objects and work of the New York State Medical Association, serving on its council and contributing to its scientific work. His thorough scholarship, with a somewhat classical bias, rendered his medical contributions not only valuable, but pleasant, reading.

Many members of the Association will recall the humourous, but at the same time learned, versification of the medicine of the Pharaohs, as voiced by a revived mummy, which was read at the annual banquet of the meeting in 1885, and the writer regrets that it was not included in the volume of his poems recently issued.

In the midst of all his activities, there often came from his pen poetic gems of rare merit. Poesy with him was not, and could not be, a pursuit, but rather a diversion, and ofttimes an expression of the conceptions that came to him in his introspective moods. The press gladly welcomed his contributions, and we find a large number of them in several poetical works of note.

In Dr. Clark the religious sentiment was profound and all pervading. The universe to him was the handiwork of a beneficent Creator, the Father of us all, and all mankind were therefore brothers. The minute details of creed, upon which many lay so much stress, did not interest him, save as a subject of mental gymnastics whose products are as varied as are the people who engage in them.

We find expression given to his religious aspirations in all the products of his pen, from his early years to the closing scenes of his life. Here is a sample, from a poem contributed to the Buffalo *Courier* several years ago, when it was edited by the late David Gray:

> "Heaven grant that I so purely live and love,
> That when I tire of this, my uncrowned race,
> Those who behold may see the light above
> Reflected in my face."

And here is a stanza, of three breathing the same religious fervour, whose tone, in connection with the date at which they were written, suggests that the writer had almost a premonition of his release from the cares of life. It was found on the back of a business letter, dated December 18, and was doubtless written at a leisure moment in his study, only the evening before he was stricken with apoplexy:

> "If I should rest some day,
> I then should know
> This life had passed away
> With all its woe."

His final summons came while in the discharge of his professional work, in caring for the inmates of the county almshouse. From the time of his attack until his death he lay unconscious, and finally passed away on December 24, 1891.

It certainly is well with our departed friend and brother. He had no fear of death; and so often had he profitably meditated upon the problem of the unseen life, which he believed to be the only real life, that it was but a step for him from the activities of the present to the realm beyond.

By W. G. RUSSELL, M. D., of Kings County.

JOSEPH CREAMER, M. D., was born in Halifax, Nova Scotia, on February 10, 1830, and died in Brooklyn, of pneumonia, January 6, 1893, after an illness of five days. He had been a physician thirty-three years, and during that time practised almost exclusively in the Eastern District of Brooklyn, where he made many friends, and where he was regarded not only as a skilful physician and surgeon, but as a gentleman who always did the fullest justice to his patients, was enthusiastic in their behalf, and loyal at all times to their interests. There was little in his early life that was worthy of note, except that the sturdy independence of his character was prominent even in his school-days.

He was a pupil in boyhood at St. Mary's Academy in his native town, and later began the study of medicine under Dr. Jennings, a prominent physician of that place. Recognising the benefit of a degree from a prominent medical institution, young Creamer came to New York and attended lectures at the College of Physicians and Surgeons of that city, graduating from that institution in 1860. Soon after that event he moved to the Eastern District of Brooklyn, where he engaged in active practice. The remainder of his professional life, with the exception of three years which he spent in Cape Breton, was devoted to the service of the people in Brooklyn. He took an active interest in politics in that city, and while he never aspired to an elective office, he held many important appointments. He was for a time county physician, police surgeon, and for many years and under many coroners, held the post of post-mortem examiner. Dr. Creamer was one of the earliest practitioners on

28

the attending staff of the Eastern District dispensary, and also served, with credit to himself and profit to the patients, as visiting surgeon in the Eastern District hospital.   He was bluff and brusque in manner, but left behind him the reputation of a skilful physician, and one who was true to his friends and the profession which he ornamented.

MEMOIR OF CALEB GREEN, M. D.

By J. G. Orton, M. D., of Broome County.

Dr. Caleb Green died at his late home, Homer, May 10, 1898, in the seventy-fourth year of his age.

Dr. Green was born in Lafayette, Onondaga county, November 14, 1819. English and Scottish blood mingled in his veins. His grandfathers both bore their part in the War of the Revolution, and his father was a soldier of the War of 1812, so that patriotism and love of American institutions were inborn in him. He was born a farmer's son, and his boyhood days were spent on the farm, where he assisted his father in the work, and gained strength, stability of character, and habits of frugality.

His earliest educational training was gained in the common school. He also enjoyed the advantages of the Lafayette high school, and of Cortland Academy in the days of Dr. Samuel B. Woolworth, then one of the leading educators of the state. In the winter of 1840-'41, he commenced the study of medicine in his native village, at the same time teaching a select school there as a means of self-support. He afterwards pursued his studies in the office of Dr. Frank H. Hamilton, the eminent surgeon. He attended three courses of lectures at the Geneva Medical College, in which institution Dr. Hamilton was professor of surgery. He received his degree of M. D. from that college, January 23, 1844, and in the March following he went to the village of Homer, where he practised his profession until failing strength incapacitated him.

In 1845, Dr. Green married Miss Roxanna R. Parsons, of Northampton, Mass., who for several years was a teacher in Mt. Holyoke Female Seminary at South Hadley, Mass., under its noble founder, Mary Lyon. Three children were born to them, the first dying in infancy, the second in the sixth

year of its life, and the third, Dr. Frank Hamilton Green,
now practising medicine in Homer.   Mrs. Green was a lady
of lovely Christian character, and departed this life in 1885.

Dr. Green brought solid attainments and enthusiastic love
of his noble profession to his work.   As an undergraduate,
in 1843 he had published in the Boston *Medical and Surgical Journal* an able essay on " Epidemic Influenza, with
Special Reference to the Epidemic of 1843," which he had
studied clinically.   He also published in the same journal, in
1845, his thesis " On the Functions of the Oblique Muscles
of the Eye," the result of original investigations.

He took an active part in the organisation of the Medical
Association of Southern New York in 1847, issuing the call
for the convention for the purpose of such organisation.
From 1849 to 1855 he was its recording secretary, and edited
its Transactions.   In 1848, at the request of the president of
the association, he read a report on vital statistics, with special reference to the climatic and hygienic conditions of the
valley of the Tioughnioga.   In 1849 he presented a notable
essay on the " Qualifications Requisite for Commencing the
Study of Medicine," one of the earliest essays published in
this country on this subject.   This paper was published in
the Transactions, and reviewed with favour in some of the
journals.

He became a member of the Cortland County Medical
Society in 1845, and was elected its president in 1852.   The
subject of his annual address in 1853 was " The Physician a Naturalist."   The address was communicated to the
state medical society by vote of the county society, and was
published in its Transactions for 1853.   The doctor took
much interest in the natural sciences, especially botany, geology, and entomology, and collected many valuable specimens, still preserved in his office.   He was a warm lover of
nature, and spent many hours of leisure in studying her
beautiful forms and wonderful manifestations.   Many former
students of Homer Academy remember with pleasure the doctor's lectures given occasionally upon biological subjects.

In 1854 he was elected state delegate to the state medical
society for four years, and in 1858 became a permanent member of that society. He was again made president of the
county medical society in 1862. At an earlier date, he also
became a member of the American Medical Association., In
1860, 1870, and 1880 he was a delegate from the state
society to the national convention for revising the United
States Pharmacopoeia, a convention which met decennially
at Washington, D. C. In 1881-'82 he was elected president
of the Central New York Medical Association. In 1884,
upon the organisation of the New York State Medical Association, he was chosen recording secretary. From 1869 to
1889 he filled the position of secretary of the county medical
society, which office is now held by his son, Dr. Frank H.
Green. From 1855 to 1858 he held the professorship of materia medica and general pathology in Geneva Medical College, and from 1858 to March, 1862, the professorship of
physiology and pathology. In 1862 he resigned his professorship, and in 1872, when the medical department of Syracuse university was instituted, he was offered a chair in that
college, but declined, preferring to devote himself to his
large practice.

The honorary degree of Master of Arts was conferred upon
him many years ago by Madison University. He was also
honoured by election as honorary member of the Buffalo
Natural History Society and of the American Society of
Microscopists. He was also a member of the American
Association for the Advancement of Science, and of the Central New York Microscopical Club.

In local affairs Dr. Green was always helpful, a loyal and
an interested and wise promoter of things worthy. He served
for twenty-four years as trustee of the old Cortland Academy,
and as a member of the board of education of Homer Academy, and Union School.

Thus briefly the achievements of· Dr. Green's active professional and public life are summarised; but the life of this
true-hearted gentleman among his patients to whom he skil-

fully administered, and among his friends in daily life with
whom he came into close and intimate relations, is still fuller
and richer in gentle triumphs of the heart. In the children
and youth he was ever interested, and ready to aid and
encourage those who sought better things. He was a faithful,
helpful member of the Baptist church for many years, and
beloved by the church people, as he was by all who came to
know him in intimate relations of friendship. Few family
physicians have been more beloved, or more faithful and
worthy the love and esteem of those to whom they wisely min-
istered. He needs no eulogy in the community where he
faithfully followed his noble calling for nearly a half century, for his best eulogy is written in the hearts of hundreds
of warm and loving friends.

The following resolutions of respect were passed by the
Cortland County Medical Society at their annual meeting,
June 8, 1898:

WHEREAS, In the dispensation of Divine Providence our worthy and
beloved friend and brother in the medical profession, Dr. CALEB GREEN,
has been removed from our midst, from our society, and from his large
sphere of usefulness; therefore,

Resolved, That we recognise in Dr. Green a man of elevated moral
character, sympathetic nature, and refined manner, a friend of a charitable and amiable disposition, who had endeared himself to a large circle by his kind and gentlemanly deportment.

Resolved, That Dr. Green was the true type of the high-minded,
trained, and skilful physician, ever ready to respond cheerfully to the
calls of rich and poor alike, relieving their sufferings by his assiduity
and skill, and aiding his professional brethren by his wise counsels.

Resolved, That by his death medical science has lost one of its most
earnest cultivators, our society and medical profession one of their oldest and most devoted members, the poor have lost a comforter in their
hour of need, and we have all lost a friend.

Resolved, That as a practitioner Dr. Green was kind, attentive, accurate, and conservative. In society he was social, amiable, benevolent,
truthful, and charitable.

Resolved, That we sincerely deplore his loss, and tender our heartfelt
sympathies with his family and friends in their bereavement.

Resolved, That a copy of these resolutions be transmitted to the members of his family and other near relatives, and the county papers.

H. O. JEWETT,
Chairman of Committee.

MEMOIR OF JAMES HALSEY HUNT, M. D.

BY MILTON C. CONNER, M. D., of Orange County.

Time, in his flight, leaves not untouched anything we call life. It may be measured by months, hours, weeks, days, years, seasons, or centuries, but the manifestations which we call life, so far as we know it in physical conditions, always end; therefore, we yield to the inevitable, and are once more called to mourn the loss of one of our active Original members, DR. JAMES HALSEY HUNT, of Port Jervis, Orange county, who died at Salt Lake City, Utah, on the 20th day of December, 1892.

Dr. Hunt was born at Centreville, Sullivan county, in 1848, being forty-four years of age at death. His early education was received at his home, and his academic education at the Travis Institute at Newton, N. J., where, just prior to its completion, when he expected to enter a literary college, he was injured by a snow-ball so that he was unable to continue his education for a period of about two years, after which he decided to study medicine without a further literary course, except such as he could obtain in Port Jervis, where his father had moved in 1866. He now began his medical education under the preceptorship of his father, the late Dr. Isaac Hunt, a thorough-going physician and surgeon of rather the old-school type.

He became a student in Bellevue Hospital Medical College in about the year 1869. After the completion of this college course in 1872, he entered the hospital as interne, serving the usual term of about eighteen months.

He went to Europe, to further perfect his education in the hospitals of England and Germany, and while there he became very much impressed with the favourable results observed with treatment of typhoid fever by means of cold baths, which he followed strictly until his death, with very good results.

His hospital service, both at home and abroad, proved of inestimable service when he came to locate in Port Jervis in 1874, bringing with him the most modern treatment in a surgical way, among surgeons who were of an older type, and who at that time had not so closely followed aseptic and antiseptic surgery, and the surgical teachings of the great masters. He readily and rapidly made a place for himself, both among the doctors, the surgeons, and the people in three states, viz., New York, New Jersey, and Pennsylvania.

Possessing natural tact and ability, together with a courage born of success and confidence in this ability, linked with a natural diffidence, and a kindly heart, especially towards children, he gained a foothold in the homes and hearts of the people of Port Jervis and vicinity not usually gained by any physician in so short a time.

A lover of travel, he found time, in spite of an exceedingly busy professional life, to visit Europe several times.

A sportsman in its truest sense, he each year tried to find time to visit in the Adirondacks for a trip, or Canada for a hunt, the incidents of which are described in a little souvenir volume, lately published, and given by the doctor to some of his intimate personal friends. His income became very large from his extensive professional work.

In 1888 he received the appointment of surgeon for the Erie Railroad Company at Port Jervis. Recognising at once the need of a hospital in such work, he established the Hunt Memorial hospital. This, in its complete adaptation to its purpose, stands now as a monument likely to last, under the management of his successors, Drs. Cuddeback and Swartwout. His marked success no doubt was largely due to his wonderful magnetic influence, whereby he inspired confidence in his ability, fidelity, and sterling good sense in his dealings with patients and the public.

In March, 1892, Dr. Hunt, feeling that his large practice and hospital work were too much for his health, decided to sell his hospital and leave town, travelling for a time west of the Mississippi.

Directly after leaving Denver, he, with others, went on a nine days hunt. The over-exertion and exposure incidental thereto proved too much for his impaired and weakened constitution. Having already developed some kidney trouble, the exposure brought on broncho-pneumonia, from the effects of which he died in a short time.

When attacked by his last illness he was in Salt Lake City, on his way to San Francisco, stopping at the Krutsford hotel. He was immediately removed to St. Luke's hospital, where he was watched with great care, as he developed some cerebral symptoms with his kidney and lung trouble.

As a man of business he was highly esteemed in Port Jervis, having done much to promote the public interests. He never married. He leaves an invalid mother, a brother, and three sisters, who mourn his loss as only those can mourn who meet with a great loss. But while mourned as lost to us, he is not dead, but living in kindly deeds and our thoughts of the past.

We, as an Association, miss him, as he was wont to be one of us, occasionally giving us something from his stored observation, and always supporting on every occasion, both in season and out of season, the code of ethics of this Association and of the American Medical Association.

MEMOIR OF FRANCIS UPTON JOHNSTON, M. D.

By Mr. L. M. Johnstone, Stapleton, Richmond County.

Francis Upton Johnston, M. D., the subject of this sketch, was born in New York city, April 8, 1826. His father, Francis Upton Johnston, M. D., son of Judge John Johnston, of Dutchess county, was a famous practitioner of that city in the first half of the present century, and attending and consulting physician of the New York hospital for thirty years, and until his death in 1858.

His mother, Mary Williamson, was a daughter of John Williamson, of Charleston, S. C., and niece of that well known patriot and physician, Hugh Williamson, M. D., LL. D., one of the framers of the United States Constitution, representing North Carolina, and at one time governor of that state, ending his days in New York in 1819, being at the time a governor of the New York hospital.

The practice of medicine came to Dr. Johnston as a family inheritance, for not only were his father and great-uncle physicians, but also his great-grandfather, Samuel Bard, M. D., LL. D., at one time president of the College of Physicians and Surgeons, attending physician to the New York hospital for twenty-three years, and one of its founders, and his great-great-grandfather, John Bard, M. D., also one of the founders of that hospital (both family physicians to Washington), and even the first of the family to come to this country, John Johnston, M. D., who landed in Perth Amboy, N. J., from Edinburgh, Scotland, 1685, besides filling most important political offices in the colonies of New Jersey and New York, practised medicine there until his death, a son, Lewis, taking the degree of M. D. under the celebrated Boerhaave, at Leyden. This family bias is further intimated by the fact that Dr. Johnston's son, Henry Cortlandt Johnston, M. D., is at present practising on Staten Island.

Dr. Johnston's education was acquired in the excellent private schools which abounded in New York during his youth, and the careful teaching of the Rev. William Berrian, D. D., of Trinity church, and the Rev. Henry Anthon, D. D., of St. Mark's, together with home examples, early formed his religious character, which was so marked a feature of his whole life, apparently increasing in strength from year to year, to the day of his death, making him most prominent in the active life of the Episcopal church in every parish and diocese in which he resided.

His elder brother, John Williamson Johnston, having chosen the profession of medicine, Dr. Johnston chose that of law, beginning its study in 1846, and after graduating, was admitted to the bar and commenced practice in New York city. In 1849, however, his brother John having died in 1844, he yielded to the evident, though unexpressed, desire of his father, and reluctantly abandoning the profession he had chosen, and for which he always felt he had a strong predilection, began the study of medicine in the College of Physicians and Surgeons, then located in Crosby street. He graduated in 1852, and having served for some time as a walker in the New York hospital and resident physician of the New York asylum for lying-in women, he began private practice with his father, who then resided at 28 East 14th street.

In 1853, Dr. Johnston married Margaret A. Babcock, daughter of John Cortlandt Babcock, of New York, who, with seven children, survives him. Shortly after, he located at 10 East 29th street, where he soon built up a large and lucrative practice, and continued there until 1860, when, his health breaking down, he was obliged for a time to retire, and, leaving the city, settled on a farm near Cooperstown, devoting his time to' the recuperation of his health and watching over the education and happiness of his young family.

When the Rebellion broke out, he at once took a strong and active part in its suppression, raising supplies and forwarding troops until 1863, when he was appointed sanitary inspector by the sanitary commission, Washington, D. C.; and while carrying out his duties of inspecting and improving the hygienic condition of the troops of New York state, in the field, accompanied the head-quarters of the Army of the Potomac, under Gen. Joe Hooker, in its famous Mud Campaign, which ended so ingloriously. After the Battle of Chancellorsville he volunteered for surgical duty at the front, and took charge for weeks, with other New York surgeons, of the Emergency hospitals, located near Fredericksburg, for the care of the thousands of wounded soldiers hastily treated on the field and sent to the rear for further attention.

In 1866, Dr. Johnston moved to Hyde Park, Dutchess county, and occupied the old family mansion erected by his grandfather, Judge John Johnston, in the last quarter of the eighteenth century, renewing friendship with the relatives and ancient allies of his family, who had resided for generations in that lovely section of the state. In 1871 he returned to Cooperstown and purchased property there, which he always retained as a summer retreat. In 1878 he located on Staten Island, where, in 1880, he acquired the extensive clientage of the late W. C. Anderson, M. D., who had gone abroad on account of impaired health. He at once became one of the most prominent figures in the professional and social life of the island, being a member of the County Medical Society from 1879, one of the medical staff of S. R. Smith Infirmary from 1881, a commissioner of lunacy for the state, and a promoter and sustainer of the Staten Island Diet Kitchen, a most useful and successful charity.

His diagnosis of disease was almost intuitive, and his manner in the sick-room so bright, cheerful, and reassuring, that one of his confrères told the writer of this sketch that, on calling him in consultation, it would not only restore his own confidence, but he had absolutely seen it renew the spirit of hope in his patient to such an extent that a recovery was effected as much by that as by the medicines administered. In obstetrics he was so universally successful that it might almost be said of him, as it had been of his father, that he had never lost a case that was wholly in his charge.

He was unalterably opposed to the attempt of the New York State Medical Society, in 1883, to alter the code of ethics in regard to consultations, holding that it was an effort of those who had already benefited pecuniarily by violating the code, and who were tired of paying to the medical profession even the modest tribute which vice is said to pay to virtue, "Hypocrisy." He was often heard to say, "Abolish the code altogether, if you will, but do not deal dishonestly with it;" and now this has already been accomplished.

His most happy and useful life was terminated November 20, 1892;—happy, in that he had been surrounded all his life by the most constant love and affection of a large family, until lately composed of four generations, the hardly less strong feeling of a host of friends attached to him through social and professional acts by the uprightness, conscientiousness, and sweetness of his character, the all but adoration of the poor and friendless, and the esteem and regard of his professional brethren; useful, in that he had, to the utmost of his ability and strength, performed every Christian, civil, or professional duty entrusted to him,—a noble example to all that a man need not leave his own fireside to impress on the world his hereditary and acquired virtues and abilities, if he will only earnestly, faithfully, fearlessly, and honestly strive to accomplish those duties which Providence places at the door of each one of us.

By S. B. W. McLeod, M. D., of New York County.

DR. MATHEWS was preëminently a New York man. He was born in Sullivan county, and educated in an academy there; graduated from the College of Physicians and Surgeons in 1860; enlisted in the War of the Rebellion, and served as surgeon of the One Hundred and Forty-third regiment of volunteers; engaged in private practice in Monticello, and after a few years removed to this city, where he practised for about twenty years, and where, on April 16, 1877, he was appointed one of the surgeons of police, and continued in office up to the time of his death. He was also attending physician to the Catholic Orphan Asylum.

In addition to these varied medical labours, he always maintained an interest in the general affairs of the profession, being a member of the New York County and New York State Medical associations and of the Medico-Legal Society.

Dr. Mathews was plain and unassuming in his manner, kind in his disposition, careful and attentive in his practice. His wife, formerly Miss Mary Lynch, of New York city, died three years before her husband.

After a short illness, at the close of a labourious and useful life, be died, July 9, 1891, in the sixty-first year of his age.

MEMOIR OF WILLIAM D. WOODEND, M. D.

By GEORGE B. BANKS, M. D., of Westchester County.

WILLIAM D. WOODEND, M. D., was born in Portsmouth, Va., in May, 1832. He received his preliminary education in the schools and academy of his native place, and when about eighteen years old he began the study of medicine in the Naval hospital at Norfolk. He remained there three years, and then entered the University of Pennsylvania at Philadelphia, from which he graduated in 1855. He spent nearly two years in Philadelphia after he graduated from the university. In February, 1857, he removed to Huntington, L. I., and commenced his life-work in the practice of medicine, as successor to the late Dr. Charles Sturgis. Unlike most young men starting in a new place, he began with a large practice, which he continued to successfully maintain and conduct in all the years following. He had an agreeable and familiar manner, a free and easy habit in conversation, easily made new acquaintances, and thus formed and continued to keep many firm and sincere friendships. His practice, as in all country places, included a large number of the poor, to whom he was ever kind-hearted and generous.

Innocent of the plans and ways of a successful financier, he failed to accumulate where another might have secured a competence.

He was strong and intense, fearless and outspoken in his political opinions. He took an active interest in the New York State Medical Association when that was formed by the division of the state society. He was a regular attendant at the meetings, as well as at the meetings of the Fifth District Branch Association. He kept himself well informed on the leading topics of the day, while not neglecting the investigations going on and the consequent changes recommended in the practice of the medical profession.

In April, 1859, Dr. Woodend married Miss Wood, of Huntington. They had four children, two of whom died in childhood. Mrs. Woodend and two children, a son and a daughter, are living. The son, William E. Woodend, M. D., graduated from Bellevue Hospital Medical College, and is now a practising physician in Harlem.

Dr. Woodend kept in active practice in Huntington from the time of his first settlement in the place, in 1857, until October, 1889, when he had an attack of apoplexy, from which he partially recovered, but did not regain sufficient strength to meet the active demands of former years. He gradually gave up his work, and went to spend the winter of 1892-'93 with his married daughter at Islip, L. I. Early in March, 1893, he went to Washington. He had long anticipated this trip to witness the inauguration of Mr. Cleveland. While on this visit, March 7, three days after the inauguration, he had another attack of apoplexy, and died the day following. He was buried at Huntington, where his many friends will long mourn their loss and cherish his memory.

THE FESTIVITIES OF THE FIRST DECENNIAL MEETING.

The social part of the first decennial celebration of the foundation of the New York State Medical Association was of a nature to merit permanent record in this volume of Transactions.

One hundred Fellows contributed a fund to be devoted to conviviality. On the first night of the meeting, Monday, October 9, a collation was partaken of after the session; on the following Wednesday, October 11, a banquet; and on Thursday, October 12, the Association went on an excursion to the island hospitals, by invitation of the commissioners of charities, a copious luncheon having been served on board the steamer *Minnehanonck*. The banquet, given at the Hotel Brunswick, was all that could be desired: the tables were tastefully ornamented, the viands were admirably prepared and served in the best style, the wines were excellent, and the good cheer general, from the oysters to the coffee. At the appointed time the President, after some remarks appropriate to the occasion, in which he happily referred to the history of the first decennium as represented in the work of certain of the Fellows of the Association, called out the Secretary to act as toast-master, who said,—

Mr. Chairman: I am very happy to act as butler in putting on tap the wisdom and the wit of the evening. I will call upon Dr. Austin Flint as the first to respond to the sentiment,—

The New York State Medical Association:
Half a score of years agone she came forth, fully formed and equipped to cope with and solve problems the most intricate. May her scientific laurels be as luxuriant in the coming as in the past decade!

Dr. FLINT.—*Mr. President and Fellow-Members of the Association:* I, for one, have never heard a speech made in response to a toast unless that speech began with an apology. I am not going to make an apology. I was notified that I should be called upon to respond in two or three minutes to one of the toasts I have read to-night, but I had no idea that it was to be "The New York State Medical Association." I had no idea that I was to have the first speech, and I only feel justified in saying anything by the conviction that there are some others to follow me who are better able to do justice to this subject.

Still there are reminiscences, memories—shadowy until this moment—which come before me now, of when, nearly ten years ago (it will be ten years on the 4th of February, 1894), I, with some others, met in Albany and presided at the birth of this, which can justly be called great, Medical Association. What a contrast between now and then!

29

There were those in our conference who thought it unwise, perhaps, to organise this Association. I did not. Those who thought it unwise have long since seen their mistake. We founded a State Association, born through dissensions, and this Association was founded with a view of advancing the science of medicine, in the hope that it would never be the theatre of dissensions (which it never has been), and I believe, not only that the next decade will show as grand scientific results as the ten years that have passed, but that we will go onward and onward, doing ourselves full credit, and show the path to others, as we have in many instances.

I, perhaps, was certainly as enthusiastic as any one in the formation of this Association. Happily the causes which brought it into being ceased altogether when it was brought into being, and they are not to be mentioned now; they should never be the subject of discussion again.

I volunteered to edit the first volume of the Transactions of this Association, and I know very well what it was and who were represented, and I can cite from memory now many who were represented who, in the course of time, have passed away. It would be invidious to mention any individual contributions that have been made to science under the auspices of this Association, but we cannot but look back upon certain of those who have passed away who were represented in the first volumes—Clark and Gay, and Rochester and Gray, and one whose name I bear, and others contributed to the first volume, as respectable, as dignified, as useful a volume as I have ever seen issued by any association. [Applause.] That this will continue I have no doubt.

The first volume contained a list of a few more than five hundred members. To-day we have eight hundred members, an increase of about sixty per cent. The number of pages in our volumes has increased about one half of that proportion, or about twenty-eight per cent.; but of the value of these discussions it is not for me to speak. All of them will be recited to you, most probably, by those who have been appointed to make a careful analysis of these things. But there is one point in which this Association has been the pioneer, I think, in this country, which has in its carrying out given more value to those discussions than any other idea that has been advanced, and I think that this was the notion of my friend and co-laborer at that time, one who has been most earnest in the advancement of the interests of this Association (I refer to Dr. Gouley), that is, the presentation of questions for carefully prepared discussions. I do not believe in the value of extemporaneous discussions, or statements upon scientific subjects that come from persons who are unprepared. Every one who has done scientific work, however great his experience, knows that when this experience is tabulated before him in black and white, it is often different from what he expected it would be. I do not believe much in solicited contributions to medical societies. A man is urged to write a paper; he does not feel the sacred call himself; it is nothing that he wants to do, and, as a general proposition, if he yields to the solicitation to write a paper, he does something that is hurried, that is incomplete, that has not its full value. Our discussions have been filled with papers that were voluntary, with papers that had value, because their authors had something to present, and desired to present them. And this will continue. There are more papers now, as I understand it, offered than can conveniently be disposed of in the time that is set for us to meet.

I have always believed, and I can say it without local vanity, that New York is the place where these meetings should be held, and that a large measure of the success that the society has met with has been due to the fact that it has met here in the city of New York, where every one wants to come, and no one wants to go away from if he can help it.

I trust you will pardon me for this imperfect address, and I will repeat, Mr. President, that I did not expect to occupy on the programme the important position that seems to have been forced upon me to-night.

The TOAST-MASTER.—It is very fitting that extremes should meet. We have heard from one of our Fellows residing in the great seaport of New York, and now, to respond to this same toast, we will ask one residing at that greater seaport at the other extreme of the state, Dr. John Cronyn, of Buffalo.

Dr. CRONYN.—*Mr. President and Fellows of the Association :* Dr. Flint has just said that he never knew a man to commence without first making an apology. I saw stated in a newspaper, or somewhere else, the other day, that a man never spoke extemporaneously, that he was always sure to think about what he was going to say a great while before. I believe it is true to a certain extent. Before I came to New York I did not know that I was going to be asked to make a speech to-night, but it will be so short and pleasant that I am quite sure none of you will take exception.

The doctor also said, in the inception of this great Association there were others beside himself. I happen to be one of them. I have been at the bedside of about three thousand obstetrical cases in my experience, but I was never so proud of being at the birth of any child as I am of this great Association as it presents itself to-night.

Now reading the toast would almost be a speech of itself, and when combined with the objects of the Association, I think I will have made as long a speech as you will care to hear. Let me read the toast over again, Mr. Toast-Master.

" Half a score of years agone she came forth, fully formed, and equipped to cope with and bravely solve problems the most intricate. May her scientific laurels be as luxuriant in the coming as in the past decade !"

Now speaking of that birth, I would like to say something about a man, the one over yonder in the corner, but I know he would be vexed at me for it, he had so much to do with this extraordinary birth. He was so busy he was not very accessible until the child was born. It is true he said he conferred with a great many others before his own good intentions were carried out. I started in to tell a story, but I won't tell it, because he wouldn't like it. But the objects of the Association,—

"The Cultivation and Advancement of the Science of Medicine." Now, I would ask the gentlemen who are in any doubt about the success of the first object, to consult the Transactions of this Association. They are all in the library, and if there is anything in them from the beginning to the end that would not be considered more or less scientific and a means of advancing the special science that we are always trying to promote, I would like to find it out.

"The Promotion of Public Health." As to that, if the evidence that we have given in disposing of everything on those tables is not sufficient, I do n't know what is.

The third and most important, "The Maintenance of the Honour and Character of the Medical Profession." To my knowledge, a very large proportion are busy all the time, busy at every opportunity, making the profession more respected, more honoured among its Fellows, among the people, and infusing in them a very different respect for one another, than any other association I know anything of. It will stand unrivalled, and I would say its Transactions have been praised in the English medical journals and in the home journals; lately it has been considered one of the best, if not the best, in the country. Some two years ago the *Lancet* made a notice of it, saying its Transactions were a credit to any society, either in Europe or America.

The fourth object of this Association—" The Establishment and Preservation of Cordial Professional Relations between the Medical Societies of this State and of other States of the United States and Foreign Countries, through the Medical Associations of Such States and Countries." Now, if we have accomplished so much at the end of ten years, it will require but a very short time to establish it; but there is every evidence that we have almost completed the object for which we were first organised. All we have to do is to increase our efforts and to continue labouring as we have done, with the same energy which we have hitherto manifested. I have been to medical banquets before, but there was always something wrong. Now here there is nothing wrong, except, perhaps, the tobacco smoke—but I am not in a very good humour to-night. I am speaking to you as one of the oldest members; I was in at the birth of the organisation, and I hope I shall continue every now and then to renew my life with a fit of sickness, and I expect to be here and to be able to speak to you encouragingly of the future, which there is no question at all about. From my own city there are several who intended to be here who are not here; they will be very sorry for it, but they know it requires money to come to New York. One gentleman said, when they come here they do n't want to go away; but some of them cannot go away without borrowing from their neighbours.

Gentlemen, it is a very great honour to be here as one of your ex-presidents. I never had a greater honour conferred on me in my life. Recently they conferred some honour on me from another quarter, but it was very tame compared with being here to-night. I hope that next year we may meet again in as good health and spirits as to-night; that the Association will not be eight hundred but twelve hundred—there will certainly be a thousand at our next meeting. The fees are small; as soon as it is very much larger we can have a banquet every year; but, as I said before, New York is a terrible place without you have money. '

Thanking you very kindly for the privilege of saying these few things, I hope we shall meet again, not at a banquet probably, but at the Association, with our numbers increased, next year. [Applause.]

TOAST-MASTER—The next toast in order is,—

The Guests of the Association:
The heartiest greeting and the warmest welcome attend the eminent labourers in the field of medicine who are here from distant regions to contribute their quota of wisdom and learning.
May these honoured brothers again assemble, to join in the debates and convivialities of the next decennial meeting.

Before I call upon the first to respond to this toast, I wish to present this communication, which was handed to me as I came into the room this evening, from one who was with us this afternoon and who intended to be with us this evening, but was called away by a message telling of the illness of a member of his family:

"NEW YORK, October 11, 1893.

"*Dear Dr. Ferguson:*—You will kindly tender to the brethren my great regret at being suddenly called away. The meeting has been a great success, and I wish you every possible degree of prosperity in your devotion to the science and practice of our noble profession.

"Sincerely yours,
"J. A. GRANT."

Our brothers from over the Canadian border are always welcome. The brotherhood may not be entirely complete, but it is a little closer than through Adam, although we may not have succeeded in destroying that little difference which exists between us—a simple geographical line. We recognise that we have with us a worthy representative of the nation of which Sir James is a member, and we feel very happy that time and tide have brought him to us this evening. We have watched his wanderings through our country for some little time back, and we have all been happy to have him with us; we have all been proud of the service that he has rendered to humanity and to the medical profession during the last few months he has sojourned in the United States.

We will now be very happy to listen to Mr. Ernest Hart, in response to the toast,—

The Guests of the Association:

Mr. HART.—*Mr. President and Gentlemen:* With you, I greatly deplore the absence of our esteemed friend (I will say my dear old friend), Sir James Grant. It seems particularly unfortunate, for I came through

Canada last year, and the same accident prevented me from meeting him. He is always welcome with us in England. The toast-master said he deplored the difference separating Canada from the United States. I shall only call to mind, without recounting it, the old story of the coloured preacher, who, in referring to a little difference of a certain kind, said, "Thank God for the difference!" We are delighted at the resemblance, but we are not altogether sorry that they do not confound us with one another, but allow us to enjoy a reciprocal friendship, which is all the more delightful for the difference which exists.

As to myself, I can only say that it affords me, as you may suppose, peculiar delight to be here, quite accidentally, through the courtesy of the President, at this meeting of this Association, which I only heard of late last night. I feel that the bonds of friendship, the indissoluble ties of common interest and common objects, which unite the association of which I have the honor to be an humble representative, the British Medical Association, with this Association, that those ties are such that I reproach myself that we have not until now taken steps to render that connection closer, and make our opportunities for meeting—as I hope they will be henceforth—more numerous, and professionally more important. The principles which led to the formation of this Association, and the principles which from the first actuated the British Medical Association and which have strengthened it and led it to its present degree of prosperity, are precisely, sir, those which underlie the formation of this important Association, and undoubtedly they are those also which led this Association to such distinguished and rapid prosperity. It has been my custom, but still not altogether without thought a part of my duty, in speaking to bodies of professional brethren here, to refer to those points of professional faith which animate our association, to those principles which guide us, to those rules which bind us, to that discipline which keeps us in order, and to those ethical rules which we think are not only important for us individually, are not only important for the whole profession, but are at least as important to our respective countries and to the general public whose interests we serve.

Now it seems to me that no man can refer to any great principle strongly without meeting with some opposition, but, for myself, I cannot but feel delighted that the addresses in which it has been my duty to make observations as to the validity of the old code, as to its ethical soundness, as to its vast service to the profession, and as to its great importance to the nation,—I cannot help feeling delighted-that they met with such unanimous concurrence, or, at least, with almost absolutely no dissension at Washington from the great representative audiences from every part of the country to whom they were delivered. And I cannot help feeling satisfied, as I feel that it must be satisfactory to this Association, which has made sacrifices so great on behalf of the code; I cannot help feeling gratified that in every great city of America, in every great medical centre which I have had the opportunity of not only visiting but of conversing with all the leading members of the profession,—at Baltimore, at Philadelphia, and at Detroit—I have never heard one person who raised his voice against it. I believe there is a small faction in this city (at any rate it is not an important factor), which, I am delighted to find, is opposed by the whole body of the profession in the United States of America.

I can say that because, in the course of recent peregrinations, through the generosity of Uncle Sam, I have been addressed by the university representatives in every medical centre in the East and West on the subject, who have always taken occasion to testify to their strong and unanimous acceptance of these principles. There has been one solitary exception; but there is no rule without an exception, and often the exception is the best expression of the rule.

As to this society and its future, sir, I am reminded of a statement by one of the old examiners of our London corporation. He was examining a student, and said, "Well, what are you going to give? What are you going to do?" and the student gave some elaborate prescription. "Yes," said the examiner, "that is a very good prescription. Is there anything else?" and the student gave another, still more elaborate. "Well," said he, "is there anything else?" and the student exhibited his whole pharmacopoeia. "My dear sir," said the examiner, "you have left out the most important part,—give her time." And so I say of this Association. It started with principles that are impregnable in their strength. It has started on a straight course, with a clear objective point; with all the means, with all the determination, and with all the knowledge necessary to attain that end. It needs nothing more than a gradual development of the normal prosperity, a firm hold, and a firm determination not only to adhere to the principles but to propagate them everywhere.

We, like you, have a volunteer body, whose motto is "Defence, not Defiance." That is a very good motto, but, for myself, I am not a fighting man. I have lived a life of peace, and never fight unless I am compelled to. I prefer the motto of our Scotch friends, "Nemo me impune lacessit." That, gentlemen, is a motto which you might well unite with your motto, "Defence, not Defiance."

I thank you, gentlemen, for the unexpected privilege of being here to-night, and I can assure you, that if on our side of the water the British Medical Association, or any of its eighteen thousand members, can do anything to show their respect and affection to the members of this Association, I know I am authorised to speak for them, and to say that it will be a delight to convert mere words into any form of action that may be most acceptable or agreeable to you. [Applause.]

TOAST-MASTER.—The idea of the marine residence of each of the first two speakers has just suggested to my mind that I can state that the gentleman whom I am about to call upon to continue in response to the toast, "The Guests of the Association," also has a marine residence, and it is a curious fact, which only a little time ago came to my observation, that great as is the tonnage that floats on the waters of the Mersey, still greater is the tonnage that floats on the waters of the Detroit river. We will now be happy to listen to Dr. Donald McLean, of Detroit.

Dr. McLEAN.—*Mr. President, Toast-Master, and Gentlemen:* I was really shocked and seriously frightened this afternoon when I was informed, by himself, that my friend, Sir James Grant, would not be able to be here; because, knowing him as I do and as most of you do, I felt sure that this toast would be in good hands as long as he was here. I was not aware that I had another and equally—to say the least of it—able ally in my friend, Mr. Hart. Therefore I felt somewhat relieved, and I now feel that the dignity of this great toast has been fully taken care of, and that, so far as I am concerned, I am a free lance and at liberty to treat the matter in any way that I please.

I thank the Toast-Master for the very kind and complimentary, and no less truthful, reference he has made to the city in which I live. It is a very curious fact, and an interesting fact, which I am always delighted to show my friends from across the water, when I take them to the banks of the Detroit river and tell them that they can sit there on any one spot, from the first of May to the first of December, and see, on an average, one great ship pass every three minutes, night and day; that the tonnage passing through the Detroit river exceeds that of the Mersey, exceeds that of London, exceeds that of New York and Baltimore and Boston combined. Whether I treat this toast respectably or not, you will understand, at all events, that I come from a respectable city. [Laughter.]

I am a great believer in medical societies. Not that I think the scientific work done there amounts to so very much. It is often hurried, haphazard, and imperfect; for example, I came here to read a great paper, which I expected would take two or three days to discuss, and there was no discussion at all. Nevertheless, I am a believer in medical societies,—not so much, I say, from that point of view, as from the social, congenial, and convivial standpoint. [Cries of Hear, hear, hear!] I stand up for the medical societies that meet and do a little scientific work just for the appearance of the thing [laughter], wind up with a good, solid, convivial meeting afterward,—anything short of absolute intoxication; even that I would not object to if it was not for the effects the next morning.

I believe in concerted action, and my only hope for the future of the human race is in the medical societies and combinations, the concerted action of the medical profession; and I believe the best work of the medical profession is done as we are doing it now—on the occasion of a banquet.

I believe that there is a great future before the human race. In the words of the poet,—

"When I dip'd into the future far as human eye could see;
Saw the vision of the world, and all the wonders that would be."

And I see the time when things will be far different from what they are now: when, for instance, there will be no such thing as a marriage contract without the consent of the medical profession; when the breeding of the human race will be conducted on even more scientific principles than those now applied to the horse and dog. I look forward to the time when every detail of city arrangements—the pavements, the drainage, everything—will be arranged by the concerted action and the combined wisdom of the medical profession. I look forward to the time when every detail of dress, instead of being governed by idle and frivolous fashion, shall be determined by the scientific principles evolved from the wisdom of the medical profession. When that time comes, Mr. President, there will be no necessity any longer for armies or for navies, or for lawyers, or even for ministers; everything will be so arranged—arranged on such wise, such solid, such complete, plans and methods—that it will be absolute perfection. Then there will be realised the dream of the poet, the time when—

"'Till the war-drum throbb'd no longer, and the battle-flags were furled,
    In the Parliament of man, the Federation of the world!"

That time, I say, will come when the medical profession has control of everything. And when that time does come, my honest conviction is, that of the sections, the battalions, the regiments, of that great army, the wise, the brilliant, the generous, the hospitable, city of New York will be about the head of the affair. And when that time comes, God grant that I may find myself there, as I do to-night, ever your thankful, grateful guest. [Prolonged applause.]

TOAST-MASTER,—In continuing the responses to this toast, we will pass away from the waters of New York bay, from the near proximity to the roar of Niagara, beyond the busy scenes of Detroit, to the peaceful flow of the Ohio, at Cincinnati, and ask our guest, Dr. Dandridge, to make a response to the toast.

Dr. DANDRIDGE.—*Mr. President and Fellows of the Association:* I am sure that I feel very grateful indeed for this honour. The Toast-Master concealed from us the fact that the guests of the Association were expected to contribute of their knowledge, wisdom, and learning for this entertainment. Certainly if we had understood that this was expected of us,—I speak for others as well as for myself—we would certainly have felt that the task was a very appalling one. And if one contributes in any way to the success of the meeting, we certainly should feel that we are taking away very much more than we give. We have felt, I am sure, that we will return to our homes, not only with our scientific horizon very much enlarged, very much broadened, but, after the meeting to-night, after the opportunity that we have had to associate with and meet the Fellows of this Association, we will return to our professional work with what is, perhaps, more important, with enlarged ideas of the manhood of our profession. This, I think, is one of the great purposes of a meeting of this sort; and certainly, of all the meetings that I have attended, no meeting has fulfilled its purpose better than this decennial meeting. I am very thankful to you for the honour that you have given me, and the distinction which I feel that you have conferred upon me personally in making me a guest and a speaker here to-night. [Applause.]

TOAST-MASTER.—The next toast on the list is one in which, as poor doctors, we all may possibly take a personal interest.

The Charities of the State and City of New York.
May the Empire State ever continue her bountiful provision of shelter and sustenance for her wards—the poor, the maimed, and the sick.
May the city's liberality be as enduring, and through her enlightened commissioners may she always preserve her existing relations with the profession in the cause of higher medical education.

I will call upon Mr. Commissioner Porter to respond to the toast.

COMMISSIONER PORTER.—*Mr. President and Gentlemen :* There has been but one drawback to this delightful occasion to me, and that was when I was told that I was expected to respond to a toast, and such a toast! I am utterly incapable of doing justice to it. You certainly ought to have Chauncey Depew, or Joseph H. Choate, or some such individual; and I shall content myself with saying to you, gentlemen, that it has always given our board great pleasure to do what we could for the promotion of the interests of the medical profession, and we will do so as long as we are permitted to remain there. I hope you will excuse me from any further remarks, and to-morrow I expect to see you all on our steamboat, the *Minnehanonck.* I thank you for this honour. [Applause.]

TOAST-MASTER.—Another one of the commissioners of charities, who is also a Fellow of our Association, is present. We shall be very glad to hear from Dr. Simmons.

Dr. SIMMONS.—*Mr. Chairman and Gentlemen :* I came here to-night to occupy this seat of honour with the understanding that I would be entirely free to enjoy the banquet and not be called upon for a speech. I do not quite understand why the good faith was not kept. I prefer to make that condition, gentlemen, when I am invited to a dinner, that I am not to be called upon; but I do n't see how I can escape it now. I recognise the fact that I am called upon because I happen to be one of the commissioners. I do not know that I can say anything in regard to the charities of the city of New York that most of the profession do not fully appreciate and understand. Perhaps some who have not lived in the city, who have not received their medical education here, cannot fully appreciate and understand the extent of the charities of New York.

If they will consider that the board of charities and corrections representing the city of New York takes care of seventeen to eighteen thousand people constantly, furnishing them with everything that they need, from the smallest article used in the household to the largest; that it cares for all classes of people,—criminal, insane, paupers, almost every class that comes under the name of helpless—they will understand, perhaps, the great work that the city is doing. Very few outside of the medical profession appreciate the work that is done by physicians here in looking after and helping these people who come under the care of the commissioners. Our most distinguished physicians contribute gratuitously their best knowledge to the care of these unfortunates. The great majority of the seventeen thousand come under the care of a physician who gives his time and knowledge to their care. No other body of men, probably, in the land contributes so much to charity as the medical profession through the bureau of the department of charities and corrections. As Mr. Porter has said, the charities not only extend to the taking care of the sick, but also to everything in our power to help the medical profession and furnish them with clinical means through the hospitals for educating the many young men who come to the city to study in our medical schools, and we hope to-morrow to show the gentlemen who will honour us with a visit, something of the work that is done. I think that we can show it much better than we can speak of it.

TOAST-MASTER.—It has just occurred to me, that possibly the type-setter, in setting up the next subject, may have omitted a comma, because there is a distinction of idea in its use or omission. It is not always a fact that Law and Justice are one, but to-night we all feel and believe that they are, and not divorce them with a comma.

May the strong bond of union of the legal and medical professions be perpetuated, and further the ends of law and justice.

I will call upon Hon. Charles W. Dayton, first, to respond to the toast.

MR. DAYTON.—*Mr. President and Gentlemen:* The first speaker of the evening succeeded in robbing every other speaker of his principal point, namely, an apology. I was greatly interested in listening to the distinguished representative of the British Medical Association. To my lay mind it conveyed an import regarding this Association that did not exist before I heard him. In his polished English he conferred, in my judgment, as a representative of eighteen thousand associates, a compliment upon this Association and its scientific work well worthy of remembrance and commemoration.

I listened with peculiar gratification to the distinguished gentleman from Detroit, who, like myself, is a lover of that exquisite gem of Tennyson's, "Locksley Hall," but never did it occur to me that those beautiful lines could be woven into such a dream of the future as he portrayed. To think that every politician, to think that every clergyman, to think that every lawyer, is to be wafted into nebular space and only doctors left to rule the world, is one of the most appalling propositions that ever fell upon the minds of men. [Laughter and applause.] Why, sirs, if he had made that speech in Tammany Hall or in a Democratic convention, I do not know that he would have had time to get out of the place.

But seriously, gentlemen, I am not entirely inappropriate here. My grandfather on my mother's side was a physician, his son was a physician, my father studied medicine in Europe, and my brother is a physician. In the course of my life I have had to call upon physicians, and there is a reciprocity existing between myself and your profession that is as binding as any feeling that I can have toward my own profession. I recall, with both pleasant and sad memories, many hours of their attendance, and I often think of those hours with a mournful pleasure: how they, with tender hands and almost tearful eyes, have watched by the bedside of those I love, some of whom have passed to the beyond. And there is here to-night one of your number who stood at the bedside of my child as he went out from the world, and to him, and to you all, I pay the tribute of a man who knows you, who believes in you, and who believes that in your prosperity, in the increase in your scientific knowledge, in the glorious work in which you are engaged, there is no greater recompense, nothing that leads more to the benefit of mankind, than in your greater advancement from now on. [Applause.]

TOAST-MASTER.—The voice that I am about to call up now is not unfamiliar to the members of this Association, and very pleasant memories indeed are associated with it. In continuation of the last toast I will call upon Hon. C. H. Truax. [Applause.]

JUDGE TRUAX.—*Mr. President and Gentlemen :* It is with more than diffidence that I rise to address you; it is with fear and trembling. I fear and I tremble, because all through the dinner I have seen you doctors eye me with a professional eye. Did I drink of the rich red wine, Ferguson *looked gout ;* did I eat of the roast, Brockway said, "His liver is gone." I believe that each lay guest here has been invited for clinical purposes only, and I shall consider myself fortunate if I get away from here without being placed on the table instead of under the table, where a gentleman should be at this time of the evening. [Laughter.] I have no doubt that some of you will look at my tongue, some of you will feel my pulse, others of you will thump me, all of you prescribe for me, and all of you send in a bill.

It is written in the sixth section of the sixteenth chapter of the sixtieth book of the Talmud—or somewhere else—that the Jehovah, the Compassionate, the Merciful, gave to Satan, after the unfortunate and unsuccessful termination of the conflict with Job, the power of inflicting on the human race one great evil, and Satan, after mature deliberation, invented after-dinner speaking. Any of you who have attended three or four public dinners have realised the full force of his malignity, and if not, you probably will before I have finished. Our guest (or, your guest), Dr. Cronyn, remarked that New York was a dear place. It is a dear place, dear to a great many of us, but it shall not be dear to him to-night, for I think I can safely promise that after he has left this hall of festivity he may go where he wants to, and may do what he wants to, without any fear of anything more than a ten-dollar fine. [Laughter.] And if he shall feel that a ten-dollar fine is too much for him, perhaps we can arrange it for him so that he will have a holiday of ten days with his friends, the commissioners of charities and corrections, at their beautiful palace in the East river.

Mr. Hart referred incidentally to a little difference. He did not tell the story, nor shall I,—because I do not know it; that is a good reason for not telling a story—but his remark reminded me of the time when the ladies sent a committee to Washington to endeavor to induce congress to pass some law that would enable ladies to vote. Mrs. Claflin and her sister, Mrs. Woodhull, were on the committee. Mrs. Woodhull was *spokesman*. She turned to "Cock-eyed Ben" and she said, "What is the difference between you and me?" Ben twisted his eye a little toward her, and said, "I can't conceive." [Laughter and applause.]

Gentlemen, Medicine and Justice are kindred sciences, for Justice is a kind of moral medicine; that is, Justice bears the same relation, or a similar relation, to the moral body that Medicine does to the physical body. It is the object of the doctor to cure the physical body and keep it in health, while it is the object of the jurist to cure the body-politic and keep it in good condition. Perhaps Justice may be better compared to Surgery than to Medicine, for Justice cures by cutting off the diseased member of the body-politic. In the language of the sentiment attached to the toast, Justice endeavours to lessen the number of the unjust; but neither Justice nor Medicine is an exact science, for you doctors may at times diagnosticate wrongfully and apply the remedy for one disease when you should have applied the remedy for another disease. So we at times make a wrong diagnosis of our cases. This counts for nothing against either science, and but little against the individuals who apply the sciences. It grows out of the difficulty of ascertaining the exact facts of the case.

Nobody knows that better than a man who has been on the bench and has heard two doctors testify. [Laughter and applause.] It would require more than the wisdom of Solomon for any judge or jury to diagnosticate a case where you have an expert on one side testifying for his client, and another expert on the opposite side testifying for his client. I have sometimes been unable to determine whether the injured man had his back broken or had consumption. Such is the fallibility of human testimony. But I think it is the desire of your profession—as I know it is the desire of our profession—to deal exact justice to all, and I think we are members of the only two professions that do endeavour to deal exact justice. We diagnosticate the cases according to the best of our ability, and we apply the remedies, I think honestly and conscientiously, that we find the diseases need.

Gentlemen, I thank you very much for your kindness, not in calling upon me here to-night, for if you had not called upon me vital forces that I have used in addressing you would have been used in digesting what I have eaten; but I here express my willingness to dine with you at each one of your annual meetings for the next decade, or longer, provided you hold out. [Prolonged applause.]

Toast-Master.—The privileges which we may receive through Judge Truax are greater than we had anticipated: that the punishment for our offences might be lessened in the court; and then, possibly, the information to our friends out of the city might be held in the post-office through the courtesy of the post-master, who has favoured us with his presence. These are important facts.   We come to the last toast,—

The Press.

To this mighty engine Medical Science owes its great development and now looks for the diffusion and popularisation of preventive medicine. May the directors of the public Press never cease to instruct the people in the art of preventing disease.

I will call upon Dr. Charles A. Leale.

Dr. LEALE.—*Mr. President and Gentlemen:* Article I of the amended constitution of the United States informs us that congress shall make no law abridging the freedom of speech, or of the press, and now the press exerts a most powerful influence on all the doings of man.   In times of war the general is greatly aided by his war correspondent.   In the peaceful political congresses of nations the press is the medium whereby the laws and the results of arbitration are given to the public.   During epidemics the press conveys the news of danger, and at the congresses of religion the press gives to the humble and lowly the opportunities of reading the reports on the sublimest of human desires.

In medicine the press spreads broadcast the latest theories and the results of our efforts for the control of sickness and death.   In that special branch, preventive medicine, little can be done without the assistance of the press.   The press is everywhere, and at all times has its representatives on the alert to discover, record, and place before its readers accounts of all the affairs of men.   It demonstrates to the inhabitants of far distant countries their needs, both their good and their bad qualities, and with its cables encircling the world enables the peoples of both hemispheres either to join in one accord or leads contending armies on the battle-fields.

The greatest forward strides that have been made in the civilisation of the world began with the Toleration act, when the censorship of the press was abolished in 1695, and history informs us that it was to King William's merit that, fond as he was of power, he recognised the fact that he could not rule except so far as he carried the good will of the nation with him.

Among my family relics I found a copy of a New York paper published in 1783, showing the desires of its honourable editor.   "He hopes that gentlemen of ability and leisure will lend him their assistance.   Everything that has a tendency to improve the mind, reform the manners, promote literature, will be gratefully received."

Notwithstanding this lofty ambition of more than one hundred years ago, the press of to-day has advanced its illuminating power proportionally as much as the light of a wax candle is overcome by that of the incandescent carbon.   At this end of the century the editors, correspondents, and reporters of the press are recruited from the brightest and most learned of our college graduates, and I know of no better school for the qualified and ambitious young man than a proper connection on the staff of a first-class newspaper. There he is brought in contact with righteousness and sin, thrift and indolence, and has unusual opportunities to see the bright and dark sides of life. He sees the beneficence of preventive medicine, and by endeavours to solve the problem of man's highest aim, claims and receives our grateful thanks.

As president of St. John's Guild, an institution annually caring for more than 44,000 of the sick poor children and their weary mothers found in New York city, I speak with earnestness of the power of the press in aiding us to accomplish our great work of charity.

The thousands of well children whose lives are preserved by the Fresh Air Fund, the thousands visited in their abodes of sickness and toil, the thousands receiving the cup of cold water by the free distribution of ice in midsummer, attest the honourable desires of the press.

We can never forget the agitation of the press against the pollution of our Croton water, and that New York city now has one of the purest supplies of water on the continent. Our profession teaches us that to live well and be happy we must keep healthful, by having good air, pure water, wholesome food, proper raiment, healthful habitations, and the enactment of good laws.

TOAST-MASTER.—That, Mr. Chairman, completes the list of toasts, and ends my term of office.

REPORTS OF THE DISTRICT BRANCHES.

FIRST DISTRICT BRANCH.

The ninth annual meeting of the First District Branch was held at the Girvan House, Little Falls, on Thursday, July 20, 1893.

The meeting was called to order by the President at 11:30 a. m.

The minutes of the last meeting were read and approved.

The Treasurer then presented his report, which showed a balance of $2 in the treasury. The report was accepted and approved.

On motion, Dr. E. T. Rulison was elected a member of the Executive Committee in place of Dr. H. M. Leach, who had removed from the state.

The President then read his address, in which he urged the higher standard of medical education.

The following papers were then read, viz.:

"Cholera, Historical and Aetiological," by Ezra Graves, M. D., of Montgomery county.

"A Case of Foreign Body in the Air Passages," by C. H. Glidden, M. D., of Herkimer county.

"Indigestion," by W. D. Garlock, M. D., of Herkimer county.

"Some Remarks on the Male Catheter and Mode of Introduction into the Bladder," by Douglas Ayres, M. D., of Montgomery county.

"Forty-eight Operations on the Uterine Cervix for Lacerations," by J. B. Harvie, M. D., of Rensselaer county.

"Recurring Uterine Polypus, with Fungous Degeneration of the Endometrium," by W. H. Robb, M. D., of Montgomery county.

"Concerning Medical Ethics," by E. T. Rulison, M. D., of Montgomery county.

"Appendicitis," by R. N. Cooley, M. D., of Oswego county.

"A Case of Extra-Uterine Pregnancy," by E. D. Ferguson, M. D., of Rensselaer county.

The papers were well received, and generally discussed.

Through an assessment on the members present, the sum of $8 was raised for the Treasurer.

The next regular meeting was appointed to be held at Amsterdam, on the call of the President and Secretary.

On motion, the present Secretary was continued in office, and the Executive Committee, with the change before noted.

Adjourned.

R. N. COOLEY, *President.*
EZRA GRAVES, *Secretary.*

SECOND DISTRICT BRANCH.

The ninth annual meeting of the Second District Branch of the New York State Medical Association was held in Saratoga Springs, at the Worden hotel, on Thursday, June 22, 1893.

The meeting was called to order by the President, Dr. J. C. Hannan, at 11 a. m.

Thirty-two members registered.

The address of welcome was made by Dr. T. B. Reynolds, of Saratoga Springs.

After the President had delivered his address, the scientific work was taken up.

Dr. W. W. Seymour read three papers,—

1. "Case of Vaginal Extirpation of the Uterus; recovery. Death from recurrence."

2. "A Case of Coeliotomy during quiescent stage of Recurrent Appendicitis; recovery."

3. "Three Cases of Cholecystotomy, two for gall-stones, with remarks on surgery of the gall-ducts."

Remarks on Cholecystotomy were made by Drs. E. D. Ferguson and D. J. Fitzgerald.

Dr. W. H. Hodgman reported an interesting case of floating kidney in a girl nineteen years old.

Her condition was discussed by Drs. E. D. Ferguson and D. W. Houston.

Dr. J. B. Harvie gave a report of "Forty-eight Operations on the Uterine Cervix for Laceration."

Remarks were made by Dr. Hodgman.

Dr. Hodgman presented two cases in which there was delayed union of bones. The first was a fracture of the radius in two places. The fracture was put in splints for four weeks, but resulted in no union. The bones were rubbed, splints applied again for two weeks; still they did not unite. The fractured bones were then wired together, and union resulted. The second case was a comminuted fracture of both bones of the leg. Reduced, and put in plaster of Paris for four weeks. No union. The bones were rubbed, and the limb again put in plaster of Paris for three weeks. Still no union. The bones were then wired, and union resulted.

Discussed by Drs. Van Vranken and Harvie.

Dr. Swan read an interesting paper on "Inversion of the Uterus, with recurrence and method of holding it in place."

Remarks were made by Dr. J. B. Harvie.

Dr. Ferguson read "An Additional Note in the Treatment of Exophthalmic Goitre."

Remarks were made by Drs. Houston and Palmer.

30

Dr. Ferguson then reported some very interesting recent surgical operations.

Dr. D. W. Houston read two papers,—

1. "Appendicitis; operation; recovery."
Remarks were made by Drs. Hammer, Harvie, and Ferguson.

2. "Remarks on Sterilisation in Relation to Surgical Operations." Discussed by Drs. Hodgman, Finder, Harvie, and Hammer.

Dr. Finder's paper on "Some Outlines on Vaccination" opens up a good field for investigation.

Dr. Rogers read a paper on "Cholera and Quarantine."

The Committee on Nominations was appointed by the chair, to consist of Drs. Ferguson, Fitzgerald, Hammer, Hodgman, and Van Vranken.

An assessment of fifty cents was made upon each member present, for the Secretary's expenditures.

The Association received an invitation from Mr. Franklin W. Smith to visit his Pompeii.

On motion of Dr. Ferguson, a vote of thanks was to be sent to Mr. Smith for his kind invitation, and if the Association had the time, the members would accept.

A vote of thanks was also tendered to the members of the Committee of Arrangements, the physicians of Saratoga, and the managers of the Hotel Worden and its employés, for the kind manner in which the members of the Association were entertained.

On motion of Dr. Ferguson, it was voted that when the Association adjourned it be to meet on the last Thursday in June, 1894, at Troy, N. Y.

On account of the meeting of the American Medical Association in San Francisco, Cal., it was thought best to have the meeting of the Second District Branch of the New York State Medical Association a little later, and the date was finally left to the president and secretary.

The following were appointed the Executive Committee, in accordance with the report of the Nominating Committee:

L. B. Rulison, M. D., Albany County.
J. W. Lockwood, M. D., Columbia County.
O. A. Holcomb, M. D., Clinton County.
C. A. Church, M. D., Essex County.
George Conkling, M. D., Green County.
W. H. Nichols, M. D., Rensselaer County.
C. S. Grant, M. D., Saratoga County.
Charles Hammer, M. D., Schenectady County.
H. F. Kingsley, M. D., Schoharie County.
D. J. Fitzgerald, M. D., Warren County.
John Lambert, M. D., Washington County.

The new Executive Committee had an informal meeting at once, and selected the present Secretary for the ensuing year.

J. C. HANNAN, *President.*

J. E. BAYNES, *Secretary.*

The ninth annual meeting was called to order at 11 a. m., at Bundy Hall, Elmira, on Thursday, June 22, 1893, by the President, Dr. N. Jacobson.

The attendance was not large, the register showing thirty-one members, visitors, and guests present.

The reading of the minutes of the eighth annual meeting at Oswego was postponed.

The Secretary, on behalf of the Committee of Arrangements, stated that there was very little to report aside from that which the programme set forth. He would call attention to the hour for dinner; i. e., at 1:30 p. m., at the Rathbun House, and stated that it was the desire that all present, both members and invited guests, should be on hand at that hour and take dinner together.

The reading of the President's address was deferred until the afternoon session.

There were no reports from delegates to other Branches, and the Secretary for the Executive Committee read his report of their last meeting, which was accepted by the Association.

Dr. C. L. Squire, as Treasurer, then reported the amount in the treasury as a balance at the last meeting, $10; received by the Chairman of the Registration Committee, $10, making the total fund in the hands of the Treasurer, $20, and the amount of the bills presented and audited by the Executive Committee, $20.50. The report was adopted.

There was no report of special committees, and no unfinished business.

Dr. C. L. Squire made the suggestion that the date of the annual meeting be changed from June to May. The latter month seemed to him for many reasons the better month for the meeting, one reason being the cooler weather of May.

Dr. J. G. Orton made a motion, which was adopted, that the Secretary notify the parent Association through the Secretary that hereafter the third Thursday in May is the date selected by this District for its meetings, and asking that the change be duly made.

Dr. C. L. Squire moved that Dr. Orton be appointed by the Association to draft a suitable article, which should be a memorial to the late Dr. Caleb Green of Homer, and to present the same at the meeting of the State Association this fall; carried.

Dr. Lester moved that the chairman appoint a committee of three members to draft resolutions of condolence and sympathy, conveying the feelings of this Association towards Dr. Didama, in the loss he has sustained by the death of Dr. Nivison, his daughter; carried. The chairman appointed Drs. Lester, Brooks, and Ross as such committee.

From the counties represented at the meeting the following Nominating Committee was named, viz., Drs. Stephenson, Smelzer, Lester, Hills, Ross, and Brooks.

The Association then began the scientific work of the session by listening to a paper by Dr. LeRoy J. Brooks, entitled "Some Observations Concerning Underground Water Currents."

This paper grew out of some study between surface and deep-water currents, and other sanitary matters in and about Norwich, N. Y., as observed by the author. The first part of the paper described the surface of the valley in which Norwich is located, a description of the creeks, and general direction of surface drainage of the land. He described the bed of an old water-way which had been filled in, and which was now built upon, and thought to be the most desirable location for houses in Norwich. He then described the underground formations or layers, consisting of loam, gravel, clay, gravel-clay, or rock. The great beds of loam were in the old water-course as filling. It was of greatest depth in this place, and was much longer moist than the more gravelly soils. The upper layers of clay were not continuous, but broken asunder and separated in many places by the gravel beds above and below. The lower clay or rock bottom often inclined in the exact opposite direction to the inclination of the surface of the land overlying it. Sometimes there would be interruptions in the surfaces of the deep clay or rocks, which would deviate the water currents from one direction to another quite opposite. The underground currents are of varying sizes, and of slow or rapid motion according to the inclination of the bottom clay or rock formation. The irregularity of the impervious clay surfaces forms deep cesspools, in which refuse accumulates and decomposes, and from which evaporation may take place into dwellings. Experimental wells and cesspools were made in various districts, and tar water and crude oil used in them, and the same articles were found to have reached the bottom of other wells at 300 to 500 feet away in a very short time, and not to be found in others that were nearer by, owing to the break in the clay beds which allowed the charged water to sink in the gravel between the clay basins. The paper was illustrated by many drawings representing these observations. Cellar walls will turn underground water currents. As a conclusion, the doctor held that the mere surface water, if running and exposed to oxidation, was the purer water, and that the deeper waters were often the cause for disease.

DISCUSSION.

Dr. Smelzer, of Havana, said he lived in a village located in a valley situated something as Norwich. Well water is the only supply which we have. In 12 years there has been no typhoid fever and no diphtheria from that cause. It seems to me that well water is not the cause in as many instances as has been supposed.

Dr. Orton, of Binghamton, said, that 15 years ago, while he was on the State Board of Health, he had to examine into matters concerning some severe diarrhoea troubles in and about Binghamton. It was thought that the cause was the water in the public wells, and that they were made impure by the river into which the drainage from the State Insane Hospital emptied. Experts examined the water in the wells and in the river. It was found that the water from the river did not enter the wells. When the experts reported, they said that the water from the wells was pure. When it became necessary to take water from the river, the disease the same day began to stop, which would seem to show that the wells were still in' some way at fault, but in the out districts not supplied by wells, the disease stopped the same day also. So the wells might not have been at fault.

Dr. Jacobson, of Syracuse, said that ten years ago the examinations of water were made by the chemists, now by chemists and bacteriologists. Several examinations of well water in Syracuse had been made and pronounced pure by chemists, and when examined by the microscope, pronounced not pure. It was not safe to examine by chemical processes alone, but also by the microscope.

Dr. Brooks, in closing, said that it would take too much time to examine the details of experiments. He would say that one of his test wells was driven 200 feet deep, and yet he could through it detect impurities in other wells at greater or less distances.

Dr. Elias Lester read a paper upon the subject, "Some Chronic Forms of Malarial Poisoning." This was a very interesting paper, in keeping with the former on account of the remarks of the author before the reading, by giving a short description of the soil and sub-soil in his district. The author maintained that the condition of malarial poisoning may go on for years, and not show itself until the system is disturbed by some other cause, such as traumatism. Injuries in subjects of malarial poisoning do not heal well. There are some symptoms of the poisoning which he places much reliance upon. One is the pain in the spine between the shoulders.

DISCUSSION.

Dr. Orton remarked that he believed the poison could be stored up in the system of the patient, and show itself in the way which the reader had stated. He knew instances where wounds did not heal until quinine in two or more grains had been given three or four times a day.

Dr. Lester said, in closing, that the symptoms which he had attributed to the poisoning could and had been prevented by the use of quinine given to subjects passing through the Isthmus of Panama, while others contracted the disease by not taking the quinine.

Dr. E. G. Drake, of Elmira, read a paper on the subject, "When shall We Operate?" This was a complete and comprehensive paper, covering the ground upon which the surgeon is often in a dilemma. One of the examples mentioned near the close of the paper called up the subject, pro and con, in relation to appendicitis. At this point of the meeting, Dr. Squire moved that the invitation of the Association be extended to Dr. LeRoy W. Hubbard, of New York, who is present as our guest at this meeting, and to the other visitors and guests present, that they also be invited to take part in the discussion. The motion was carried.

Dr. Hubbard, of New York, said,—We may now be in a surgical craze. There is a rush to operate, because the results of modern surgery are so brilliant. Even those operations which were condemned before are undertaken, without a word in comment, other than to have a record for numbers,—to say that we have had a hundred cases, etc., leaving out the question of recovery and results. I think it may be said that we are beyond the laparotomy craze. What are the results to look back upon? There are a good many women going about to-day deprived of the chances of maternity, owing to the removal of ovaries which should not have been removed. Therefore there is no subject so important as this. I see this in my line, viz., that of orthopaedic surgery. I came from Bellevue hospital drilled in surgical work. I thought that the old rule— "When we see pus, let it out"—must always apply. I entered the Orthopaedic hospital, and found quite a different state of feeling in this matter. The best results followed the non-surgical treatment. I thus learned that rest and mechanical support will give nature the best relief, and soon the functions will be restored.

While I fear that we may be rushing along too much in the manner of a craze in most instances, in respect to the disease appendicitis, I do not believe this to be the case, and think that the operation should be done. I have known of some examples where delay was fatal. A young physician in a Philadelphia hospital was taken down, and, notwithstanding he was in the midst of the best surgical help, he was allowed to go day by day until his case was beyond relief.

Dr. Brooks, of Norwich, said,—The question is to be decided, in my mind, largely by the question of temperature. If it remains low, do not operate; if high, operate.

Dr. Lester, of Seneca Falls, said,—The physician should not be concerned about "When to operate" as much as *Who* should operate? As far as he was concerned, he thought that only those who were properly educated should operate.

Dr. Jacobson, of Syracuse, said,—I do n't think there can be a more important question raised. All the pathological conditions show that the appendix was primarily involved, and the lesions all of a serious character. The comma bacillus has a more active part in the production of the disease than all the twists, concretions, etc. The temperature should not be a ground for deciding the local conditions. The character of the pulse is a more reliable symptom. The danger of general peritonitis is great. One day there may be no rise of temperature; next day, all the signs of peritonitis. Jacoby's words express the proper thing, "Timely, not early." We cannot depend upon the percentage of cases that recover without operation; we never can know this. When the percentage of recoveries is as great as ninety per cent. from the operation, we should not fear to operate. The general practitioner is the one to do the operation: there is danger in waiting for a surgeon to arrive. In those cases where great tenderness and fever continue for thirty-six hours, I should operate. In all recurrent cases the operation should be performed during the intervening period.

Dr. F. W. Ross, of Elmira, said,—I have seen a number of cases operated upon; have seen others recover. I heard Dr. Jacobson's paper at the meeting in New York. My own opinion is on the side of timely operation. It is not good for pus to form. It may not wait for you to evacuate it. No credit can come to conservative surgery in waiting for such an event.

Dr. Drake, in closing, said,—There are two things which should be borne in mind by the general practitioner: First, he should investigate the matter, and witness the operations of surgeons as often as he has the chance. Specialists make mistakes, but even the worst mistakes, when they are witnessed, educate the general practitioner. The second thing is, to operate. Having witnessed these operations by the specialist, the general practitioner seldom permits himself to run the risk of the charge of misjudgment. His mistakes in the line of operation are fewer than those of the specialist.

Dr. Lester said he did not wish to say that he would send a case of hernia or appendicitis to the specialist, but those greater operations, where time need not be taken into account. Those he thought best to send to the places where preparations are at hand to do the operation with neatness and cleanliness.

Dr. N. Jacobson, of Syracuse, reported a case of tumor of the bladder, which he removed. Recovery was perfect, and the bladder could contain a pint of water after the operation. Had healed without fistula by the supra pubic operation.

Dr. Moroney, of Elmira, in discussing this paper, said,—I have a case very much of the same clinical history as that reported by Dr. Jacobson. The case is one of interest. What the results will be without operation are yet to be told. He was interested in the paper, as it assists materially in giving hope for the case if it should come to an operation.

Drs. Drake and Ross were both interested in the case of Dr. Jacobson, on account of a case where fistula formed and remained until death, as the result of the operation.

At this point the Association adjourned to the Rathbun House for dinner.

AFTERNOON SESSION.

The following report of the Nominating Committee was read and accepted:

At a meeting of the Nominating Committee, appointed during the morning session of the ninth annual meeting of the Third District Branch, the following members were present:

Dr. Stephenson, Onondaga County.
Dr. Smelzer, Schuyler County.
Dr. Lester, Seneca County.
Dr. Hills, Broome County.
Dr. Ross, Chemung County.
Dr. Brooks, Chenango County.

Dr. Smelzer, as clerk of the committee, reported for that body the names of the Executive Committee for the ensuing year, as follows:

Dr. J. H. Chittenden, Binghamton.
Dr. W. R. Laird, Auburn.
Dr. F. W. Ross, Elmira.
Dr. F. W. Higgins, Cortland.
Dr. W. B. Morrow, Walton.
Dr. H. D. Didama, Syracuse.
Dr. J. K. Leaning, Cooperstown.
Dr. H. C. Lyman, Sherburne.
Dr. B. T. Smelzer, Havana.
Dr. Elias Lester, Seneca Falls.
Dr. W. L. Ayer, Oswego.
Dr. W. M. Fitch, Dryden.
Dr. M. Cavana, Oneida.

The place of meeting, Syracuse, N. Y.

Dr. LeRoy W. Hubbard read a paper on the subject, "Early Diagnosis on Chronic Diseases of Joints." In this paper the author wished to show the importance of early recognising joint diseases, before lesions of a serious character were observed. He pointed out some early signs of disease of the larger joints, as well as some of the early signs of spinal bone disease. He objected to the severer measures of manipulation, and depended much upon gentle manipulation and observation of slight "muscular reflex" as a very important sign. In the diseases which, if left to a later stage before diagnosis is made, result so badly from treatment, if discovered early, the results are much better from treatment than could be expected from some less important disease by old treatment. In other words, the maximum is reduced by early diagnosis to less than the minimum of the old results. A brief outline was given for the diagnosis of diseases of the spine, hip, knee, and ankle joint. The paper was one of interest, and full of good suggestions.

Dr. F. W. Ross, of Elmira, read a paper on "Aspiration, and Injection of Iodoform in Chronic Synovitis." Three cases reported by the author were all successful in not aggravating the disease in any way, and resulted in a more rapid cure than could have been expected from any other plan of treatment. The operation must be done, of course, under great attention to cleanliness of instruments, skin of patient, and hands of operator. The initial rise of temperature amounts to nothing. Aspiration of the synovial cavity should be done as surely as in cases of pleural cavity, and be followed by as good results. Any form of retaining splint, to keep the joint at rest, is as good or better than the plaster of Paris used by most surgeons. The opening must be closed by paste or collodion.

Dr. C. L. Squire, of Elmira, read a paper on "Spinal Arthropathy," as a preface to the report of a case of Charcot's knee of three years' standing. The paper was accompanied by photographs of the diseased limb. One, a front view, showed the patient standing, the left knee diseased. The other was a back view of the patient, standing, with the left knee dislocated.

Discussion of the above subjects was not generally entered into by the members. Dr. Hubbard closed the subjects of diseases of the joints in general, aspiration, and injection of joints with iodoform mixtures, and lastly, the subject of neuropathic arthropathy in a well chosen and masterly manner.

The President's address, delivered by Dr. Nathan Jacobson, was the next paper read.

After thanking the Fellows for the honour conferred upon him personally, he spoke a word in commendation of the union of physicians into societies for scientific research. Medicine occupies a rather unique position among the professions. In the case of the attorney, certain principles are at stake. He is judged only by the manner in which he conducts his case,—his knowledge, his logic, and his thoroughness all go to make up his professional ability.

, The field of operation of the clergy is also in full view. He moulds religious thought, and his power is felt in the swaying of his congregation which is impressed by his views, and his convictions are most firmly stamped upon their minds, and it is possible to appreciate how nearly he approaches the ideal.

Not so with the physician. There is no judiciary to pass upon the character of his work, as in the case of the attorney; nor is it possible to determine a medical man's worth by the public estimate of him, as in the case of the clergy. The public cannot follow the means, but judge of the results of treatment. If it be a happy one, the results are praised; be the end otherwise,—it matters little how skilful the management—the physician is frequently blamed. Credit is often given where none is deserved, and censure follows when praise should have been bestowed. Let us judge of ourselves. We are, as Holmes says, our *real selves*, which only our Maker knows; or we are as we think ourselves to be, which often assumes greater proportions than He could justify; or we may be as we are seen by the public, which may be at our disadvantage, save in the esteem of our professional brethren. For them to be able to judge him requires a long and varied acquaintance. This is to be done by association with him at the bedside, in private life, and in medical societies. The opportunity of the society is open to all. Not all can have hospital or college appointments. There may be many barriers in the way of early attainment of a lucrative practice, which must be lived down. The motives of the public may not be understood in the selection of a medical attendant, but it cannot be changed and must be endured. Inordinate ambition may impel him to disregard medical ethics. Quackery and pretension, however, are of mushroom growth. But all this simply confirms the statement, that the popular estimate of a physician is not the true estimate of his worth. In the medical meeting the situation is changed; here the physician is appreciated for what he is. His scientific contribution reflects his study and works. His deeds are judged by a body of his peers. Dr. Jacobson urged the young physician to become actively interested in the work of medical societies. Pathology, bacteriology, and physiology are all departments in which young men have done, and will continue to do, brilliant work.   The history of medicine shows that these departments have been explored by young men.   Short histories of many young men in the profession were given, showing that some of the great advancements were made by young men.   The doctor said that it had been his intention to consider, in extenso, the tubercular affections of the genito-urinary tract, but the paper has already assumed such proportions that he could, at this time, but briefly refer to the sub- ject.   There is no structure from the prepuce to the supra renal capsules which may not be primarily affected.   In the remaining ten pages of the paper the writer reviewed the whole subject in an interesting and instruc- tive manner.   At the close of the paper, by motion of Dr. Brooks, a vote of thanks was extended to Dr. Hubbard and Dr. Jacobson for the inter- esting and valuable papers presented for this occasion.

Dr. Stephenson, of Syracuse, read a voluntary paper on the subject of "Melancholia," with reports of cases and treatment.   Dr. John Moro- ney was invited to read a short paper which he had on the subject of "Intubation of the Larynx."   He exhibited a new instrument, one of his own invention, which was claimed to possess many advantages over the O'Dwyer tubes. . No other papers or business being before the meet- ing, the Association adjourned.

N. JACOBSON, *President.*

C. L. SQUIRE, *Secretary.*

EXECUTIVE COMMITTEE.

A meeting of the Executive Committee, called for Wednesday, June 21, 1893, at 8 p. m., was not held, enough members not being present to organise.   A second meeting was called for 10 a. m. of the following day, at Bundy hall, the place of general meeting.

At this meeting of the Committee, the following members and alter- nates were present: Drs. Jacobson, Orton, Lester, Ross, Brooks, and Squire,—Dr. Jacobson the chairman.

Drs. Hills, Wales, and Smelzer were appointed Registration Committee for this ninth annual meeting of the Association.

Drs. Squire and Ross were appointed a Committee of Arrangements.

Bills were presented and audited as follows: For use of room, $7; for printing, $8; for postage, $5.50; total, $20.50.

An assessment of one dollar on each Fellow present was made, to defray the expenses of the session.

The Secretary announced the death of Dr. Caleb Green, and Dr. Jacob- son announced the death of Dr. Nivison, the daughter of Dr. Didama, a Fellow of the Association.

It was decided that some action should be taken during the session touching the above circumstances.

The bills audited were ordered paid, and the Secretary authorized to make such payments from the funds of the Association in his hands.

Adjourned.

C. L. SQUIRE, *Secretary.*

At a meeting of the new Executive Committee, held at Elmira on the close of the morning session of the annual meeting of the Third Branch, for 1893, the following members were present: Drs. Chittenden, Ross, Smelzer, Lester, and Dr. Stephenson representing Onondaga county.

On motion, Dr. F. H. Stephenson was elected Secretary of the Branch for 1894.

B. T. SMELZER, *Clerk.*

FOURTH DISTRICT BRANCH.

The ninth annual meeting of the Fourth District Branch was held at the rooms of the Genesee Valley Club, Rochester, Tuesday, May 9, 1893. The meeting was called to order at eleven o'clock a. m., by the President, Dr. Z. J. Lusk.

The minutes of the last meeting were read by the Secretary, and upon motion were approved.

President Lusk delivered the annual address, subject, "The Treatment of Intestinal Haemorrhage in Typhoid Fever, with Cases."

The Treasurer presented his annual report, showing receipts of $40.28, expenditures, $12.25; balance on hand, $28.03.

The Treasurer recommended that no assessment be levied this year.

Upon motion of Dr. E. M. Moore, the report of the Treasurer was received, filed, and approved.

Upon motion of the Secretary, it was voted to proceed with the scientific programme before adjournment.

Dr. J. Dunn, of Steuben county, presented a paper upon "Some Hints in Relation to the Application of the Plaster Jacket for Curvature of the Spine."

The paper was discussed by Drs. E. M. Moore, Chittenden, and O'Hare.

Dr. Goler, for the Committee on Arrangements, reported that at the close of the morning session all present were requested to partake of a lunch served in the adjoining room, upon the invitation of Dr. E. M. Moore, Jr.

President Lusk announced that immediately upon adjournment the members present from each county should appoint one Fellow to serve as a member on the Nominating Committee.

AFTERNOON SESSION.

The meeting was called to order by the President.

Dr. DeLancey Rochester, of Erie county, presented "A Résumé of the Treatment of Acute Follicular Tonsilitis," which was discussed by Drs. E. M. Moore, Goler, Young, and Townsend.

The Nominating Committee reported by Dr. Townsend, chairman, in favour of the following Executive Committee for the ensuing year:

Dr. James A. Stephenson, Alleghany County.
Dr. S. J. Mudge, Cattaraugus County.
Dr. R. T. Rolph, Chautauqua County.
Dr. A. H. Briggs, Erie County.
Dr. A. P. Jackson, Genesee County.
Dr. G. H. Jones, Livingston County.
Dr. G. W. Goler, Monroe County.

Dr. W. Q. Huggins, Niagara County.
Dr. J. H. Allen, Ontario County.
Dr. J. H. Taylor, Orleans County.
Dr. D. J. Chittenden, Steuben County.
Dr. Darwin Colvin, Wayne County.
Dr. A. G. Ellinwood, Wyoming County.
Dr. W. Oliver, Yates County.

Upon motion of Dr. Young, the report of the Nominating Committee was accepted and adopted.

Dr. G. W. Goler then presented two patients, showing the results of trephining.

The next paper was read by Dr. G. W. Goler, upon "The Uses of the Intra-Peritonaeal Iodoform Tampon."

The paper was discussed by Dr. E. M. Moore.

Dr. E. M. Moore then exhibited a number of very interesting pathological specimens, and discussed the subject of "Fracture of the Neck of the Femur."

The meeting then adjourned.

Z. J. LUSK, *President.*
WILLIAM H. THORNTON, *Secretary.*

FIFTH DISTRICT BRANCH.

The ninth annual meeting of the Branch was held at 315 Washington street, Brooklyn, on Tuesday, May 23, 1893. The morning session was called to order by the President, Dr. S. B. W. McLeod, at 11: 20 a. m. The Secretary read the minutes of the last meeting, which were approved.

The report of the Committee of Arrangements was read and approved- The Secretary announced that Drs. William Govan and A. D. Ruggles had been appointed to act with the Secretary as Registration Committee. The names of the invited guests and delegates from the Kings County Medical Association to this meeting were then read, and upon motion, they all were extended a cordial welcome and were invited to full privileges of the floor, as recommended by the Executive Committee.

The President next read his address. There were no reports of delegates to other branches.

There was no formal report from the Executive Committee, but the Secretary read their minutes for the year past.

The report of the Treasurer, in the form of his annual statement, was read, and upon explanation by the President that it, together with the detailed accounts, had been duly audited and found correct, it was approved.

Report of Special Committees was called for. The Secretary, as Committee on Necrology, announced officially the deaths of five Fellows for the year,—

Dr. F. U. Johnston,
Dr. W. D. Woodend,
Dr. Joseph Creamer,
Dr. J. H. Hunt,
Dr. W. R. Ballou.

The biographical sketches were then called for, and in the absence of three of the writers the Secretary read the sketches of the late Drs. F. U. Johnston, W. D. Woodend, and Joseph Creamer. As Drs. E. Potts and W. T. White had not yet presented their sketches and were not present, the Secretary was authorised by the meeting to receive all sketches on the deceased Fellows and refer them to the Committee on Necrology of the State Association for publication in the Transactions.

There being no unfinished or new business, the scientific business was taken up.

Dr. Edward R. Squibb read the paper of the morning on "Chloroform in 1893" (published in the *Ephemeris*, Vol. IV). Several valuable and interesting points were brought out and answered in the discussion by Drs. J. G. Truax, E. V. Delphey, and the reader. Upon motion, permission was granted to the reader to publish his paper as he preferred.

The next order of business was choosing a Nominating Committee to nominate members for an Executive Committee for the ensuing year. The Secretary called off the counties of the district in alphabetical order, and members present from each county nominated a member for their county to form the following Nominating Committee:

Dr. I. D. LeRoy, Dutchess County.
Dr. William McCollom, Kings County.
Dr. A. D. Ruggles, New York County.
Dr. J. O. Davis, Orange County.
None present from Putnam County.
      "   Queens County.
Dr. H. C. Johnston, Richmond County.
Dr. William Govan, Rockland County.
None present from Suffolk County.
      "   Sullivan County.
Dr. H. Van Hoevenberg, Ulster County.
Dr. H. E. Schmid, Westchester County.

This committee was requested to meet in the coming intermission, so that their report might be offered at the afternoon session.

On motion, adjournment was taken for lunch at 1:10 p. m.

The afternoon session was called to order by the President at 2:15 p. m., and the scientific business resumed by Dr. L. A. W. Alleman reading his paper on "The Prevention of Blindness from Ophthalmia Neonatorum" (published in the *Brooklyn Medical Journal*, Vol. VII, p. 660).

Discussed by Dr. Lawrence Coffin, of Brooklyn (an invited guest), and Drs. T. H. Burchard, H. C. Johnston, and E. R. Squibb, and closed by the reader.

The second paper of the afternoon was by Dr. Edward J. Bermingham on "Chronic Nasal Catarrh, and what the General Practitioner Can Do for It." This was interestingly illustrated with an improved air pump and reservoir for the local application of medicaments, together with adaptations of the simple forms of burners and light, by means of reflectors and bull's-eyes to the special use. The trouble and care taken by the reader to make the subject plain and useful were fully appreciated by the meeting.

Discussed by Drs. Robert Newman, T. H. Burchard, E. R. Squibb, and closed by the reader.

Dr. Charles Phelps then read his paper on "The Treatment of Certain Forms of Fracture" (published in the *New York Medical Journal*, Vol. LVIII, p. 57).

Discussed by Drs. T. H. Manley, H. L. Taylor (invited guest), and closed by the reader.

Dr. A. B. Judson next read his paper on "The Management of Hip Disease" (published in the *New York Medical Journal*, Vol. LVII, p. 577).

Discussed by Dr. H. L. Taylor and Dr. Manley, and closed by the reader.

The final paper was offered by Dr. T. H. Manley on "The Aetiology, Clinical History, Symptomatology, Morbid Anatomy, Diagnosis, and Treatment of Gonorrhoeal Rheumatism or Arthritis" (published in the *American Journal of Medical Sciences*), which was read by title.

The Nominating Committee then made its report for members of Executive Committee, to represent

Dr. I. D. LeRoy, Dutchess County.
Dr. J. D. Rushmore, Kings County.
Dr. Robert Newman, New York County.
Dr. M. C. Conner, Orange County.
Dr. G. W. Murdock, Putnam County.
Dr. E. G. Rave, Queens County.
Dr. F. E. Martindale, Richmond County.
Dr. William Govan, Rockland County.
Dr. Wallie Lindsay, Suffolk County.
Dr. C. W. Piper, Sullivan County.
Dr. H. Van Hoevenberg, Ulster County.
Dr. H. E. Schmid, Westchester County.

On motion, the report was accepted and approved, and the Committee discharged.

The president then called a meeting of this new Executive Committee for immediately after adjournment, as provided by the by-laws, to elect a Secretary for the ensuing year; but as a quorum was seen not to be present, a meeting was not held.

A motion to adjourn was carried at 5 p. m., to meet one year from this date.

The Register recorded thirty-nine Fellows, two candidates for Fellowship, and two delegates from Kings County Medical Association present, together with some invited guests who failed to register.

S. B. W. McLEOD, President.
E. H. SQUIBB, Secretary.

EXECUTIVE COMMITTEE.

A called meeting of the Executive Committee was held at 315 Washington St., Brooklyn, on Tuesday, May 23, 1893.

In the absence of the President, Dr. S. B. W. McLeod, the Secretary called the meeting to order at 10:35 a. m.

Present: Drs. H. E. Schmid, M. C. Conner, William Govan, H. Van Hoevenberg, I. D. LeRoy, S. B. W. McLeod (later), E. H. Squibb.

Seven members present, seven absent (two deceased).

Upon motion, Dr. Van Hoevenberg was requested to take the chair until the arrival of the President.

The Secretary read the minutes of the last meeting, which were approved as read.

The Secretary reminded the members of the circular vote, dated January 18, 1893, to appoint a Committee of Arrangements for the ninth annual meeting, and announced the result of eleven in the affirmative, no vote from two, and one vacancy by death.

The report of the Committee of Arrangements was then read as follows:

REPORT OF THE COMMITTEE OF ARRANGEMENTS FOR THE ANNUAL MEETING, APRIL 29, 1893.

Your undersigned Committee beg leave to report that little work was necessary this year in making the necessary arrangements, as those of last year were so satisfactory that they have been exactly repeated, and the hour of 11 a. m. was decided upon for opening the morning session.

Respectfully submitted:

[Signed]
R. M. WYCKOFF, *Chairman.*
J. C. BIERWIRTH.
T. M. LLOYD.
WILLIAM MCCOLLOM.
GEORGE WIEBER.
S. B. W. MCLEOD, *President.* } *Ex-Officio.*
E. H. SQUIBB, *Secretary.*

April 29, 1893.

The Chair then appointed Dr. William Govan to act with the Secretary as Registration Committee, together with another Fellow from the general meeting later.

The Secretary, as the Committee on Necrology, reported the death of five Fellows of our district for the year past,—

Dr. F. U. Johnston.
Dr. W. D. Woodend.
Dr. Joseph Creamer.
Dr. J. H. Hunt.
Dr. W. R. Ballou.

The first two were members of this committee.

The following communication was then offered, and ordered spread on the minutes:

Mr. Chairman, since our last meeting we have sustained a great loss in the death of two of our number, Drs. F. U. Johnston and W. D. Woodend, both founders of our Association. They have long. represented their respective counties in this Committee, and show a good record in attendance. They have freely shared the responsibilities of furthering the welfare of the Branch, and have repeatedly given wise counsel, not only to the Committee itself at its meetings, but to the Secretary individually at other times. It is therefore fitting that we spread on the Minutes this slight expression of our esteem for them both, and our great loss in parting with them.

31

The Treasurer next read his itemized expense account for the year, and presented his annual statement as follows:

TREASURER'S ANNUAL STATEMENT, MAY 24, 1892, TO MAY 22, 1893.

Fifth District Branch New York State Medical Association,
with E. H. Squibb, Treasurer.

Dr.		*Cr.*	
To balance cash as per		By rent of meeting rooms	
statement May 24, 1892,	$123.51	for eighth annual meeting	$10.00
Assessments collected	30.00	Catering for eighth annual	
Interest collected	67.40	meeting	55.00
		Postage	10.00
		Stationery and printing	13.25
		Cash at interest	72.40
		Balance cash on hand	60.26
	$220.91		$220.91

PERMANENT FUND ACCOUNT.

Dr.		*Cr.*	
To total amount of fund		By investment in railroad	
as per statement May		bonds, 5 per cent. inter-	
24, 1892,	$1,090.00	est	$830.00
Contributions to fund to		Balance on hand at inter-	
date	50.00	est	310.00
	$1,140.00		$1,140.00

The cash book, statement, and vouchers were presented for verification, and the Chair named Dr. Conner to audit the accounts.

Upon motion it was then decided to hold the next (10th) annual meeting in Brooklyn, on the fourth Tuesday (22d) in May, 1894.

Under the head of unfinished business, the Secretary reminded the Committee, that as a quorum was not present when a meeting was called by the By-Laws last year to elect a Secretary, the present incumbent had held over.

Under new business, the following named gentlemen were announced as invited guests at the request of Dr. A. B. Judson:

Dr. C. Fayette Taylor, New York City.
Dr. H. L. Taylor, New York City.
Dr. J. C. Schapps, of Brooklyn.

Also the following Delegates from the Kings County Medical Association:

Dr. F. C. Raynor.
Dr. H. C. Riggs.
Dr. A. Wieber.
Dr. C. F. Barber.
Dr. R. H. Sullivan.
Dr. J. Scott Wood.

On motion, a cordial welcome was extended to all these gentlemen, and they were invited to full privileges of the floor.

The Secretary was next directed to look after the publication of all the papers offered, and to keep track of them until published.

The Treasurer was directed to send out the regular annual $1.00 assessment bills to all the Fellows of the District, except the subscribers to the Permanent Fund, extending the usual invitation to voluntarily join that Fund upon payment of $5.00, and thus be exempted from future assessments.. Those in arrears to the extent of $6.00 are not to be accorded this privilege until the arrears be paid up.

Upon motion, 21 Fellows who had recently joined were exempted from assessments for the ensuing year.

Dr. Conner, having examined the Treasurer's accounts, here reported that the vouchers corresponded with the items charged, and that the cash book was in good order. Upon motion for approval of the report, it was unanimously carried.

A motion to adjourn was carried at 11:03 a. m.

E. H. SQUIBB, *Secretary*.

NEW YORK COUNTY MEDICAL ASSOCIATION.

ANNUAL REPORT.

In presenting this report to be incorporated with the Transactions of the decennial meeting of the State Association, it may not be amiss to recall the following historical facts, viz.:

This County Association was founded at an informal meeting held December 14, 1883. At this meeting officers were elected, Dr. WILLIAM DETMOLD being the first President. The first meeting at which scientific exercises were observed was held in the College of Physicians and Surgeons, on January 14, 1884. Without interruption, regular monthly meetings have been held from that time to the present, except during July, August, and September, when, by the By-Laws, all meetings are suspended. What has been our success during this period of constant service, may better be left to our successors to determine. "Time proves all things," and may supply the best evidence that the work of the Association has not been in vain.

We hope that the recent change in the Constitution of the State Association, which permits the Local or County Associations to be represented by delegates therein, will be promotive of still greater efficiency—will enlarge the sphere of coöperation, and secure to the National Association an increased membership in consequence of the right we *now* possess of sending delegates directly thereto.

We can only present abstracts—some of them very brief—of the useful and excellent papers read and discussed during the past year. Many of them have been published in the various medical journals, and some of them in full in reprints therefrom.

PRACTICE OF MEDICINE.—At the meeting October 17, 1892, Dr. CHAS. A. LEALE read a paper on "Cholera, its Propagation and Treatment," and Dr. J. LEWIS SMITH on "Choleriform Disease in Infants and Young Children." At the same meeting, Dr. EDWARD K. DUNHAM addressed the Association on the "Bacteriological Diagnosis in the cases which have recently occurred in New York." This was illustrated by lantern demonstrations and specimens under the microscope.

November 21, Dr. J. MOUNT BLEYER read a paper on "Diet and Digestion, their Influence on the Voice," with observations useful to all voice users. Discussion by Drs. J. R. MacGregor, F. J. Quinlan, and T. H. Tyndale, closed by Dr. Bleyer, who illustrated the alcoholic voice by the phonograph.

On January 16, 1893, Dr. G. T. Hunter wrote on the subject of "Digestion and Digestive Ferments." His paper was discussed by Drs. Tyndall and Valentine, and was closed by Dr. Hunter.

At the meeting April 17, Dr. PEDRO J. SALICRUP read a paper on "Small-Pox and Vaccine," which was discussed by Dr. A. L. Gihon, U. S. Navy, by invitation, and by Drs. J. Lewis Smith, J. A. Campbell, and Antranig Ayvazian, and by Dr. Salicrup in closing.

On June 19, Dr. THOS. H. BURCHARD presented a paper on "Suspended Animation, its Pathology and Treatment." Discussion by Dr. J. B. White, and Dr. Burchard in closing.

SURGERY.—At the meeting March 20, 1893, Dr. STEPHEN SMITH's paper was on the subject of "Shot Wounds of the Orbital Region, and the Value of Girdner's Telephonic Bullet Probe in Locating the Ball." Discussed by Drs. Callan and Girdner by invitation, and by Drs. J. D. Bryant and N. J. Hepburn, being closed by Dr. Smith.

On May 15, 1893, Dr. SAMUEL E. MILLIKEN read his paper on "Diagnosis and Treatment of Hernia in Children." Discussion by Drs. Von Dönhoff, Erdman, Oberndorfer, and Truax, Dr. Milliken closing.

At the meeting June 19, 1893, Dr. VON DÖNHOFF presented a case of fracture of both bones of the forearm in a child, illustrating the advantage of abandoning fixed apparatus in fractures as soon as formation of protective calus had occurred.

GYNAECOLOGY.—November 21, 1892, Dr. JAMES STAFFORD presented a paper on "Cervical Dilatation," and exhibited and described a new instrument having a vagino-uterine curve. Paper was discussed by Drs. Geo. T. Harrison, H. J. Boldt, J. G. Truax, and S. B. W. McLeod, and discussion closed by Dr. Stafford.

On December 19, 1892, Dr. JAMES A. CAMPBELL's paper was on the "Conservative Surgery of the Uterus and Appendages," with description of cases. Discussion by Drs. Janvrin, Von Dönhoff, and Valentine, closed by Dr. Campbell.

On February 20, 1893, a paper was presented by Dr. SIMON MARX on "Cervical Incision," for the purpose of bringing prompt delivery in cases of eclampsia, concealed haemorrhage, and in other emergencies. Discussion by Drs. Van Ramdohr and Ettinger, and closed by Dr. Marx.

On May 15, 1893, Dr. EDWARD SANDERS presented a paper on "Chronic Oöphoritis, and Treatment by Electricity." Paper discussed by Drs. Newman, Tull, and Goelet, and discussion closed by Dr. Sanders.

MATERIA MEDICA.—At the meeting December 19, 1892, Dr. A. M. Fernandez read a paper on "The Great Influence Exerted by the Size of Dose in Changing Therapeutic Action." Discussion by Drs. Thompson, Valentine, Bleyer, Tyndale, and Farries, Dr. Fernandez closing.

INSANITY.—On April 17, 1893, Drs. WILLIAMS and MATTHEW D. FIELD addressed the meeting on the subject of "Medication in Lieu of Physical Restraint in Treatment of the Insane," this being the theme of a paper expected from Dr. TRAUTMAN, who was absent.

SYPHILIS.—Meeting March 20, 1893. Dr. L. D. BULKLEY read a paper on "Chancre of Tonsils," with description of fifteen cases; discussed by Drs. Burchard, Valentine, and Oberndofer.

On May 15, 1893, Dr. E. W. RUSSELL presented the case of a boy five years of age suffering with chancre of the tongue.

474   NEW YORK STATE MEDICAL ASSOCIATION.

PUBLIC HEALTH.—At the meeting October 17, 1892, Dr. JOHN GOD-
FREY, of United States Marine Hospital service, addressed the Association on "The Probable Advantages of Quarantine, and the Proper
Methods of Conducting It." He was followed by Dr. WILLIAM PEPPER,
of Philadelphia, who delivered an address on "The Pan-American Congress, and Its Influence on Sanitation and Quarantine." These subjects,
and the papers on "Cholera" and "Bacteriology" already noticed,
were discussed by Drs. George M. Sternberg and A. L. Gihon, United
States Navy.

At the meeting June 19, 1893, a paper on the "Climate of South
Africa" was read by Dr. JAMES L. CAMPBELL. At the same date Dr.
VON DÖNHOFF read a paper on "The Efficiency of Nature's Remedial
Processes."

This gives an epitome of the scientific work in formal papers and discussions classified under the headings, Practice of Medicine, Public
Health, Materia Medica, Surgery, Syphilography, Gynaecology, Insanity,
and general subjects.

In addition, pathological specimens have been shown at several
meetings.

November 21, 1892. A specimen from "Case of Penetrating Gun-Shot
Wound of Thorax," and another from a "Case of Strangulated Hernia,"
both by Dr. MANLEY. February 20, 1893, he introduced a patient on
whom was performed the operation of resection of tibia and fibula for
compound comminuted fracture of leg, and presented the specimen of
bone removed. In this case there was a good recovery and a very useful limb. Also a hernial sac which had been operated on under cocaine,
1 per cent. solution. Also an ovary and Fallopian tube for a child three
months old, removed through vulva, into which it had become prolapsed;
no bad effects; ovary showed signs of cystic degeneration. These were
presented by Dr. MANLEY.

March 20, 1893, Dr. GEORGE LINDINMEYER exhibited a specimen of
Cardiac Thrombosis with characteristics of so called Heart Polypus.

April 17, 1893, Dr. VON DÖNHOFF showed a specimen of Adeno Sarcoma from a female breast.

On November 21, 1892, Dr. MANLEY proposed a resolution for the
appointment of a Committee on Public Health, Hygiene, and Sanitary
Affairs, with certain specified duties, and that at the annual meeting or
on other occasions a report be made to the Association. The resolution
was adopted, and Drs. T. H. Manley, J. Lewis Smith, J. Blake White,
Alvah H. Doty, and J. R. MacGregor were appointed as that committee.

On December 19, 1892, in accordance with a call of the Committee of
the American Medical Association, a paper was adopted on the matter
of the Code of Ethics, approving of the Code as it is and desiring its
maintenance in its present form. This paper was duly transmitted to
Dr. H. D. Holton of Vermont, chairman of the National Committee.

The Committee on Legislation has been enlarged, and as now constituted consists of Drs. S. S. Purple, A. D. Ruggles, Samuel W. Smith,
Louis W. Schultz, and Charles E. Simmons.

The meeting of January, 1893, was the annual meeting, and was devoted to the election of officers and reading annual reports. At that meeting the following were chosen:

President—Dr. S. B. W. McLEOD.
Vice President—Dr. BENJAMIN F. VOSBURGH.
Recording Secretary—Dr. P. BRYNBERG PORTER.
Corresponding Secretary—Dr. A. D. RUGGLES.
Treasurer—Dr. JOHN H. HINTON.
Member of Executive Committee—Dr. N. J. HEPBURN.

At the meeting February 20, 1893, the President delivered the annual address, the theme of which was "Certain Mental Endowments Tending to Success in the Practice of Medicine, and the Importance of International Consultations." The address closed with a comparison of Rome and New York as medical centres.

It has long been our custom to partake of a collation at the close of each monthly meeting, and at the end of our June assembly to indulge in short postprandial addresses, expressive of our less serious thoughts but more lively feelings of good will towards each other as we separate until the close of our summer vacation. This custom was most cordially observed at the meeting June 17, 1893.

The membership continues to increase, and the attendance at the meetings is large. At the close of the month of June, 1893, the total membership was nine hundred and twenty (920).

Let the last record of this annual report be of those who have died, and whose memory we desire to cherish—Drs. Ross, Greene, Leaning, Elmore, Price, Ballou, Ingraham, George E. Hubbard, Doubleday, Weyman, O'Rorke, and W. T. White. Some of these were to some of us dear, personal friends, some intimate professional friends, and our own medical advisers. The memory of all of them we honor as having been faithful members of our Association.

S. B. W. McLEOD, *President.*

KINGS COUNTY MEDICAL ASSOCIATION.

ANNUAL REPORT.

The Kings County Medical Association has to report the following as its list of officers for the year 1893:

President—Dr. T. M. ROCHESTER.
Vice-President—Dr. R. M. WYCKOFF.
Recording Secretary—Dr. F. C. RAYNOR.
Corresponding Secretary—Dr. H. C. RIGGS.
Treasurer—Dr. E. H. SQUIBB.

These officers, together with the following, constituting the Executive Committee—Dr. E. R. SQUIBB, Dr. J. D. RUSHMORE, Dr. JONATHAN WRIGHT, Dr. T. M. LLOYD.

There have been nine regular meetings of the Association, at which the following papers have been read and discussed before the members:

January, 1893. "The Modern Urethroscope," with demonstrations, by Dr. W. K. OTIS. Followed by a paper on "Diagnosis and Treatment of the Antrum of Highmore," by Dr. F. S. MILLBURY.

February, 1893. "Clinical Observations on Appendicitis, with a Report of Cases Illustrating Different Forms of the Disease," by Dr. J. D. SULLIVAN.

March, 1893. "Our Dispensaries, Hospitals, Philanthropy, Frauds, and the Necessity for Medical Reform," by Dr. L. F. CRIADO.

April, 1893. "The Case of the Inebriate," by Dr. C. F. BARBER. "Inebriety," by Dr. L. D. MASON.

May, 1893. "Scarlatinoid Eruptions," by Dr. GEORGE A. OSTRANDER.

June, 1893. "Restraining Haemorrhage," by Dr. GEORGE G. HOPKINS.

October, 1893. "Philosophy of Differentiation, with Especial Reference to the Practice of Medicine," by Dr. G. H. PIERCE.

November, 1893. "Biology of the Brooklyn Water Supply," by Dr. SMITH ELY JELLIFFE.

December, 1893. "Induced Labour as Related to Puerperal Eclampsia," by Dr. H. C. RIGGS.

This summary shows a total of eleven scientific papers read at nine stated meetings of the Association for the year 1893. These papers indicate commendable activity on the part of the members individually, and a lively interest in the Association and its work.

[Signed]   H. C. RIGGS, *Corresponding Secretary.*

PROCEEDINGS.

TENTH ANNUAL MEETING

OF THE

NEW YORK STATE MEDICAL ASSOCIATION,

HELD AT THE MOTT MEMORIAL HALL, 64 MADISON AVENUE, NEW
YORK CITY, OCTOBER 9, 10, 11, and 12, 1893.

INTRODUCTORY SESSION.

MONDAY·EVENING, OCTOBER 9, 1893.

The meeting was called to order by the PRESIDENT at 8:30 p. m.

The report of the Committee of Arrangements was presented by the Chairman, Dr. JOHN G. TRUAX, and, upon motion, the report was accepted and adopted.

After the delivery of the PRESIDENT'S address, and an address by Dr. JOHN SHRADY, on "The Medical Work of the Association During Its First Decade," the Association, on motion, adjourned to partake of a collation.

FIRST DAY, TUESDAY, OCTOBER 10, 1893.
MORNING SESSION.

The meeting was called to order by the PRESIDENT at 10 a. m.

The annual report of the Council was then read by the SECRETARY, and on motion, the report was accepted.

Dr. JOHN CRONYN then moved that the thanks of the Association be tendered to the SECRETARY and TREASURER for the thoroughness and care with which he had managed the affairs of the Association during the past ten years. Seconded, and carried unanimously.

Due notice having been given of a proposed amendment to the constitution (see Vol. IX, Transactions, p. 776), the SECRETARY moved that this amendment be made a part of the constitution. Seconded. Carried. This amendment gives Kings County Association and New York County Association the right to send delegates to the State Association, and consequently to the American Medical Association.

The annual reports of the Presidents of the Branch Associations, and the annual report of the President of the Kings and the New York County Medical Associations, were then read by title, after the reading of papers and discussion.

At the close of the session, the PRESIDENT appointed Dr. JAMES G. PORTEOUS, of Dutchess county, member at large on the Nominating Committee.

On motion, the Association adjourned at 11: 45 a. m.

AFTERNOON SESSION.

The meeting was called to order by the SECRETARY at 1: 45 p. m.

The SECRETARY then announced the following Nominating Committee:

First District, Dr. DOUGLAS AYRES, Dr. W. H. ROBB.
Second District, Dr. THOMAS WILSON, Dr. R. B. BOUTECOU.
Third District, Dr. C. W. GREEN, Dr. E. LESTER.
Fourth District, Dr. A. P. JACKSON, Dr. H. J. DEAN.
Fifth District, Dr. M. C. CONNER, Dr. J. W. S. GOULEY.
Member at Large, Dr. J. G. PORTEOUS.

After the scientific work, on motion, the Association adjourned at 5 p. m.

EVENING SESSION.

The meeting was called to order by the PRESIDENT at 8 p. m.

The session was devoted entirely to scientific papers, and, on motion, the Association adjourned at 9: 45 p. m.

SECOND DAY, WEDNESDAY, OCTOBER 11.
MORNING SESSION.

The meeting was called to order by the PRESIDENT at 10 a. m.

The SECRETARY said he had received a communication from the American Medical Association, asking for an expression of opinion from this State Association regarding the advisability of amending the Code of Ethics of the American Medical Association. He therefore moved that the following reply be sent:

" In reply to the notice that the American Medical Association had requested the State Medical organisations in affiliation with that body to express their wishes in reference to any change in the Code of Ethics, the New York State Medical Association has to state that it has made that Code one of its foundation stones, and that it is entirely opposed to any alteration therein. This is the result of a full re-consideration of the subject, and after an experience of ten years of organisation under the Code."

Seconded. Carried unanimously.

At the close of the scientific work, the Association adjourned at 12: 30 p. m.

AFTERNOON SESSION.

The meeting was called to order at 2 p. m. by the SECRETARY.

The afternoon was devoted to the reading and discussion of scientific papers.

On motion, the Association adjourned at 4:30 p. m.

In the evening there was a banquet at the Hotel Brunswick.

———

THIRD DAY, THURSDAY, OCTOBER 12,
MORNING SESSION.

The meeting was called to order by the PRESIDENT at 10 a. m.

The Nominating Committee reported as follows:

President:

    Fourth District, Dr. THOMAS D. STRONG, of Chautauqua County.

Vice-Presidents:

    First District, Dr. ISAAC DE ZOUCHE.

    Second District, Dr. J. C. BENHAM.

    Third District, Dr. HOMER O. JEWETT.

    Fifth District, Dr. J. D. RUSHMORE.

On motion, the SECRETARY was authorised to cast an affirmative ballot for those mentioned in the above report.

Report of the Committee Appointed to Secure Legislation for the Establishment of Hospitals for Chronic Inebriates.

Dr. H. ERNST SCHMID reported that the other members of the Committee, Drs. Brush and Granger, ably assisted by Dr. Peterson, of New York City, had drafted a bill which he had himself engineered through the legislature, securing its passage through both houses. He did not approach the governor, because he had been assured privately that the governor would sign it. However, the governor unexpectedly vetoed it. Under these circumstances, he asked that the Committee be continued, for he felt sure the bill could be passed this winter.

The SECRETARY—I move that this Committee be continued for the ensuing year. Seconded. Carried.

The scientific portion of the programme having been completed, and there being no further business before the meeting, the PRESIDENT said, It would be unjust to myself if I did not again thank you for the honor of being elected PRESIDENT of this Association, as well as for the many kindly expressions and courtesies that have been extended to me since I have had the honour of presiding over your deliberations at this time.

Inasmuch as Dr. THOMAS D. STRONG is not here to be formally introduced to you as your presiding officer, it only remains for me to announce the fact that he will be recognised as PRESIDENT of this Association from the close of this meeting until the end of his term.

On motion of the SECRETARY, the tenth annual meeting was adjourned at 12 m. The members of the Association, however, were enabled to spend a profitable and pleasant afternoon in a trip to the charitable institutions on "The Islands," under the direction and through the courtesy of the Commissioners of Charities. During this trip, at an informal meeting, the SECRETARY was directed to communicate the thanks of the members of the Association for the valuable privilege of the trip.

[Signed]   E. D. FERGUSON, *Secretary.*

ANNUAL REPORT OF THE COUNCIL

AND

MINUTES OF THE SESSION OF THE COUNCIL,

FOR THE YEAR 1898.

The Council met in its tenth annual session at the Mott Memorial Library on Monday evening, October 9, 1898.

The session opened at 8 p. m.

Present: The Chairman, Dr. McLeod, and Drs. Ferguson, Gouley, Hannan, Jewett, Shrady, Strong, Truax, and Wilson.

The Secretary reported the following list of applicants for Fellowships, who had been appointed members by circular vote since the last meeting of the Council, viz.,—

William E. Beardsley, S. Oppenheimer, A. B. Judson, James K. King, E. D. Leffingwell, E. Gould Woodruff, Theodore Godell Wright, Thomas H. Hull, Charles W. Jackson, L. A. W. Alleman, Edward E. Hicks, M. K. Hogan, William M. Kemp, John E. Richardson, Charles E. Simmons, Alexander Dallas, Henry C. Johnston, Lewis B. Andrews, J. S. Brandt, Albert H. Little, Alpheus Prince, DeLancey Rochester, Charles Reitz, Justin H. Schopp, Edward Von Dönhoff, Charles A. Wall, Neil J. Hepburn, F. E. Stewart, F. C. Raynor, Louis L. Seaman, Lawrence Coffin, Max Einhorn, Austin Flint, Jr., Joseph F. Gray, George W. Newman, Henry J. Allen, Adelbert Hewitt, J. F. Humphrey, F. A. Smith, A. A. Swanick, Amos W. Thompson, Miles E. Varney, G. S. Hulette.

The following applicants were then appointed Fellows, viz.,—

William O'Meagher, Frank R. Pratt, Donald Maclean (non-resident), Cyrus J. Strong, E. T. Sabal (non-resident), David St. John (non-resident), Alfred C. McDaniel (non-resident), Almon H. Cooke, Thomas H. Hannan.

The Secretary then presented the

Report of the Committee on Publications.

It is with profound regret that the Committee on Publications finds it necessary to offer a report by the hand of another than its Chairman, Dr. A. L. Carroll, who for some months has been unable on account of illness, to give any attention to the affairs of the Association.

The high value and unselfish character of the service that has been given by Dr. Carroll in the interests of the Association, together with the esteem and affection in which he is held by his associates in the Council, render his illness a subject of personal grief to each of us.

The ninth volume of our Transactions was edited by Dr. O. C. Ludlow, and printed by the Fless & Ridge Printing Company, of New York city. The type and paper resulted in a heavier volume than was necessary or desirable. An edition of one thousand copies was printed.

The total disbursements connected with printing, editing, and distributing the volume have been about $1,850.

[Signed]   E. D. FERGUSON, *Secretary.*

The report was accepted and adopted.

This was followed by the

ANNUAL REPORT OF THE TREASURER FROM NOVEMBER 1, 1892, TO OCTOBER 1, 1893.

RECEIPTS—GENERAL FUND.

Balance from last report	$1,677.11	
Dues	2,190.00	
Initiation fees	285.00	
Sale of Transactions	14.00	
Interest on deposit	30.00	
		$4,196.11

DISBURSEMENTS.

Sundries, including printing the Transactions	$2,125.57	
Postage stamps	94.50	
Expressage and freight	27.43	
		$2,247.50

Balance in the General Fund, October 1, 1893 . . . . . $1,848.61

LIBRARY AND BUILDING FUND.

Balance from last report	$2,582.41	
Interest for a portion of the year	61.00	
		$2,643.41

Total funds in the treasury, October 1, 1893 . . . . . $4,492.02

The foregoing statement shows an increase in the funds of the Association of $232.50, and though this increase is less than for the preceding two years, still, in view of the size of the volume of Transactions, and the monetary troubles, which have had their effects even in our ranks, the Treasurer feels that the showing is fairly gratifying.

[Signed]   E. D. FERGUSON, *Treasurer.*

The report was accepted.

The Directors of the Library then presented the

Ninth Annual Report of the Library Committee of the New York State Medical Association.

October 9, 1893.

The ninth annual report of the Library Committee shows only a slight increase during the current year in the number of volumes, but, in addition, many pamphlets, reports, medical journals, and transactions of societies are regularly received. On the 14th of November, 1892, there were nine thousand and twelve (9,012) volumes in the library; since that date thirty-three (33) books have been received, making a total of nine thousand and forty-five (9,045) volumes. The medical journals that have been received during the past two years are not included in this statement of the number of volumes now in the library. During the years 1892 and 1893 there were made seven hundred and forty-two visits to the library by Fellows of the Association, other physicians, medical students, and non-medical persons.

The library was organised at the morning session of the second day, November 19, 1884, of the first annual meeting of the Association, the first publication in possession of the committee being a bound volume of forty-three printed pages, bearing the title of "Minutes of a Convention held in the city of Albany, February 4th and 6th, 1884, at which the New York State Medical Association was organised on a Permanent Basis." These "Minutes" were reprinted in the first volume of the Association's Transactions. The library was not open to visitors until the first day of June, 1885, and on the 19th of November of the same year the number of volumes had increased to three thousand four hundred and forty-eight (3,448). Every successive year has shown some increase up to the grand total of nine thousand and forty-five (9,045) volumes. The shelves are over-crowded, and more extended accommodations are much needed.

J. W. S. GOULEY, M. D.,
Director of the Library and Chairman of the Committee.

The report was accepted.

The Secretary presented the following communication:

PHILADELPHIA, September 25, 1893.

Secretary of the New York State Medical Association:

MY DEAR DOCTOR: At our recent session, June, 1893, the following were adopted:

Resolved, That the respective state medical societies entitled to representation in this Association, and through them their affiliated local societies, are hereby requested to consider the matter of revision of the Code of Ethics, and report to this Association at its next annual meeting, and if any alteration be deemed advisable, each state society so deciding to specially indicate the part to be changed and write out in full the new form proposed.

Resolved, That the state medical societies in such states as do not have now legal boards for the examination of persons desiring to become practitioners in such states, are requested by this Association to use their influence to have the states create such boards by statute.

Resolved, That the several state medical societies are hereby requested to use their influence to have statutory restraint in their respective states placed upon the sale of poisonous and mischievous medicines, except when prescribed by legally qualified persons.

Dear Doctor, please acknowledge the receipt of this communication, and in due time inform me of the action taken by your Association.

Yours very truly,

W. B. ATKINSON, *Permanent Secretary.*

The matter was referred to the general meeting of the Association.

The Secretary presented a communication from the Smithsonian Institution, calling attention to the offer of prizes of $1,000, $2,000, and $10,000, for prize essays on Atmospheric Air, by Thomas George Hodgkins, Esq.

A bill of expenditures by the Committee of Arrangements, amounting to $55.22, was audited and allowed.

The Council then adjourned.

E. D. FERGUSON, *Secretary.*

The new Council met on board the steamer during the trip to " The Islands," on the adjournment of the annual meeting, October 12, 1893.

The following applicants were appointed Fellows, viz.: William R. Pryor, C. D. Van Etten, Charles H. Andrews, J. B. Noyes, and N. P. Dandridge (non-resident).

On the nomination of Drs. Gouley, Truax, and Ferguson, Sir James A. Grant, M. D., K. C. M. G., of Ottawa, Canada, and Mr. Ernest Hart, F. R. S., of London, England, were presented for Honourary Fellowship, the election to lie over for one year under the rule.

On motion, the Treasurer was authorised to pay $100 to the trustees of the Mott Memorial Library, in addition to the annual sum of $100.

The members of the Council of the Second District were appointed the Committee on Publications, with the Secretary as Chairman and Editor.

The members of the Council in the Fifth District were appointed a Committee of Arrangements for the next annual meeting, with power to add to their number.

The next annual meeting was fixed for October 9, 10, 11, 1894.

On motion, the Council adjourned.

E. D. FERGUSON, *Secretary.*

The members of the Council of the New York State Medical Association deeply mourn the loss of their beloved, erudite, scholarly, and gentle colleague, Alfred Ludlow Carroll, M. D., who has laboured so well and so assiduously for the Association, for the profession, and for the people, as the editor of the Association Transactions, as a prolific contributor of scientific material, as a promoter of the honour, dignity, and advancement of medical science, and as one of the foremost sanitarians of the land.

The Council has, therefore, resolved that their high appreciation of the noble qualities, and of the scientific accomplishments, of their late gifted and lamented colleague be recorded in this volume of Transactions, and in the medical journals, and that a copy of the above be transmitted to the family of the deceased.

E. D. FERGUSON, M. D.,
Secretary.

Done by the Council,
November 4, 1893.

LIST OF FELLOWS.

BY DISTRICT AND COUNTY.

FIRST OR NORTHERN DISTRICT.

FRANKLIN COUNTY.

Founder. Gillis, William. Fort Covington.

1

FULTON COUNTY.

Original. Blake, Clarence R. Northville.
Founder. de Zouche, Isaac. Gloversville.
Drake, D. Delos. Johnstown.
Edwards, John. Gloversville.

4

HAMILTON COUNTY.

McGann, Thomas. Wells.

1

HERKIMER COUNTY.

Casey, J. E. Mohawk.
Douglass, A. J. Ilion.
Garlock, William D. Little Falls.
Original. Glidden, Charles H. Little Falls.
Greene, H. H. Paine's Hollow.
Original. Potter, Vaughan C. Starkville.
Original. Sharer, John P. Little Falls.
Original. Southworth, Mark A. Oakland, Cal.
Original. Young, John D. Starkville.

9

JEFFERSON COUNTY.

Founder. Abell, Ira H. Antwerp.
Founder. Crawe, J. Mortimer. Watertown.
Original. Johnson, Parley H. Adams.

3

LEWIS COUNTY.

Crosby, Alexander H. Lowville.
Douglass, Charles E. Lowville.
Joslin, Albert A. Martinsburgh.
Kelley, John D. Lowville.
Kilborn, Henry F. Crogham.

5

MONTGOMERY COUNTY.

Original. Ayres, Douglas, Fort Plain.
Caldwell, Nathan A. Hageman's Mills.
French, S. H. Amsterdam.
Original. Graves, Ezra. Amsterdam.
Original. Johnson, Richard G. Amsterdam.
Klock, Charles M. St. Johnsville.
Original. Leach, H. M. Charlton City, Mass.
Parr, John. Buel.
Parsons, W. W. D. Fultonville.
Founder. Robb, William H. Amsterdam.
Simons, Frank E. Canajoharie.
Smyth, Arthur V. H. Amsterdam.

12

ONEIDA COUNTY.

Armstrong, James A. Clinton.
Babcock, H. E. New London.
Original. Bagg, Moses M. Utica.
Barnum, D. Albert. Cassville.
Original. Blumer, G. Alder. Utica.
Bond, George F. M. Utica.
Original. Booth, Wilbur H. Utica.
Original. Brush, Edward N. Towsen, Md.
Churchill, Alonzo. Utica.
Clarke, Wallace. Utica.
Dodge, Amos P. Oneida Castle.

Douglass, James W. Booneville.
Ellis, J. B. Whitesborough.
English, G. P. Booneville.
Flandrau, Thomas M. Rome.
Fraser, Jefferson C. Ava.
Fuller, Earl D. Utica.
Gibson, William M. Utica.
Holden, Arthur L. Utica.
Hughes, Henry R. Clinton.
Original. Hunt, James G. Utica.
Kuhn, William. Rome.
Munger, Charles. Knoxboro.
Nelson, William H. Taberg.
Palmer, Henry C. Utica.
Palmer, Walter B. Utica.
Phelps, George G. Utica.
Founder. Porter, Harry N. Washington, D. C.
Quin, Hamilton S. Utica.
Reid, Christopher C. Rome.
Russell, Charles P. Utica.
Scully, Thomas P. Rome.
Sutton, H. C. Rome.
Sutton, Richard E. Rome.
Swartwout, Leander. Prospect.
Tefft, Charles B. Utica.
West, Joseph E. Utica.
37

OSWEGO COUNTY.

Bacon, Charles G. Fulton.
Bates, Nelson W. Central Square.
Cooley, F. L. Oswego.
Cooley, R. N. Hannibal Centre.
Original. DeWitt, Byron. Oswego.
Huntington, John W. Mexico.
Johnson, George P. Mexico.
Marsh, E. Frank. Fulton.
Todd, John B. Parish.
9

St. LAWRENCE COUNTY.

Cook, Guy Reuben. Louisville.
1

SECOND OR EASTERN DISTRICT.

ALBANY COUNTY.

Abrams, H. C. Newtonville.
Founder. Bailey, Theodore P. Albany.
Haynes, John U. Cohoes.
Founder. Peters, Samuel. Cohoes.
Rulison, L. B. West Troy.
Founder. Sabin, William B. West Troy.
Original. Van Vranken, Adam T. West Troy.
Witbeck, Charles E. Cohoes.
Zeh, Merlin J. West Troy.
9

CLINTON COUNTY.

Founder. Dodge, Lyndhurst C. Rouse's Point.
Holcomb, O. A. Plattsburgh.
Founder. Lyon, E. M. Plattsburgh.
3

COLUMBIA COUNTY.

Original. Benham, John C. Hudson.
Bradley, O. Howard. Hudson.
Clum, Franklin D. Cheviot.
Fritts, Crawford Ellsworth. Hudson.
Original. Lockwood, J. W. Philmont.
Original. Smith, H. Lyle. Hudson.
Vedder, George W. Philmont.
Wheeler, John T. Chatham.
Founder. Wilson, Thomas. Claverack.
Woodruff, R. Allen. Philmont.
Woodworth, T. Floyd. Kinderhook.
11

ESSEX COUNTY.

Founder. Barton, Lyman. Willsborough.
Barton, L. G. Willsborough.
Church, Charles A. Bloomingdale.
Original. D'Avignon, Francis J. Au Sable Forks.
Original. LaBell, Martin J. Lewis.

Original. Rand, Hannibal W. Keene.
Original. Riley, Andrew W. Au Sable Forks.
Original. Robinson, Ezra A. Jay.
Original. Turner, Melvin H. Moriah.

9

GREENE COUNTY.

Original. Conkling, George. Durham.
           Getty, A. H. Athens.
           Howland, George T. Norwich, Conn.
           Huestis, W. B. Kiskatom.
Original. Selden, O. G. Catskill.
Original. Selden, Robert. Catskill.

6

RENSSELAER COUNTY.

Original. Allen, Amos. Grafton Centre.
Founder. Allen, Charles S. Greenbush.
           Allen, William L. Greenbush.
           Baynes, Joseph E. Troy.
           Bissell, James H. Troy.
           Bonesteel, H. F. Troy.
Founder. Bonesteel, William N. Troy.
Original. Bontecou, Reed B. Troy.
           Boyce, Elias B. Averill Park.
Founder. Burbeck, Charles H. Troy.
Founder. Burton, Matthew H. Troy.
           Cahill, John T. Hoosick Falls.
           Church, Thomas C. Valley Falls.
Original. Cooper, William C. Troy.
           Crounse, Andrew C. Melrose.
           Dickinson, M. D. Troy.
           Dickson, Thomas Gordon. Troy.
Founder. Ferguson, E. D. Troy.
Founder. Finder, William. Troy.
           Greenman, C. E. Troy.
Founder. Hannan, James C. Hoosick Falls.
           Hannan, Thomas H. Hoosick Falls.
Founder. Harvie, J. B. Troy.
Original. Heimstreet, Thomas B. Troy.
Original. Houston, David W. Troy.
           Hull, William H. Poestenkill.

	Keith, Halbert Lyon. Upton, Mass.
Original.	Lyon, George E. St. Louis, Mo.
	Lyons, Edward L. Troy.
Original.	Magee, Daniel. Troy.
	Marsh, James P. Troy.
Founder.	Mitchell, Howard E. Troy.
Founder.	Nichols, Calvin E. Troy.
Founder.	Nichols, William H. West Sand Lake.
	Phelan, Michael F. Troy.
Original.	Rogers, S. Frank. Troy.
Founder.	Rousseau, Zotique. Troy.
Founder.	Seymour, W. Wotkyns. Troy.
Original.	Skinner, Smith A. Hoosick Falls.
	Tompkins, Fred J. Lansingburgh.
Original.	Traver, Richard D. Troy.
	Ward, R. H. Troy.

42

SARATOGA COUNTY.

	Allen, Henry J. Corinth.
Founder.	Comstock, George F. Saratoga Springs.
Original.	Crombie, Walter C. Mechanicsville.
	Curtis, P. C. Round Lake.
Original.	Dunlop, John J. Waterford.
	Gow, Frank F. Schuylerville.
Founder.	Grant, Charles S. Saratoga Springs.
Original.	Hall, William H. Saratoga Springs.
	Hewitt, Adelbert. Saratoga Springs.
Founder.	Hodgman, William H. Saratoga Springs.
	Hudson, George. Stillwater.
	Humphrey, J. F. Saratoga Springs.
	Inlay, Erwin G. Conklingville.
Original.	Johnson, Ianthus G. Greenfield Centre.
	Keefer, Charles W. Mechanicsville.
	Kniskern, A. C. Mechanicsville.
Founder.	*McEwen, Robert C. Saratoga Springs.
	Moriarta, D. C. Saratoga Springs.
Original.	Murray, Byron J. Saratoga Springs.
	Palmer, F. A. Mechanicsville.
	Parent, J. S. Birchton.
Original.	Preston, John R. Schuylerville.
Founder.	Reynolds, Tabor B. Saratoga Springs.

* Deceased.

           Rice, George. Mechanicsville.
           Sherer, John D. Waterford.
           Sherman, F. J. Ballston.
           Smith, F. A. Corinth.
Original. Stubbs, Roland H. Waterford.
           Swan, William E. Saratoga Springs.
           Swanick, A. A. Saratoga Springs.
           Sweetman, J. T., Jr. Ballston.
           Thompson, Amos W. Saratoga Springs.
           Varney, Miles E. Saratoga Springs.
           Webster, W. B. Schuylerville.
           Zeh, Edgar. Waterford.
                 35
                 •

SCHENECTADY COUNTY.

           Fuller, Robert. Schenectady.
           Hammer, Charles. Schenectady.
Original. McDonald, George E. Schenectady.
           McDougall, R. A. Duanesburgh.
Original. Reagles, James R. Schenectady.
Original. Van Zandt, Henry C. Schenectady.
           Veeder, Andrew T. Schenectady.
                 7

SCHOHARIE COUNTY.

Original. Hagadorn, William. Gilboa.
Original. Kingsley, Henry F. Schoharie.
                 2

WARREN COUNTY.

           Fitzgerald, David J. Glens Falls.
Original. Martine, Godfrey R. Glens Falls.
                 2

WASHINGTON COUNTY.

           Lambert, John. Salem.
           Long, Alfred J. Whitehall.
                 2

THIRD OR CENTRAL DISTRICT.

BROOME COUNTY.

Allen, S. P. Whitney's Point.
Founder. Chittenden, Joseph H. Binghamton.
Dudley, Dwight. Maine.
Original. Ely, Henry Oliver. Binghamton.
Farnham, LeRoy D. Binghamton.
. Farrington, John M. Binghamton.
Forker, Frederick L. Binghamton.
Fitzgerald, John F. Binghamton.
• Greene, Clark W. Chenango Forks.
Original. Hills, Lyman H. Binghamton.
Hough, F. P. Binghamton.
Ingraham, Charles W. Binghamton.
Knapp, W. H. Union Centre.
Meacham, Isaac D. Binghamton.
Moore, William A. Binghamton.
Founder. Orton, John G. Binghamton.
Pierce, Edward A. Binghamton.
Pierson, G. E. Kirkwood.
Place, John F., Jr. Binghamton.
Founder. Putnam, Frederick W. Binghamton.
Original. Race, W. F. Kearney, Neb.
Founder. Richards, Charles B. Binghamton.
. Rogers, Harris C. Binghamton.
Seymour, Ralph A. Whitney's Point.
Slater, Frank Ellsworth. Binghamton.
Wagner, Charles Gray. Binghamton.
Wells, E. H. Binghamton.
27

CAYUGA COUNTY.

Allison, Henry E. Auburn.
Original. Kenyon, M. Moravia.
Original. Laird, William R. Auburn.
Founder. Sawyer, Conant. Auburn.
Original. Tripp, John D. Auburn.
5

CHEMUNG COUNTY.

Original. Brown, Charles W. Washington, D. C.
Drake, E. G. Elmira.

Original. Ross, Frank W.   Elmira.
           Squire, Charles L.   Elmira.
Original. Wales, Theron A.   Elmira.
                      5

CHENANGO COUNTY.

Original. Blair, Louis P.   McDonough.
Original. Brooks, Leroy J.   Norwich.
           Copley, Herman D.   Bainbridge.
           Douglas, George.   Oxford.
           Guy, John D.   Coventry.
           Hand, S. M. Norwich.
           Hayes, Philetus A.   Afton.
Original. Johnson, Leonard M.   Greene.
Original. *Lyman, Elijah S.   Sherburne.
Original. Lyman, H. C.   Sherburne.
           Noyes, James B.   New Berlin.
           Packer, Thurston G.   Smyrna.
           Smith, Samuel L.   Smithville.
           Thompson, R. A.   Norwich.
           Van·Wagner, L. A.   Sherburne.
           Williams, George O.   Greene.
                      16

CORTLAND COUNTY.

           Bradford, George D.   Homer.
Original. Clark, DeWitt.   Marathon.
           Didama, E. A.   Portland.
           Halbert, M. L.   Cincinnatus.
Founder.   Hendrick, Henry C.   McGrawville.
           Higgins, F. W.   Cortland.
Founder.   Jewett, Homer O.   Cortland.
           Kenyon, Benjamin.   Cincinnatus.
                      8

DELAWARE COUNTY.

           Drake, James B.   Hancock.
           Morrow, William B.   Walton.
           Smith, George C.   Delhi.
           Travis, Edward M.   Eagle Grove, Ia.
                      4

* Deceased.

MADISON COUNTY.

Original. Birdsall, Gilbert. N. Brookfield.
Burhyte, O. W. Brookfield.
Cavana, Martin. Oneida.
Original. Carpenter, Henry W. Oneida.
Drake, Frank C. Oneida.
Huntley, James F. Oneida.
Original. Nicholson, A. R. Madison.

7

ONONDAGA COUNTY.

Original. Aberdein, Robert. Syracuse.
Founder. Allen, Henry B. Baldwinsville.
Brown, Ulysses H. Syracuse.
Campbell, A. J. Syracuse.
Founder. Dallas, Alexander J. Syracuse.
Founder. Didama, Henry D. Syracuse.
Original. Donohue, Florence O. Syracuse.
Earle, George W. Tully.
Original. Edwards, Amos S. Syracuse.
Original. Edwards, George A. Syracuse.
Flanigan, John R. Syracuse.
Frazee, A. Blair. Elbridge (Altoona, Pa.).
Original. Hatch, C. A. Syracuse.
Founder. Head, Adelbert D. Syracuse.
Original. Jacobson, Nathan. Syracuse.
Founder. Kneeland, Jonathan. South Onondaga.
Magee, Charles M. Syracuse.
Original. McNamara, Daniel. Syracuse.
Original. Munson, W. W. Otisco.
Founder. Parsons, Israel. Marcellus.
Original. Saxer, Leonard A. Syracuse.
Sears, F. W. Syracuse.
Stephenson, F. Halleck. Syracuse.
Founder. Van de Warker, Ely. Syracuse.
Original. Whitford, James. Onondaga Valley.

25

OTSEGO COUNTY.

Original. Barney, C. S. Milford.
Church, B. A. Oneonta.
Ford, M. L. Oneonta.

Founder.   Leaning, John K.   Cooperstown.
Original.   Martin, John H.   Otego.
Original.   Merritt, George.   Cherry Valley.
Original.   Sweet, Joseph J.   Unadilla.
        Sweet, Joshua J.   Unadilla.
8

SCHUYLER COUNTY.

King, James K.   Watkins.
Roper, P. B.   Alpine.
Leffingwell, E. D.   Watkins.
Smelzer, Baxter T.   Havana.
Stewart, F. E.   Watkins.
Woodruff, E. Gerald.   Watkins.
6

SENECA COUNTY.

        Bellows, George A.   Waterloo.
        Blaine, Myron D.   Willard.
Founder.   Lester, Elias.   Seneca Falls.
Original.   Pilgrim, Charles W.   Willard.
        Seaman, Frank G.   Seneca Falls.
        Welles, S. R.   Waterloo.
6

TIOGA COUNTY.

Original.   Ayer, W. L.   Owego.
        Cady, George M.   Nichols.
2

TOMPKINS COUNTY.

Founder.   Beers, John E.   Danby.
        Biggs, Chauncey P.   Ithaca.
Founder.   *Fitch, William Dryden.
        Flickinger, John.   Trumansberg.
4

* Deceased.

FOURTH OR WESTERN DISTRICT.

ALLEGHANY COUNTY.

Original.   Wakely, Benjamin C.   Angelica.

1

CATTARAUGUS COUNTY.

Eddy, John L.   Olean.
Ellsworth, Victor A.   Wellsville.
Lake, Albert D.   Gowanda.
Mudge, Selden J.   Olean.
Original.   Tompkins, Orren A.   East Randolph.

5

CHAUTAUQUA COUNTY.

Founder.   Ames, Edward.   Kalamazoo, Mich.
Bemus, Morris N.   Jamestown.
Bemus, William Marvin.   Jamestown.
Founder.   Dean, Harmon J.   Brocton.
Richmond, Nelson G.   Fredonia.
Rolph, R. T.   Fredonia.
Founder.   Strong, Thomas D.   Westfield.

7

ERIE COUNTY.

Andrews, Charles H.   Holland.
Founder.   Andrews, Judson B.   Buffalo.
Original.   Atwood, H. L.   Collins Centre.
Original.   Banta, Rollin L.   Buffalo.
Original.   Bartlett, Frederick W.   Buffalo.
Original.   Bartow, Bernard.   Buffalo.
Bergtold, W. H.   Buffalo.
Original.   Boies, Loren F.   East Hamburgh.
Original.   Briggs, Albert H.   Buffalo.
Brown, George L.   Buffalo.
Bryant, Percy.   Buffalo.
Burghardt, Francis Augustus.   Buffalo.
Cohen, Bernard.   Buffalo.
Congdon, Charles E.   Buffalo.
Founder.   Cronyn, John.   Buffalo.
Original.   Dagenais, Alphonse.   Buffalo.

Original. Daniels, Clayton M. Buffalo.
    Dayton, C. L. Buffalo.
Original. Dorland, Elias T. Buffalo.
    Fell, George E. Buffalo.
    Fowler, Joseph. Buffalo.
    Frederick, Carlton C. Buffalo.
    Gould, Cassius W. Buffalo.
    Green, Stephen S. Buffalo.
Original. Greene, DeWitt C. Buffalo.
Founder. Greene, Joseph C. Buffalo.
Original. Greene, Walter D. Buffalo.
Original. Harrington, D. W. Buffalo.
    Hartwig, Marcell. Buffalo.
    Hayd, Herman E. Buffalo.
    Heath, William H. Buffalo.
    Himmelsbach, George A. Buffalo.
    Howard, Charles F. Buffalo.
Founder. Hoyer, F. F. Tonawanda.
    Hubbell, Alvin A. Buffalo.
    Hunt, H. L. Orchard Park.
    Ingraham, Henry D. Buffalo.
    Jackson, William H. Springville.
Original. Johnson, Thomas M. Buffalo.
    Jones, Allen A. Buffalo.
    Lapp, Henry. Clarence.
    Long, Ben. G. Buffalo.
    Macfarlane, William A. Springville.
Original. Murray, William D. Tonawanda.
    Park, Roswell. Buffalo.
Original. Pettit, John A. Buffalo.
    Phelps, William C. Buffalo.
    Pohlman, Julius. Buffalo.
Original. Putnam, James W. Buffalo.
    Rochester, DeLancey. Buffalo.
    Stockton, Charles G. Buffalo.
    Strong, Orville C. Colden.
    Taber, R. C. Tonawanda.
    Thornton, William H. Buffalo.
Founder. Tremaine, William S. Buffalo.
    Trull, H. P. Williamsville.
    Twohey, John J. Buffalo.
    Wall, Charles A. Buffalo.
    Wheeler, Isaac G. Marilla.
    Whipple, Electa B. Buffalo.

Willoughby, M. Buffalo.
Founder. Wyckoff, Cornelius C. Buffalo.

62

GENESEE COUNTY.

Andrews, Lewis B. Byron.
Original. Crane, Frank W. Corfu.
Founder. Jackson, Albert P. Oakfield.
Prince, Alpheus. Byron.
Stone, Frank L. Le Roy.
Founder. Townsend, Morris W. Bergen.

6

LIVINGSTON COUNTY.

Original. Briggs, Wm. H. Hemlock Lake.
Brown, J. P. Tuscarora.
Dodge, Frank H. Mount Morris.
Jones, George H. Fowlerville.
Kneeland, B. T. Dalton.
Original. Menzie, R. J. Caledonia.
Original. Moyer, Frank H. Moscow.

7

MONROE COUNTY.

Original. Backus, Ogden. Rochester.
Briggs, C. M. Fairport.
Original. *Buckley, Charles. Rochester.
Original. Buckley, James. Rochester.
Original. Burke, John J. A. Rochester.
Curtis, D. F. Rochester.
Original. Dunning, J. D. Webster.
Fenno, Henry M. Rochester.
Goler, George W. Rochester.
Founder. Hovey, B. L. Rochester.
Jones, S. Case. Rochester.
Maine, Alva P. Webster.
McDougall, William D. Spencerport.
Founder. Moore, Edward M. Rochester.
Original. Moore, Edward M., Jr. Rochester.
Original. Moore, Richard Mott. Rochester.
Nold, John B. Rochester.
Original. O'Hare, Thomas A. Rochester.

* Deceased.

Original. Pease, Joseph. Hamlin.
Reitz, Charles. Webster.
Schopp, Justin H. Rochester.
Snook, George M. Parma.
Stockschlaeder, P. Rochester.
23

NIAGARA COUNTY.

Eddy, George P. Lewiston.
Huggins, William Q. Sanborn.
2

ONTARIO COUNTY.

Original. Allen, Duncan S. Seneca.
Original. Allen, James H. Gorham.
Founder. Bentley, Francis R. Cheshire.
De Laney, John Pope. Geneva.
Original. Hicks, W. Scott. Bristol.
Founder. ' Nichols, H. W. Canandaigua.
Pratt, Frank R. Manchester.
Founder. Simmons, E. W. Canandaigua.
Original. Vanderhoof, Frederick D. Phelps.
9

ORLEANS COUNTY.

Original. Bailey, William C. Knoxville, Tenn.
Founder. Chapman, James. Medina.
Curtis, Daniel. Jeddo.
Original. Taylor, John H. Holley.
Founder. Tompkins, H. C. Knowlesville.
5

STEUBEN COUNTY.

Chittenden, Daniel J. Addison.
Original. Dunn, Jeremiah. Bath.
Original. Ellison, Metler D. Canisteo.
Gilbert, Horatio. Hornellsville.
Hubbard, Chauncey G. Hornellsville.
Hunter, Nathaniel P. Jasper.
Original. Jamison, John S. Hornellsville.
Original. Perry, Nathaniel M. Troupsburgh.
Wallace, Edwin E. Jasper.
9

WAYNE COUNTY.

Founder. Arnold, J. Newton. Clyde.
          Brandt, J. S. Ontario Centre.
Founder. Colvin, Darwin. Clyde.
          Horton, David B. Red Creek.
Original. Ingraham, Samuel. Palmyra.
Original. Landon, Newell E. Newark.
          Nutten, Wilbur F. Newark.
Original. Sprague, John A. Williamson.
          Sprague, L. S. Williamson.
Original. Young, Augustus A. Newark.
                              10

WYOMING COUNTY.

Original. Ellinwood, A. G. Attica.
          Fisher, John C. Warsaw.
          Hulette, G. S. Arcade.
          Lusk, Zera J. Warsaw.
Original. Palmer, George M. Warsaw.
Original. Rae, Robert. Portageville.
          Rudgers, Denton W. Perry.
                              7

YATES COUNTY.

          Oliver, William. Penn Yan.
                              1

FIFTH OR SOUTHERN DISTRICT.

DUTCHESS COUNTY.

          Baker, Benjamin N. Rhinebeck.
Original. Barnes, Edwin. Pleasant Plains.
          Barton, Thomas J. Tivoli.
Original. Bates, Xyris T. Poughkeepsie.
Original. Bayley, Guy Carleton. Poughkeepsie.
Founder. Codding, George H. Amenia.
Founder. Cramer, William. Poughkeepsie.
Original. Fletcher, Charles L. Wing's Station.
          Julian, John M. Moore's Mill.
Founder. Kittredge, Charles S. Fishkill-on-Hudson.
          32

Founder.   Leroy, Irving D.   Pleasant Valley.
Founder.   Porteous, James G.   Poughkeepsie.
Founder.   Pultz, Monroe T.   Stanfordville.
           Van Etten, Cornelius.   Rhinebeck.
Original.   Van Wyck, Richard C.   Hopewell Junction.
Original.   *Young, John.   Fishkill-on-Hudson.
                        16

KINGS COUNTY.

           Alleman, L. A. W.   Brooklyn.
           Baker, Frank R.   Brooklyn.
Founder.   Baker, George W.   Brooklyn, E. D.
           Beardsley, William E.   Brooklyn.
           Benton, Stuart H.   Brooklyu.
           Bierwirth, Julius C.   Brooklyn.
Original.   Biggam, William H., Jr.   Brooklyn.
Original.   Brundage, Amos H.   Brooklyn.
Original.   Conway, John Francis.   Brooklyn.
           Coffin, Laurence.   Brooklyn.
           Creamer, Joseph, Jr.   Brooklyn, E. D.
           Criado, Louis F.   Brooklyn.
           Feeley, James F.   Brooklyn, E. D.
           Gardiner, William F.   Brooklyn.
           Hicks, Edward A.   Brooklyn.
           Hughes, Peter.   Brooklyn.
           Hull, Thomas H.   Brooklyn.   ˙
Original.   Ilgen, Ernst.   Brooklyn.
Original.   Jenkins, John A.   Brooklyn, E. D.
           Jewett, F. A.   Brooklyn.˙
Original.   Leighton, Nathaniel W.   Brooklyn.
           Little, Frank.   Brooklyn.
Original.   Lloyd, T. Mortimer.   Brooklyn.
Original.   Lung, Jesse B.   Brooklyn.
Original.   McCollom, William.   Brooklyn.
Original.   Minard, E. J. Chapin.   Brooklyn.
           Newman, George W.   Brooklyn.
Original.   North, Nelson L.   Brooklyn.
           Ostrander, George A.   Brooklyn.
Original.   Paine, Arthur R.   Brooklyn.
Original.   Pray, S. R.   Brooklyn.
           Price, Henry R.   Brooklyn.
           Raynor, F. C.   Brooklyn.
                        * Deceased.

Reed, Henry B. Brooklyn.
Richardson, John E. Brooklyn.
Risch, Henry F. W. Brooklyn.
Rochester, Thomas M. Brooklyn.
Founder. Rushmore, John D. Brooklyn.
Original. Russell, William G. Brooklyn.
Founder. Segur, Avery. Brooklyn.
Original. Shepard, A. Warren. Brooklyn.
Original. Sizer, Nelson Buell. Brooklyn.
Founder. Squibb, Edward H. Brooklyn.
Founder. Squibb, Edward R. Brooklyn.
Original. Steinke, Carl Otho Hermann. Brooklyn.
Sullivan, John D. Brooklyn.
Thwing, Clarence. Fort Wrangel, Alaska.
Waterworth, William. Brooklyn.
Original. Wieber, George. Brooklyn.
Original. Williams, William H. Brooklyn.
Founder. Wyckoff, Richard M. Brooklyn.
51

NEW YORK COUNTY.

Adams, Calvin Thayer. New York.
Agramonte, E. V. New York.
Original. Allen, S. Busby. New York.
Allen, Thomas H. New York.
Andrews, John L. New York.
Arango, Augustin. New York.
Original. Arcularius, Lewis. New York.
Armstrong, S. T. New York.
Original. Arnold, Edmund S. F. New York.
Arnold, Glover C. New York.
Baldwin, F. A. New York.
*Ballou, William R. New York.
Bermingham, Edward J. New York.
Original. Biggs, Herman M. New York.
Founder. Bozeman, Nathan. New York.
Bozeman, Nathan G. New York.
Brodrick, William P. New York.
Original. Bryant, Joseph D. New York.
Original. Buchanan, Alexander. New York.
Original. Bull, Charles Stedman. New York.
Bull, William T. New York.
Original. Burchard, Thomas H. New York.

Campbell, Clarence G. New York.
Founder. *Carroll, Alfred Ludlow. New York.
Original. Carter, H. Skelton. New York.
Original. Chauveau, Jean F. New York.
Original. Chrystie, T. M. Ludlow. New York.
Collins, Stacy B. Seaford, Sussex Co., Del.
Comfort, John E. New York.
Founder. Conover, William S. New York.
Conway, John R. New York.
Cook, Almon H. New York.
Original. Curry, Walker. New York.
Dallas, Alexander. New York.
Daniels, F. H. New York.
Davis, J. Griffith. New York.
Davis, Robert C. New York.
De Garmo, W. B. New York.
Delphey, Eden V. New York.
Original. Denison, C. Ellery. New York.
Original. Denison, Ellery. New York.
Founder. Dennis, Frederic S. New York.
de Quesada, Gregorio J. New York.
Original. Du Bois, Matthew B. New York.
Dudley, A. Palmer. New York.
Dunham, Edward K. New York.
Original. Eastman, Robert W. New York.
Einhorn, Max. New York.
Original. Eliot, Ellsworth. New York.
Enders, Thomas Burnham. New York.
Erdmann, John F. New York.
Farrington, Edward S. New York.
Farrington, Joseph O. New York.
Field, Matthew D. New York.
Founder. Flint, Austin. New York.
Flint, Austin, Jr. New York.
Founder. Flint, William H. New York.
Foster, George V. New York.
Frankenberg, Jacob H. New York.
Original. Furman, Guido. New York.
Gleitsmann, J. W. New York.
Goldthwaite, Henry. New York.
Founder. Gouley, John W. S. New York.
Grauer, Frank. New.York.
Gray, Joseph F. New York.

* Deceased.

Gulick, A. Reading. New York.
Gulick, Charlton R. New York.
Hammond, Frederick Porter. New York.
Original. Harrison, George Tucker. New York.
Haubold, H. A. New York.
Hepburn, Neil J. New York.
Hillis, Thomas J. New York.
Founder. Hinton, John H. New York.
Founder. Hodgman, Abbott. New York.
Hogan, M. K. New York.
Holmes, Martha C. New York.
Hubbard, Dwight L. New York.
Hubbard, George E. New York.
Founder. Hubbard, Samuel T. New York.
Jackson, Charles W. New York.
Founder. Janeway, Edward G. New York.
Janvrin, J. E. New York.
Jenkins, William T. New York.
Judson, A. B. New York.
Kemp, William M. New York.
King, Ferdinand. New York.
Kneer, F. G. New York.
Knipe, George. New York.
Founder. Leale, Charles A. New York.
Lewis, Robert. New York.
Little, Albert H. New York.
Lockwood, Charles E. New York.
Ludlow, Ogden C. New York.
Lukens, Anna. New York.
Founder. Lusk, William T. New York.
Lynch, Patrick J. New York.
MacGregor, James R. New York.
Mackenzie, J. C. New York.
McAlpine, D. Hunter. New York.
McBurney, Charles. New York.
McGillicuddy, T. J. New York.
McGowan, John P. New York.
McIlroy, Samuel H. New York.
McLeod, Johnston. New York.
Founder. McLeod, S. B. Wylie. New York.
Original. McLochlin, James A. New York.
Original. McNamara, Laurence J. New York.
Founder. Manley, Thomas H. New York.
Marshall, Francis F. New York.

Meier, Gottlieb, C. H.   New York.
Original.   Miller, William T.   New York.
Milliken, S. E.   New York.
Original.   Miranda, Ramon L.   New York.
Original.   Mitchell, Hubbard W.   New York.
Moran, James.   New York.
Mott, Valentine.   New York.
Original.   Murphy, John.   New York.
Original.   Murray, Sandford J.   New York.
Original.   Newman, Robert.   New York.
Founder.   Nicoll, Henry D.   New York.
Original.   Obendorfer, Isidor P.   New York.
O'Brien, Frederick William.   New York.
O'Brien, M. Christopher.   New York.
Ochs, Benjamin F.   New York.
O'Meagher, William, New York.
Oppenheimer, H. S.   New York.
Oppenheimer, S.   New York.
Palmer, Edmund J.   New York.
Original.   Parsons, John.   New York.
Perry, John Gardner.   New York.
Phelps, Charles.   New York.
Original.   Pooler, Hiram A.   New York.
Original.   Porter, P. Brynberg.   New York.
Pritchard, R. L.   New York.
Pryor, William R.   New York.
Founder.   Purple, Samuel S.   New York.
Ransom, H. B.   New York.
Rau, Leonard S.   New York.
Read, Ira B.   New York.
Original.   Ricketts, Benjamin M.   Cincinnati, Ohio.
Roth, Julius A.   New York.
Ruggles, Augustus D.   New York.
Original.   Sabine, Gustavus A.   New York.
Sanders, E.   New York.
Founder.   Sayre, Lewis A.   New York.
Sayre, Reginald H.   New York.
Seaman, Louis L.   New York.
Shaw, Henry B.   New York.
Shea, Dennis L.   New York.
Shrady, John.   New York.
Shrady, John Eliot.   New York.
Shunk, Albert.   New York.
Silver, Henry M.   New York.

Simmons, Charles E. New York.
Smeallie, James A. New York.
Original. Smith, J. Lewis. New York.
Original. Smith, Samuel W. New York.
Original. Smith, Stephen. New York.
Spicer, Walter E. New York.
Strong, Cyrus J. New York.
Founder. Thomas, T. Gaillard. New York.
Thompson, Von Beverhout. New York.
Tiemann, Paul E. New York.
Truax, J. G. New York.
Founder. Tucker, Carlos P. New York.
Van Fleet, Frank. New York.
Vincent, Ludger C. New York.
Von Dönhoff, Edward. New York.
Original. Wallach, Joseph N. New York.
Walsh, Simon J. New York.
Founder. Ward, Charles S. New York.
Warner, Frederic M. New York.
Warner, John W. New York.
Weeks, John E. New York.
Weston, Albert T. New York.
White, Charles B. New York.
White, J. Blake. New York.
Founder. White, Whitman V. New York.
Founder. *White, William T. New York.
Founder. Wiener, Joseph. New York.
Wiggin, Frederick Holme. New York.
Williams, Henry Smith. New York.
Williamson, Edward A. New York.
Woodend, William E. New York.
Original. Wyeth, John A. New York.
185

ORANGE COUNTY.

Conner, Milton C. Middletown.
Davis, J. O. Howells.
Potts, E. Port Jervis.
Swartwout, H. B. Port Jervis.
Townsend, Charles E. Newburgh.
Vanderveer, J. C. Monroe.
Vanderveer, J. R. Monroe.
7

* Deceased.

PUTNAM COUNTY.

Founder. Murdock, George W. Cold Spring.
Founder. Young, William. Cold Spring.
2

QUEENS COUNTY.

Original. Burns, William J. Sea Cliff.
Original. Rave, Edward G. Hicksville.
2

RICHMOND COUNTY.

Johnston, Henry C. New Brighton.
Martindale, F. E. Port Richmond.
Walser, William C. West New Brighton.
3

ROCKLAND COUNTY.

Founder. Govan, William. Stony Point.
1

SUFFOLK COUNTY.

Original. Chambers, Martin L. Port Jefferson.
Hamill, Edward H. Newark, N. J.
Hulse, William A. Bay Shore.
Original. Lindsay, Walter. Huntington.
4

SULLIVAN COUNTY.

Original. Bennett, Thomas W. Jeffersonville.
Crocker, Edwin. Narrowsburgh.
DeKay, William H. Parksville.
Johnston, N. C. Barryville.   •
McWilliams, F. A. Monticello.
Original. Munson, J. A. Woodbourne.
Piper, Charles W. Wurtsborough.
7

ULSTER COUNTY.

Original. Chambers, Jacob. Kingston.
Original. HoornBeek, Philip Du Bois. Wawarsing.

Founder. Hühne, August. Rondout.
Original. Hühne, Frederick. Rondout.
Original. Van Hovenberg, Henry. Kingston.
· Ward, John J. Ellenville.
6

WESTCHESTER COUNTY.

Acker, Thomas J. Croton-on-Hudson.
Original. Banks, George B. Hartsdale.
Original. Brush, Edward F. Mount Vernon.
Original. Coutant, Richard B. Tarrytown.
Original. Furman, J. Henry. Tarrytown. ·
Granger, William D. Mount Vernon.
Original. Huntington, Henry K. New Rochelle.
Original. Lyons, G. A. New Rochelle.
Original. Schmid, H. Ernst. White Plains.
Small, John W. New Rochelle.
Original. Southworth, Richmond Joseph. Washington, D. C.
Original. Wells, William L. New Rochelle.
12

SUMMARY OF FELLOWSHIP BY DISTRICTS.

First District, ... 82
Second District, ... 128
Third District, ... 128
Fourth District, ... 154
Fifth District, ... 296
Non-resident, ... ·. . . 8

Total Fellowship, ... 791

ALPHABETICAL LIST OF FELLOWS.

Abell, Ira H., Antwerp, Jefferson Co. Founder.
Aberdein, Robert, Warren and Fayette Sts., Syracuse, Onondaga Co. Original.
Abrams, H. C., Newtonville, Albany Co.
Acker, Thomas J., Croton-on-Hudson, Westchester Co.
Adams, Calvin Thayer, 8 W. 33d St., New York, New York Co.
Agramonte, E. V., 267 W. 45th St., New York, New York Co.
Alleman, L. A. W., 64 Montague St., Brooklyn, Kings Co.
Allen, Amos, Grafton, Rensselaer Co. Original.
Allen, Charles S., Greenbush, Rensselaer Co. Founder.
Allen, Duncan S., Seneca, Ontario Co. Original.
Allen, Henry B., Baldwinsville, Onondaga Co. Founder.
Allen, Henry J., Corinth, Saratoga Co.
Allen, James H., Gorham, Ontario Co. Original.
Allen, S. Busby, 164 E. 89th St., New York, New York Co.
Allen, S. P., Whitney's Point, Broome Co.
Allen, Thomas H., 52 W. 45th St., New York, New York Co.
Allen, William L., Greenbush, Rensselaer Co.
Allison, Henry E., Asylum for Insane Criminals, Auburn, Cayuga Co.
Ames, Edward, 123 E. Lovell St., Kalamazoo, Mich. Founder.
Andrews, Charles H., Holland, Erie Co.
Andrews, John L., 323 E. 86th St., New York, New York Co.
Andrews, Judson B., State Hospital, Buffalo, Erie Co. Founder.
Andrews, Lewis B., Byron, Genesee Co.
Arango, Augustin, 125 E. 36th St., New York, New York Co.
Arcularius, Lewis, 121 E. 25th St., New York, New York Co. Original.
Armstrong, James A., Clinton, Oneida Co.
Armstrong, S. T., 166 W. 54th St., New York, New York Co.
Arnold, Edmund S. F., 64 Madison Ave., New York, New York Co. Original.
Arnold, Glover C., 115 E. 30th St., New York, New York Co.
Arnold, J. Newton, Clyde, Wayne Co. Founder.
Atwood, H. L., Collins Centre, Erie Co. Original.
Ayer, W. L., Owego, Tioga Co. Original.
Ayres, Douglas, Fort Plain, Montgomery Co. Original.
Babcock, H. E., New London, Oneida Co. Original.
Backus, Ogden, 67 S. Fitzhugh St., Rochester, Monroe Co. Original.
Bacon, Charles G., Fulton, Oswego Co. (Retired list.)

Bagg, Moses M., Utica, Oneida Co. Original. (Retired list.)
Bailey, Theodore P., 95 Eagle St., Albany, Albany Co. Founder.
Bailey, William C. Original. Knoxville, Tenn.
Baker, Benjamin N., Rhinebeck, Dutchess Co.
Baker, Frank R., 540 Bedford Ave., Brooklyn, E. D., Kings Co.
Baker, George W., 540 Bedford Ave., Brooklyn, E. D., Kings Co. Founder.
Baldwin, F. A., 329 W. 23d St., New York, New York Co.
*Ballou, William R., Oakland Heights Sanitarium, Asheville, N. C.
Banks, George B., Hartsdale, Westchester Co. Original. (Retired list.)
Banta, Rollin L., 330 Elk St., Buffalo, Érie Co. Original.
Barnes, Edwin, Pleasant Plains, Dutchess Co. Original.
Barney, Charles S., Milford, Otsego Co. Original.
Barnum, D. Albert, Cassville, Oneida Co.
Bartlett, Frederick W., 528 Delaware Ave., Buffalo, Erie Co. Original.
Barton, Lyman, Willsborough, Essex Co. Founder. (Retired list.)
Barton, L. G., Willsborough, Essex Co.
Barton, Thomas J., Red Hook, Dutchess Co.
Bartow, Bernard, 220 Franklin St., Buffalo, Erie Co.
Bates, Nelson W., Central Square, Oswego Co.
Bates, Xyris T., Poughkeepsie, Dutchess Co. Original.
Bayley, Guy Carleton, Poughkeepsie, Dutchess Co. Original.
Baynes, Joseph E., 2419 5th Ave., Troy, Rensselaer Co.
Beardsley, William E., 101 Taylor St., Brooklyn, Kings Co.
Beers, John E., Danby, Tompkins Co. Founder.
Bellows, George A., Waterloo, Seneca Co.
Bemus, Morris N., Jamestown, Chautauqua Co.
Bemus, William Marvin, Jamestown, Chautauqua Co.
Benham, John C., Hudson, Columbia Co. Original.
Bennett, Thomas W., Jeffersonville, Sullivan Co. Original.
Bentley, Francis R., Cheshire, Ontario Co. Original. (Retired list.)
Benton, Stuart H., 1063 Bergen St., Brooklyn, Kings Co.
Bergtold, W. H., 56 Allen St., Buffalo, Erie Co.
Bermingham, Edward J., 7 W. 45th St., New York, New York Co.
Bierwirth, Julius C., 187 Montague St., Brooklyn, Kings Co.
Biggam, William H., Jr., 1095 Dean St., Brooklyn, Kings Co. Original.
Biggs, Chauncey P., 14 E. Seneca St., Ithaca, Tompkins Co.
Biggs, Hermann M., 58 E. 25th St., New York, New York Co. Original.
Birdsall, Gilbert, North Brookfield, Madison Co. Original.
Bissell, James H., 2187 5th Ave., Troy, Rensselaer Co.
Blaine, Myron D., Willard, Seneca Co.
Blair, Louis P., McDonough, Chenango Co. Original.
Blake, Clarence R., Northville, Fulton Co. Original.
Blumer, G. Alder, State Hospital, Utica, Oneida Co. Original.
Boies, Loren F., 286 Howard Ave., Buffalo, Erie Co. Original.
Bond, G. F. M., State Hospital, Utica, Oneida Co.
Bonesteel, H. F., Mill St., Troy, Rensselaer Co.

* Deceased.

Bonesteel, William N., Mill St., Troy, Rensselaer Co.   Founder.   (Retired list.)

Bontecou, Reed B., 82 4th St., Troy, Rensselaer Co.   Original.

Booth, Wilbur H., 172 Genesee St., Utica, Oneida Co.   Original.

Boyce, Elias B., Averill Park, Rensselaer Co.

Bozeman, Nathan, 9 W. 31st St., New York, New York Co.   Founder.

Bozeman, Nathan G., 9 W. 31st St., New York, New York Co.

Bradford, George D., Homer, Cortland Co.

Bradley, O. Howard, Hudson, Columbia Co.

Brandt, J. S., Ontario Center, Wayne Co.

Briggs, Albert H., 267 Hudson St., Buffalo, Erie Co.   Original.

Briggs, C. M., Fairport, Monroe Co.

Briggs, William H., Hemlock Lake, Livingston Co.   Original.

Brodrick, William P., 272 Willis Ave., New York, New York Co.

Brooks, Leroy J., Norwich, Chenango Co.   Original.

Brown, Charles W., 902 14th St., N. W., Washington, D. C.   Original.

Brown, George L., 121 Franklin St., Buffalo, Erie Co.

Brown, J. P., Nunda, Livingston Co.

Brown, Ulysses H., 312 Warren St., Syracuse, Onondaga Co.

Brundage, Amos H., 609 Madison St., Brooklyn, Kings Co.   Original.

Brush, Edward F., Mount Vernon, Westchester Co.   Original.

Brush, Edward N., Shepperd Asylum, Towsen, Md.   Original.

Bryant, Joseph D., 54 W. 36th St., New York, New York Co.   Original.

Bryant, Percy, State Hospital, Buffalo, Erie Co.

Buchanan, Alexander, 358 W. 30th St., New York, New York Co.   Original.

*Buckley, Charles, 127 E. Main St., Rochester, Monroe Co.   Original.

Buckley, James, 127 E. Main St., Rochester, Monroe Co.   Original.

Bull, Charles Stedman, 47 W. 36th St., New York, New York Co.   Original

Bull, William T., 35 W. 35th St., New York, New York Co.

Burbeck, Charles H., 91 First St., Troy, Rensselaer Co.   Founder.

Burchard, Thomas H., 7 E. 48th St., New York, New York Co.   Original.

Burghardt, Francis Augustus, 632 Elm St., Buffalo, Erie Co.

Burhyte, O. W., Brookfield, Madison Co.

Burke, John J. A., 65 East Ave., Rochester, Monroe Co.   Original.

Burns, William J., Sea Cliff, Queens Co.   Original.

Burton, Matthew H., 75 4th St., Troy, Rensselaer Co.   Founder.

Cady, George N., Nichols, Tioga Co.

Cahill, John T., Hoosick Falls, Rensselaer Co.

Caldwell, Nathan A., Hagemans's Mills, Montgomery Co.

Campbell, A. J., 332 Warren St., Syracuse, Onondaga Co.

Campbell, Clarence G., 36 W. 33d St., New York, New York Co.

Carpenter, Henry W., Oneida, Madison Co.   Original.

*Carroll, Alfred Ludlow, 30 W. 59th St., New York, New York Co.

Carter, H. Skelton, 130 E. 24th St., New York, New York Co.   Original.

Casey, J. E., Mohawk, Herkimer Co.

Cavana, Martin, Oneida, Madison Co.

Chambers, Jacob, Kingston, Ulster Co.   Original.   ·

* Deceased.

Chambers, Martin L., Port Jefferson, Suffolk Co. Original.
Chapman, James, Medina, Orleans Co. Founder.
Chauveau, Jean F., 31 W. 60th St., New York, New York Co. Original.
Chittenden, Daniel J., Addison, Steuben Co.
Chittenden, Joseph H., Binghamton, Broome Co. Founder.
Chrystie, T. M. Ludlow, 216 W. 46th St., New York, New York Co. Original.
Church, B. A., Oneonta, Otsego Co.
Church, Charles A., Bloomingdale, Essex Co.
Church, Thomas C., Valley Falls, Rensselaer Co.
Churchill, Alonzo, 189 Genesee St., Oneida Co. (Retired list.)
Clark, Dewitt C., Marathon, Cortland Co. Original.
Clarke, Wallace, 186 Park Ave., Utica, Oneida Co.
Clum, Franklin D., Cheviot, Columbia Co.
Codding, George H., Amenia, Dutchess Co. Founder.
Coffin, Lawrence, 473 Bedford Ave., Brooklyn, Kings Co.
Cohen, Bernard, 497 Niagara St., Buffalo, Erie Co.
Collins, Stacy B., Seaford, Sussex Co., Del.
Colvin, Darwin, Clyde, Wayne Co. Founder.
Comfort, John E., 1315 Franklin Ave., New York, New York Co.
Comstock, George F., Saratoga Springs, Saratoga Co. Founder.
Congdon, Charles E., 1034 Jefferson St., Buffalo, Erie Co.
Conkling, George, Durham, Greene Co. Original.
Conner, Milton C., Middletown, Orange Co.
Conover, William S., 237 W. 132d St., New York, New York Co. Founder.
Conway, John Francis, cor. Buffalo and Union Sts., Brooklyn, Kings Co. Original.
Conway, John R., 130 Lexington Ave., New York, New York Co.
Cook, Guy Reuben, Louisville, St. Lawrence Co.
Cooke, Almon H., Bellevue Hospital, New York, New York Co.
Cooley, F. L., 210 First St., Oswego, Oswego Co.
Cooley, R. N., Hannibal Centre, Oswego Co.
Cooper, William C., 81 3d St., Troy, Rensselaer Co. Original.
Copley, Herman D., Bainbridge, Chenango Co.
Coutant, Richard B., Tarrytown, Westchester Co. Original.
Cramer, William, 136 Mansion St., Poughkeepsie, Dutchess Co. Founder.
Crane, Frank W., Corfu, Genesee Co. Original.
Crawe, J. Mortimer, Watertown, Jefferson Co. Founder.
Creamer, Joseph, Jr., 168 N. 6th St., Brooklyn, E. D., Kings Co.
Criado, Louis F., 147 Fort Green Place, Brooklyn, Kings Co.
Crocker, Edwin, Narrowsburgh, Sullivan Co.
Crombie, Walter C., Mechanicsville, Saratoga Co. Original.
Cronyn, John, 55 W. Swan St., Buffalo, Erie Co. Founder.
Crosby, Alexander H., Lowville, Lewis Co.
Crounse, Andrew C., Melrose, Rensselaer Co.
Curry, Walker, 21 E. 61st St., New York, New York Co. Original.
Curtis, Daniel, Jeddo, Orleans Co.
Curtis, D. F., 95 South Ave., Rochester, Monroe Co.

Curtis, P. C., Round Lake, Saratoga Co.
Dagenais, Alphonse, 473 W. Virginia St., Buffalo, Erie Co. Original.
Dallas, Alexander, 65 W. 86th St., New York, New York Co.
Dallas, Alexander J., 48 Warren St., Syracuse, Onondaga Co. Founder.
Dandridge, N. P., 148 Broadway, Cincinnati, Ohio.
Daniels, Clayton M., 868 Main St., Buffalo, Erie Co. Original.
Daniels, F. H., 126 W. 126th St., New York, New York Co.
D'Avignon, Francis J., Au Sable Forks, Essex Co. Original.
Davis, J. Griffith, 200 W. 14th St., New York, New York Co.
Davis, J. O., Howells, Orange Co.
Davis, Robert C., 150 E. 128th St., New York, New York Co.
Dayton, C. L., 246 Dearborn St., Buffalo, Erie Co. (Retired list.)
Dean, Harmon J., Brocton, Chautauqua Co. Founder.
De Garmo, W. B., 56 W. 36th St., New York, New York Co.
DeKay, William H., Parksville, Sullivan Co.
De Laney, John Pope, Geneva, Ontario Co.
Delphey, Eden V., 358 W. 58th St., New York, New York Co.
Denison, Charles Ellery, 124 W. 13th St., New York, New York Co.
    Original.
Denison, Ellery, 124 W. 13th St., New York, New York Co. Original.
Dennis, Frederic S., 542 Madison Ave., New York, New York Co.
    Founder.
de Quesada, Gregorio J., 413 W. 43d St., New York, New York Co.
De Witt, Byron, Oswego, Oswego Co. Original.
de Zouche, Isaac, Gloversville, Fulton Co. Founder.
Dickinson, M. D., Troy, Rensselaer Co.
Dickson, Thomas Gordon, Troy, Rensselaer Co.
Didama, Emory A., Cortland, Cortland Co.
Didama, Henry D., 112 S. Salina St., Syracuse, Onondaga Co. Founder.
Dodge, Amos P., Oneida Castle, Oneida Co.
Dodge, Frank B., Mount Morris, Livingston Co.
Dodge, Lyndhurst C., Rouse's Point, Clinton Co. Founder.
Donohue, Florence O., 410 Warren St., Syracuse, Onondaga Co. Original.
Dorland, Elias T., 86 N. Division St., Buffalo, Erie Co. Original.
Douglas, George, Oxford, Chenango Co.
Douglass, A. J., Illion, Herkimer Co.
Douglass, Charles E., Lowville, Lewis Co.
Douglass, James W., Booneville, Oneida Co.
Drake, D. Delos, Johnstown, Fulton Co.
Drake, E. G., 312 W. Church St., Elmira, Chemung Co.
Drake, Frank C., Oneida, Madison Co.
Drake, James B., Hancock, Delaware Co.
Du Bois, Matthew B., 156 Broadway, Manhattan Life Ins. Co., New York,
    New York Co. Original.
Dudley, A. Palmer, 640 Madison Ave., New York, New York Co.
Dudley, Dwight, Maine, Broome Co.
Dunham, Edward K., 347 Lexington Ave., New York, New York Co.
Dunlop, John J., Waterford, Saratoga Co. Original.

Dunn, Jeremiah, Bath, Steuben Co. Original.
Dunning, J. D., Webster, Monroe Co. Original.
Earle, George W., Tully, Onondaga Co.
Eastman, Robert W., 170 W. 78th St., New York, New York Co. Original.
Eddy, George P., Lewiston, Niagara Co.
Eddy, John L., Olean, Cattaraugus Co.
Edwards, Amos S., 1506 N. Salina St., Syracuse, Onondaga Co. Original.
Edwards, George A., Catherine and Lodi Sts., Syracuse, Onondaga Co. Original.
Edwards, John, Gloversville, Fulton Co.
Einhorn, Max, 107 E. 65th St., New York, New York Co.
Eldridge, Stuart, Yokohama, Japan. (Non-resident.)
Eliot, Ellsworth, 48 W. 36th St., New York, New York Co. Original.
Ellinwood, A. G., Attica, Wyoming Co. Original.
Ellis, J. B., Whitesborough, Oneida Co.
Ellison, Metler D., Canisteo, Steuben Co. Original.
Ellsworth, Victor A., Wellsville, Cattaraugus Co.
Ely, Henry Oliver, Binghamton, Broome Co. Original.
Enders, Thomas Burnham, 163 W. 121st St., New York, New York Co.
English, G. P., Booneville, Oneida Co.
Erdmann, John F., 141 W. 34th St., New York, New York Co.
Farnham, LeRoy D., Binghamton, Broome Co.
Farrington, Edward S., Bellevue Hospital, New York, New York Co.
Farrington, John M., Binghamton, Broome Co.
Farrington, Joseph O., 1991 Madison Ave., New York, New York Co.
Feely, James F., 296 Lorimer St., Brooklyn, E. D., Kings Co.
Fell, George E., 72 Niagara St., Buffalo, Erie Co.
Fenno, Henry Marshall, 77 W. Main St., Rochester, Monroe Co.
Ferguson, E. D., 1 Union Place, Troy, Rensselaer Co. Founder.
Field, Matthew D., 115 E. 40th St., New York, New York Co.
Finder, William, Jr., 2 Union Place, Troy, Rensselaer Co. Founder.
Fisher, John C., Warsaw, Wyoming Co.
*Fitch, William, Dryden, Tompkins Co. Founder.
Fitzgerald, David J., Glens Falls, Warren Co.
Fitzgerald, John F., State Hospital, Binghamton, Broome Co.
Flandrau, Thomas M., Rome, Oneida Co.
Flanigan, John R., Syracuse, Onondaga Co.
Fletcher, Charles L., Wing's Station, Dutchess Co. Original.
Flickinger, John, Trumansburg, Tompkins Co.
Flint, Austin, 60 E. 34th St., New York, New York Co. Founder.
Flint, Austin, Jr., 252 Madison Ave., New York, New York Co.
Flint, William H., 37 E. 33d St., New York, New York Co. Founder.
Ford, M. L., Oneonta, Otsego Co.
Forker, Frederick L., Binghamton, Broome Co.
Foster, George V., 109 E. 18th St., New York, New York Co.
Fowler, Joseph, 31 Church St., Buffalo, Erie Co.
Frankenberg, Jacob H., 142 E. 74th St., New York, New York Co.

* Deceased.

Fraser, Jefferson C., Ava, Oneida Co.
Frazee, A. Blair, Altoona, Pa.
Frederick, Carlton C., 64 Richmond Ave., Buffalo, Erie Co.
French, S. H., Amsterdam, Montgomery Co.
Fritts, Crawford Ellsworth, Hudson, Columbia Co.
Fuller, Earl D., 66 Varick St., Utica, Oneida County.
Fuller, Robert, Schenectady, Schenectady Co.
Furman, Guido, 125 W. 73d St., New York, New York Co.   Original.
Furman, J. Henry, Tarrytown, Westchester Co.   Original.
Gardiner, W. F., 175 6th Ave., Brooklyn, Kings Co.
Garlock, William D., Little Falls, Herkimer Co.
Getty, A. H., Athens, Greene Co.
Gibson, William M., 187 Genesee St., Utica, Oneida Co.
Gilbert, Horatio, Hornellsville, Steuben Co.
Gillis, William, Fort Covington, Franklin Co.   Founder.
Gleitsmann, J. W., 46 E. 25th St., New York, New York Co.
Glidden, Charles H., Little Falls, Herkimer Co.   Original.
Goldthwaite, Henry, Fifth Avenue Hotel, New York, New York Co.
Goler, George W., 54 S. Fitzhugh St., Rochester, Monroe Co.
Gould, Cassius W., 1428 Main St., Buffalo, Erie Co.   ·
Gouley, John W. S., 324 Madison Ave., New York, New York Co.
    Founder.
Govan, William, Stony Point, Rockland Co.   Founder.
Gow, Frank F., Schuylerville, Saratoga Co.
Granger, William D., Bronxville (Vernon House), Westchester Co.
Grant, Charles S., Saratoga Springs, Saratoga Co.   Founder.
Grauer, Frank, 326 W. 46th St., New York, New York Co.
Graves, Ezra, Amsterdam, Montgomery Co.   Original.
Gray, Joseph F., 326 W. 31st St., New York, New York Co.
Green, H. H., Paine's Hollow, Herkimer Co.
Green, Stephen S., 426 Niagara St., Buffalo, Erie Co.
Greene, Clark W., Chenango Forks, Broome Co.
Greene, DeWitt C., 1125 Main St., Buffalo, Erie Co.   Original.
Greene, Joseph C., 124 Swan St., Buffalo, Erie Co.   Founder.
Greene, Walter D., 444 Elk St., Buffalo, Erie Co.   Original.
Greenman, C. E., 575 1st St., Troy, Rensselaer Co.
Gulick, A. Reading, 30 W. 36th St., New York, New York Co.
Gulick, Charlton R., 30 W. 36th St., New York, New York Co.
Guy, J. D., Coventry, Chenango Co.
Hagadorn, William, Gilboa, Schoharie Co.   Original.
Halbert, M. L., Cincinnatus, Cortland Co.
Hall, William H., Saratoga Springs, Saratoga Co.   Original.
Hamill, Edward H., 302 6th Ave., Newark, N. J.
Hammer, Charles, Schenectady, Schenectady Co.
Hammond, Frederick Porter, 157 E. 115th St., New York, New York Co.
Hand, S. M., Norwich, Chenango Co.
Hannan, James C., Hoosick Falls, Rensselaer Co.   Founder.
Hannan, Thomas H., Hoosick Falls, Rensselaer Co.

Harrington, D. W., 1430 Main St., Buffalo, Erie Co. Original.
Harrison, George Tucker, 221 W. 23d St., New York, New York Co. Original.
Hartwig, Marcell, 34 E. Huron St., Buffalo, Erie Co.
Harvie, J. B., 6 Clinton Place, Troy, Rensselaer Co. Founder.
Hatch, C. A., 110 E. Onondaga St., Syracuse, Onondaga Co. Original.
Haubold, H. A., 225 E. 72d St., New York, New York Co.
Hayd, Herman E., 78 Niagara St., Buffalo, Erie Co.
Hayes, Philetus A., Afton, Chenango Co.
Haynes, John U., 108 Mohawk St., Cohoes, Albany Co.
Head, Adelbert D., 322 S. Salina St., Syracuse, Onondaga Co. Founder.
Heath, William H., 415 Pearl St., Buffalo, Erie Co.
Heimstreet, Thomas B., 14 Division St., Troy, Rensselaer Co. Original.
Hendrick, Henry C., McGrawville, Cortland Co. Founder.
Hepburn, Neil J., 369 W. 23d St., New York, New York Co.
Hewitt, Adelbert, Saratoga Springs, Saratoga Co.
Hicks, Edward E., Poughkeepsie, Dutchess Co.
Hicks, W. Scott, Bristol, Ontario Co. Original.
Higgins, F. W., Cortland, Cortland Co.
Hillis, Thomas J., 51 Charlton St., New York, New York Co.
Hills, Lyman H., Binghamton, Broome Co. Original.
Himmelsbach, George A., 30 12th St., Buffalo, Erie Co.
Hinton, John H., 41 W. 32d St., New York, New York Co. Founder.
Hodgman, Abbott, 141 E. 38th St., New York, New York Co. ▼Founder.
Hodgman, William H., 108 Caroline St., Saratoga Springs, Saratoga Co. Founder.
Hogan, M. K., 226 W. 34th St., New York, New York Co.
Holcomb, O. A., Plattsburgh, Clinton Co.
Holden, Arthur L., 116 South St., Utica, Oneida Co.
Holmes, Martha C., 75 W. 126th St., New York, New York Co.
HoornBeek, Philip Du Bois, Wawarsing, Ulster Co. Original. [(Retired list.)
Horton, David C., Red Creek, Wayne Co.
Hough, F. P., Binghamton, Broome Co.
Houston. David W., 44 2d St., Troy, Rensselaer Co. Original.
Hovey, B. L., 34 N. Fitzhugh St., Rochester, Monroe Co. Founder.
Howard, Charles F., 1458 Main St., Buffalo, Erie Co.
Howland, George T., Norwich, Conn.
Hoyer, F. F., Tonawanda, Erie Co. Founder.
Hubbard, Chauncey G., Hornellsville, Steuben Co.
Hubbard, Dwight L., 344 W. 32d St., New York, New York Co.
Hubbard, George E., 257 W. 52d St., New York, New York Co.
Hubbard, Samuel T., 27 W. 9th St., New York, New York Co. Founder.
Hubbell, Alvin A., 212 Franklin St., Buffalo, Erie Co.
Hudson, George, Stillwater, Saratoga Co.
Huestis, W. B., Kiskatom, Greene Co.
Huggins, William Q., Sanborn, Niagara Co.
Hughes, Henry R., Clinton, Oneida Co.
33

Hughes, Peter, 275 Berry St., Brooklyn, Kings Co.
Hulette, G. S., Arcade, Wyoming Co.
Hühne, August, Rondout, Ulster Co. Founder.
Hühne, Frederick, Rondout, Ulster Co. Original.
Hull, Thomas H., 55 Lee Ave., Brooklyn, Kings Co.
Hull, William H., Poestenkill, Rensselaer Co.
Hulse, William A., Bay Shore, Suffolk Co.
Humphrey, J. F., Saratoga Springs, Saratoga Co.
Hunt, H. L., Orchard Park, Erie Co.
Hunt, James G., 5 Gardner Block, Utica, Oneida Co. Original.
Hunter, Nathaniel P., Jasper, Steuben Co.
Huntington, Henry K., New Rochelle, Westchester Co. Original.
Huntington, John W., Mexico, Oswego Co.
Huntley, James F., Oneida, Madison Co.
Ilgen, Ernst, 369 Herkimer St., Brooklyn, Kings Co. Original.
Ingraham, Charles W., Binghamton, Broome Co.
Ingraham, Henry D., 405 Franklin St., Buffalo, Erie Co.
Ingraham, Samuel, Palmyra, Wayne Co. Original. (Retired list.)
Inlay, Erwin G., Saratoga Springs, Saratoga Co.
Jackson, Albert P., Oakfield, Genesee Co. Founder.
Jackson, Charles W., 168 W. 81st St., New York, New York Co.
Jackson, William H., Springville, Erie Co.
Jacobson, Nathan, 430 S. Salina St., Syracuse, Onondaga Co. Original.
Jamison, John S., Hornellsville, Steuben Co. Original.
Janeway, Edward G., 36 W. 40th St., New York, New York Co. Founder.
Janvrin, J. E., 191 Madison Ave., New York, New York Co.
Jenkins, John A., 271 Jefferson Ave., Brooklyn, E. D., Kings Co. Original.
Jenkins, William T., 109 E. 26th St., New York, New York Co.
Jewett, F. A., 232 Hancock St., Brooklyn, Kings Co.
Jewett, Homer O., Cortland, Cortland Co. Founder.
Johnson, George P., Mexico, Oswego Co.
Johnson, Ianthus G., Greenfield Centre, Saratoga Co. Original.
Johnson, Leonard M., Greene, Chenango Co. Original.
Johnson, Parley H., Adams, Jefferson Co. Original.
Johnson, Richard G., Amsterdam, Montgomery Co. Original.
Johnson, Thomas M., 418 Main St., Buffalo, Erie Co. Original.
Johnston, Henry C., New Brighton, Richmond Co.
Johnston, N. B., Barryville, Sullivan Co.
Jones, Allen A., 436 Franklin St., Buffalo, Erie Co.
Jones, George H., Fowlerville, Livingston Co.
Jones, S. Case, 89 N. Fitzhugh St., Rochester, Monroe Co.
Joslin, Albert A., Martinsburgh, Lewis Co.
Judson, A. B., 38 E. 25th St., New York, New York Co.
Julian, John M., Moore's Mill, Dutchess Co.
Keefer, Charles W., Mechanicsville, Saratoga Co.
Keith, Halbert Lyon, Upton, Mass.
Kelly, John Devin, Lowville, Lewis Co.
Kemp, William M., 267 W. 23d St., New York, New York Co.

Kenyon, Benjamin, Cincinnatus, Cortland Co.
Kenyon, M., King's Ferry, Cayuga Co. Original.
Kilborn, Henry F., Croghan, Lewis Co.
King, Ferdinand, 315 W. 58th St., New York, New York Co.
King, James K., Watkins, Schuyler Co.
Kingsley, Henry F., Schoharie, Schoharie Co. Original.
Kittredge, Charles S., Fishkill-on-Hudson, Dutchess Co. Founder.
Klock, Charles M., St. Johnsville, Montgomery Co.
Knapp, W. H., Binghamton, Broome Co.
Kneeland, B. T., Dalton, Livingston Co.
Kneeland, Jonathan S., Onondaga, Onondaga Co. Founder. (Retired list.)
Kneer, F. G., 286 W. 51st St., New York, New York Co.
Knipe, George, 354 W. 24th St., New York Co.
Kniskern, A. C., Mechanicsville, Saratoga Co.
Kuhn, William, Rome, Oneida Co.
LaBell, Martin J., Lewis, Essex Co. Original.
Laird, William R., 98 Wall St., Auburn, Cayuga Co. Original.
Lake, Albert D., Gowanda, Cattaraugus Co.
Lambert, John, Salem, Washington Co.
Landon, Newell E., Newark, Wayne Co. Original.
Lapp, Henry, Clarence, Erie Co.
Leach, H. M., Charlton City, Massachusetts. Original.
Leale, Charles A., 604 Madison Ave., New York, New York Co. Founder.
Leaning, John K., Cooperstown, Otsego Co. Founder.
Leffingwell, E. D., Watkins, Schuyler Co.
Leighton, N. W., 143 Taylor St., Brooklyn, E. D., Kings Co. Original.
Le Roy, Irving D., Pleasant Valley, Dutchess Co. Founder.
Lester, Elias, Seneca Falls, Seneca Co. Founder.
Lewis, Robert, 19 E. 38th St., New York, New York Co.
Lindsay, Walter, Huntington, Suffolk Co. Original.
Little, Albert H., 230 W. 43d St., New York, New York Co.
Little, Frank, 114 Montague St., Brooklyn, Kings Co.
Lloyd, T. Mortimer, 125 Pierrepont St., Brooklyn, Kings Co. Original.
Lockwood, Charles E., 59 W. 36th St., New York, New York Co.
Lockwood, J. W., Philmont, Columbia Co. Original.
Long, Alfred J., Whitehall, Washington Co.
Long, Ben G., 1408 Main St., Buffalo, Erie Co.
Ludlow, Ogden C., 210 W. 135th St., New York, New York Co.
Lukens, Anna, 1068 Lexington Ave., New York, New York Co.
Lung, Jesse B., 382 Marion St., Brooklyn, Kings Co. Original.
Lusk, William T., 47 E. 34th St., New York, New York Co. Founder.
Lusk, Zera J., Warsaw, Wyoming Co.
*Lyman, Elijah S., Sherburne, Chenango Co. Original.
Lyman, H. C., Sherburne, Chenango Co. Original.
Lynch, Patrick J., 216 E. 13th St., New York, New York Co.
Lyon, E. M., Plattsburgh, Clinton Co. Founder.

* Deceased.

Lyon, George E., 1230 Olive St., St. Louis, Mo.   Original.
Lyons, Edward L., 298 4th St., Troy, Rensselaer Co.
Lyons, G. A., New Rochelle, Westchester Co.   Original.
Macfarlane, William A., Springville, Erie Co.
MacGregor, James R., 1118 Madison Ave., New York, New York Co.
Mackénzie, J. C., 432 W. 22d St., New York, New York Co.
Maclean, Donald, 652 Mission St., Detroit, Mich.   (Non-resident.)
Magee, Charles M., West and Seymour Sts., Syracuse, Onondaga Co.
Magee, Daniel, 116 3d St., Troy, Rensselaer Co.   Original.
Maine, Alvah P., Webster, Monroe Co.
Manley, Thomas H., 302 W. 53d St., New York, New York Co.   Founder.
Marsh, E. Frank, Fulton, Oswego Co.
Marsh, James P., 1739 5th Ave., Troy, Rensselaer Co.
Marshall, Francis F., 56 W. 56th St., New York, New York Co.
Martin, John H., Otego, Otsego Co.   Original.
Martindale, F. E., Port Richmond, Richmond Co.
Martine, Godfrey R., Glens Falls, Warren Co.   Original.
McAlpin, D. Hunter, 40 W. 40th St., New York, New York Co.
McBurney, Charles, 28 W. 37th St., New York, New York Co.
McCollom, William, 195 Lefferts Place, Brooklyn, Kings Co.   Original.
McDaniel, Alfred C., San Antonio, Texas.   (Non-resident.)
McDonald, George E., Schenectady, Schenectady Co.   Original.
McDougall, R. A., Duanesburgh, Schenectady Co.
McDougall, William D., Spencerport, Monroe Co.   (San José, Cal.)
*McEwen, Robert C., Saratoga Springs, Saratoga Co.   Founder.
McGann, Thomas, Wells, Hamilton Co.
McGillicuddy, T. J., 776 Madison Ave., New York, New York Co.
McGowen, John P., 137 E. 28th St., New York, New York Co.
McIlroy, Samuel H., 330 Alexander Ave., New York, New York Co.
McLeod, Johnston, 247 W. 23d St., New York, New York Co.
McLeod, S. B. Wylie, 247 W. 23d St., New York, New York Co.   Founder.
McLochlin, James A., 401 E. 10th St., New York, New York Co.   Original.
McNamara, Daniel, 243 W. Genesee St., Syracuse, Onondaga Co.   Original.
McNamara, Laurence J., 126 Washington Place (West), New York, New
    York Co.   Original.
McWilliams, F. A., Monticello, Sullivan Co.
Meacham, Isaac D., Binghamton, Broome Co.
Meier, Gottlieb C. H., 210 E. 53d St., New York, New York Co.
Menzie, R. J., Caledonia, Livingston Co.   Original.
Merritt, George, Cherry Valley, Otsego Co.   Original.
Miller, William T., 310 W. 27th St., New York, New York Co.   Original.
Milliken, S. E., 36 W. 59th St., New York, New York Co.
Minard, E. J. Chapin, 243 Quincy St., Brooklyn, Kings Co.   Original.
Miranda, Ramon L., 349 W. 46th St., New York, New York Co.   Original.
Mitchell, Howard E., 3 Clinton place, Troy, Rensselaer Co.   Founder.
Mitchell, Hubbard W., 747 Madison Ave., New York, New York Co.
    Original.

* Deceased.

Moore, Edward M., 74 S. Fitzhugh St., Rochester, Monroe Co. Founder.
Moore, Edward M., Jr., 74 S. Fitzhugh St., Rochester, Monroe Co.
Original.
Moore, Richard Mott, 74 Fitzhugh St., Rochester, Monroe Co. Original.
Moore, William A., Binghamton, Broome Co.
Moran, James, 352 W. 51st St., New York, New York Co.
Moriarta, Douglas C.. Saratoga Springs, Saratoga Co.
Morrow, William B., Walton, Delaware Co.
Mott, Valentine, 62 Madison Ave., New York, New York Co.
Moyer, Frank H., Moscow, Livingston Co. Original.
Mudge, Selden J., Olean, Cattaraugus Co.
Munger, Charles, Knoxborough, Oneida Co.
Munson, J. A., Woodbourne, Sullivan Co. Original.
Munson, W. W., Otisco, Onondaga Co. Original.
Murdoch, James Bissett, 4232 5th Ave., Pittsburgh, Pa. (Non-resident.)
Murdock, George W., Cold Spring, Putnam Co. Founder.
Murphy, John, 249 E. 35th St., New York, New York Co. Original.
Murray, Byron J., Saratoga Springs, Saratoga Co. Original.
Murray, S. J., 133 W. 87th St., New York, New York Co. Original.
Murray, William D., Tonawanda, Erie Co. Original.
Nelson, William H., Taberg, Oneida Co.
Newman, George W., 234 Leonard St., Brooklyn, Kings Co.
Newman, Robert, 68 W. 36th St., New York, New York Co. Original.
Nichols, Calvin E., 25 1st St., Troy, Rensselaer Co. Founder.
Nichols, H. W., Canandaigua, Ontario Co. Founder. (Retired list.)
Nichols, William H., West Sand Lake, Rensselaer Co. Founder.
Nicholson, A. R., Madison, Madison Co. Original.
Nicoll, Henry D., 51 E. 57th St., New York, New York Co. Founder.
Nold, John B., 165 North Ave., Rochester, Monroe Co.
North, Nelson L., 627 Bedford Ave., Brooklyn, Kings Co. Original.
Noyes, James B., New Berlin, Chenango Co.
Nutten, Wilbur F., Newark, Wayne Co.
Oberndorfer, Isidor P., 1037 Lexington Ave., New York, New York Co.
Original.
O'Brien, Frederick Wm., 234 E. 112th St., New York, New York Co.
O'Brien, M. Christopher, 161 W. 122d New York, New York Co.
Ochs, Benjamin F., 773 Lexington Ave., New York, New York Co.
O'Hare, Thomas A., 157 State St., Rochester, Monroe Co. Original.
Oliver, William, Penn Yan, Yates Co.
O'Meagher, William, 427 E. 84th St., New York, New York Co.
Oppenheimer, H. S., 49 E. 23d St., New York, New York Co.
Oppenheimer, S., 583 E. 120th St., New York, New York Co.
Orton, John G., Binghamton, Broome Co.
Ostrander, George A., 61 Greene Ave., Brooklyn, Kings Co.
Packer, Thurston G., Smyrna, Chenango Co.
Paine, Arthur R., 99 Lafayette Ave., Brooklyn, Kings Co. Original.
Palmer, Edmund J., 1342 Lexington Ave., New York, New York Co.
Palmer, F. A., Mechanicsville, Saratoga Co.

Palmer, George M., Warsaw, Wyoming Co. Original.
Palmer, Henry C., cor. Genesee and Hopper Sts., Utica, Oneida Co.
Palmer, Walter B., 30 South St., Utica, Oneida Co.
Parent, J. S., Birchton, Saratoga Co.
Park, Roswell, 510 Delaware Ave., Buffalo, Erie Co.
Parr, John, Buel, Montgomery Co.
Parsons, Israel, Marcellus, Onondaga Co. Founder.
Parsons, John, Kingsbridge, New York, New York Co. Original.
Parsons, W. W. D., Fultonville, Montgomery Co.
Pease, Joseph, Hamlin, Monroe Co. Original.
Perry, John Gardner, 48 E. 34th St., New York, New York Co.
Perry, Nathaniel M., Troupsburgh, Steuben Co. Original.
Peters, Samuel, 86 Mohawk St., Cohoes, Albany Co. Founder.
Pettit, John A., 519 Swan St., Buffalo, Erie Co. Original.
Phelan, Michael F., 339 Congress St., Troy, Rensselaer Co.
Phelps, Charles, 34 W. 37th St., New York, New York Co.
Phelps, George G., 239 Blandina St., Utica, Oneida Co.
Phelps, William C., 146 Allen St., Buffalo, Erie Co.
Pierce, Edward A., Binghamton, Broome Co.
Pierson, George E., Kirkwood, Broome Co.
Pilgrim, Charles W., State Hospital, Willard, Seneca Co. Original.
Piper, Charles W., Wurtsborough, Sullivan Co.
Place, John F., Jr., Binghamton, Broome Co.
Pohlman, Julius, 539 Niagara St., Buffalo, Erie Co.
Pooler, Hiram A., 34 Gramercy Park, New York, New York Co. Original. (Retired list.)
Porteous, James G., Poughkeepsie, Dutchess Co. Founder.
Porter, Harry N., 1910 Harewood Ave., Washington, D. C. Founder. (Retired list.)
Porter, P. Brynberg, 8 W. 35th St., New York, New York Co. Original.
Potter, Vaughn C., Starkville, Herkimer Co. Original.
Potts, E., Port Jervis, Orange Co.
Pratt, Frank R., Manchester, Ontario Co.
Pray, S. R., 523 Bedford Ave., Brooklyn, Kings Co. Original.
Preston, John R., Schuylerville, Saratoga Co. Original.
Price, Henry R., 485 Franklin Ave., Brooklyn, Kings Co.
Prince, Alpheus, Byron, Genesee Co.
Pritchard, R. L., 72 W. 49th St., New York, New York Co.
Pryor, William R., 15 Park Ave., New York, New York Co.
Pultz, Monroe T., Standfordville, Dutchess Co. Founder.
Purple, Samuel S., 36 W. 22d St., New York, New York Co. Founder.
Putnam, Frederick W., Binghamton, Broome Co. Founder.
Putnam, James W., 388 Franklin St., Buffalo, Erie Co. Original.
Quin, Hamilton S., 171 Genesee St., Utica, Oneida Co.
Race, W. F., 115 W. 25th St., Kearney, Neb. Original.
Rae, Robert, Portageville, Wyoming Co. Original.
Rand, Hannibal W., Keene, Essex Co. Original.

Ransom, H. B. (in care S. V. White & Co.), 36 Wall St., New York, New York Co.
Rau, Leonard S., 72 W. 55th St., New York, New York Co.
Rave, Edward G., Hicksville, Queens Co. Original.
Raynor, F. C., 163 Clinton St., Brooklyn, Kings Co.
Read, Ira B., 66 E. 126th St., New York, New York Co.
Reagles, James, Schenectady, Schenectady Co. Original.
Reed, Henry B., 12 Verona Place, Brooklyn, Kings Co.
Reid, Christopher C., Rome, Oneida Co.
Reitz, Charles, Webster, Monroe Co.
Reynolds, Tabor B., Saratoga Springs, Saratoga Co. Founder.
Rice, George, Mechanicsville, Saratoga Co.
Richards, Charles B., Binghamton, Broome Co. Founder.
Richardson, John E., 127 S. Oxford St., Brooklyn, Kings Co.
Richmond, Nelson G., Fredonia, Chautauqua Co.
Ricketts, Benjamin M., 137 Broadway, Cincinnati, Ohio. Original.
Riley, Andrew W., 207 S. 16th St., Omaha, Neb. Original.
Risch, Henry F. W., 521 3d St., Brooklyn, Kings Co.
Robb, William H., Amsterdam, Montgomery Co. Founder.
Robinson, Ezra A., Geneva, De Kalb Co., Ill. Original.
Rochester, DeLancey, 469 Franklin St., Buffalo, Erie Co.
Rochester, Thomas M., 326 De Kalb Ave., Brooklyn, Kings Co.
Rodgers, Harris C., 1 Wall St., Binghamton, Broome Co.
Rogers, S. Frank, 3161 6th Ave., Troy, Rensselaer Co. Original.
Rolph, R. T., Fredonia, Chautauqua Co.
Roper, P. B., Alpine, Schuyler Co.
Ross, Frank W., 251 Baldwin St., Elmira, Chemung Co. Original.
Roth, Julius A., 308 E. 79th St., New York, New York Co.
Rousseau, Zotique, 99 2d St., Troy, Rensselaer Co. Founder.
Rudgers, Denton W., Perry, Wyoming Co.
Ruggles, Augustus D., 289 W. 14th St., New York, New York Co.
Rulison, L. B., West Troy, Albany Co.
Rushmore, John D., 129 Montague St., Brooklyn, Kings Co. Founder.
Russell, Charles P., 198 Genesee St., Utica, Oneida Co.
Russell, William G., 27 McDonough St., Brooklyn, Kings Co. Original.
Sabal, E. T., 45 W. Monroe St., Jacksonville, Fla. (Non-resident.)
Sabin, William B., 1425 Broadway, West Troy, Albany Co. Founder.
Sabine, Gustavus A., 8 E. 24th St., New York, New York Co. Original.
Sanders, E., 126 E. 82d St., New York, New York Co.
Sawyer, Conant, Auburn, Cayuga Co. Founder.
Saxer, Leonard A., 514 Prospect Ave., Syracuse, Onondaga Co. Original.
Sayre, Lewis A., 285 5th Ave., New York, New York Co. Founder.
Sayre, Reginald H., 285 5th Ave., New York, New York Co.
Schmid, H. Ernst, White Plains, Westchester Co. Original.
Schopp, Justin H., 127 E. Main St., Rochester, Monroe Co.
Scully, Thomas P., Rome, Oneida Co.
Seaman, Louis L., 18 W. 31st St., New York, New York Co.
Seaman, Frank G., Seneca Falls, Seneca Co.

524   NEW YORK STATE MEDICAL ASSOCIATION.

Sears, F. W., 326 Montgomery St., Syracuse, Onondaga Co.
Segur, Avery, 281 Henry St., Brooklyn, Kings Co. Founder. (Retired list.)
Selden, O. G., Catskill, Greene Co. Original.
Selden, Robert, Catskill, Greene Co. Original.
Seymour, Ralph A., Whitney's Point, Broome Co.
Seymour, W. Wotkyns, 105 3d St., Troy, Rensselaer Co. Founder.
Sharer, John P., Little Falls, Herkimer Co. Original.
Shaw, Henry B., 21 E. 127th St., New York, New York Co.
Shea, Dennis L., 116 Waverly Place, New York, New York Co.
Shepard, A. Warner, 126 Willoughby St., Brooklyn, Kings Co. Original.
Sherer, John D., Waterford, Saratoga Co. Original.
Sherman, F. J., Ballston, Saratoga Co.
Shrady, John, 149 W. 126th St., New York, New York Co.
Shrady, John Eliot, 149 W. 126th St., New York, New York Co.
Shunk, Albert, 232 W. 22d St., New York, New York Co.
Silver, Henry M., 89 7th St., New York, New York Co.
Simmons, Charles E., 742 Lexington Ave., New York, New York Co.
Simmons, E. W., Canandaigua, Ontario Co. Founder. (Retired list.)
Simons, Frank E., Canajoharie, Montgomery Co.
Sizer, Nelson Buell, 336 Green Ave., Brooklyn, Kings Co. Original.
Skinner, Smith A., Hoosick Falls, Rensselaer Co. Original.
Slater, Frank Ellsworth, Binghamton, Broome Co.
Small, John W., New Rochelle, Westchester Co.
Smeallie, James A., 12 W. 40th St., New York, New York Co.
Smelzer, Baxter T., Havana, Schuyler Co.
Smith, F. A., Corinth, Saratoga Co.
Smith, George C., Delhi, Delaware Co.
Smith, H. Lyle, Hudson, Columbia Co. Original.
Smith, J.|Lewis, 64 W. 56th St., New York, New York Co. Original.
Smith, Samuel L., Smithville Flats, Chenango Co.
Smith, Samuel W., 24 W. 30th St., New York, New York Co. Original.
Smith, Stephen, 574 Madison Ave., New York, New York Co. Original.
Smyth, Arthur V. H., Amsterdam, Montgomery Co.
Snook, George M., Parma, Monroe Co.
Southworth, Malek A., 524 13th St., Oakland, Cal. Original.
Southworth, Richmond Joseph, 1220 36th St. N. W., Washington, D. C. Original.
Spicer, Walter E., 41 N. Moore St., New York, New York Co.
Sprague, John H., Williamson, Wayne Co. Original.
Sprague, L. S., Williamson, Wayne Co. (Retired list.)
Squibb, Edward H., 148 Columbia Heights, Brooklyn, Kings Co. Founder. (P. O. Box 760.)
Squibb, Edward R., 152 Columbia Heights, Brooklyn, Kings Co. Founder.
Squire, Charles L., 409 E. Church St., Elmira, Chemung Co.
Steinke, Carl Otho Hermann, 220 17th St., Brooklyn, Kings Co. Original.
Stephenson, F. Halleck, 101 Warren St., Syracuse, Onondaga Co.
Stewart, F. E., Watkins, Schuyler Co.

St. John, David, Hackensack, N. J. (Non-resident.)
Stockschlaeder, P., 186 South Ave., Rochester, Monroe Co.
Stockton, Charles G., 436 Franklin St., Buffalo, Erie Co.
Stone, Frank L., Le Roy, Genesee Co.
Strong, Cyrus J., 166 W. 105th St., New York, New York Co.
Strong, Orville C., Colden, Erie Co.
Strong, Thomas D., Westfield, Chautauqua Co. Founder.
Stubbs, Roland H., Waterford, Saratoga Co. Original.
Sullivan, John D., 74 McDonough St., Brooklyn, Kings Co.
Sutton, H. C., Rome, Oneida Co.
Sutton, Richard E., Rome, Oneida Co.
Swan, William E., Saratoga Springs, Saratoga Co.
Swanick, A. A., Saratoga Springs, Saratoga Co.
Swartwout, H. B., Port Jervis, Orange Co.
Swartwout, Leander, Prospect, Oneida Co.
Sweet, Joseph J., Unadilla, Otsego Co. Original.
Sweet, Joshua J., Unadilla, Otsego Co.
Sweetman, J. T., Jr., Ballston, Saratoga Co.
Taber, R. C., Tonawanda, Erie Co.
Taylor, John H., Holley, Orleans Co. Original.
Tefft, Charles B., Room 20, Arcade, Utica, Oneida Co.
Thomas, T. Gaillard, 600 Madison Ave., New York, New York Co.
   Founder.
Thompson, R. A., Norwich, Chenango Co.
Thompson, Amos W., Saratoga Springs, Saratoga Co.
Thompson, Von Beverhout, 111 W. 48d St., New York, New York Co.
Thornton, William H., 572 Niagara St., Buffalo, Erie Co.
Thwing, Clarence, Ft. Wrangel, Alaska.
Tiemann, Paul E., 180 W. 94th St., New York, New York Co.
Todd, John B., Parish, Oswego Co.
Tompkins, Fred J., 128 2d Ave., Lansingburgh, Rensselaer Co.
Tompkins, H. C., Knowlesville, Orleans Co. Founder. (Retired list.)
Tompkins, Orren A., East Randolph, Cattaraugus Co. Original.
Townsend, Charles E., Broadway and Grand Sts., Newburgh, Orange Co.
Townsend, Morris W., Bergen, Genesee Co. Founder.
Traver, Richard D., 14 4th St., Troy, Rensselaer Co. Original.
Travis, Edward M., Eagle Grove, Iowa.
Tremaine, Wm. S., 217 Franklin St., Buffalo, Erie Co. Founder.
Tripp, John D., Auburn, Cayuga Co. Original.
Truax, J. G., 17 E. 127th St., New York, New York Co.
Trull, H. P., Williamsville, Erie Co.
Tucker, Carlos P., 43 W. 26th St., New York, New York Co. Founder.
Turner, Melvin H., Mineville, Essex Co. Original.
Twohey, John J., 170 E. Utica St., Buffalo, Erie Co.
Vanderhoof, Frederick D., Phelps, Ontario Co. Original.
Vanderveer, J. C., Monroe, Orange Co.
Vanderveer, J. R., Monroe, Orange Co.
Van de Warker, Ely, 404 Fayette Park, Syracuse, Onondaga Co. Founder.

Van Etten, Cornelius, Rhinebeck, Dutchess Co.
Van Fleet, Frank, 158 E. 81st St., New York, New York Co.
Van Hoevenberg, Henry, Kingston, Ulster Co. Original.
Van Vranken, Adam T., 1603 3d Ave., West Troy, Albany Co. Original.
Van Wagner, L. A., Sherburne, Chenango Co.
Van Wyck, Richard C., Hopewell Junction, Dutchess Co. Original.
Van Zandt, Henry C., Schenectady, Schenectady Co. Original.
Varney, Miles E., Saratoga Springs, Saratoga Co.
Vedder, George W., Philmont, Columbia Co.
Veeder, Andrew T., Schenectady, Schenectady Co.
Von Donhoff, Edward, 210 W. 4th St., New York, New York Co.
Vincent, Ludger C., 52 W. 26th St., New York, New York Co.
Wagner, Charles Gray, State Hospital, Binghamton, Broome Co.
Wakeley, Benjamin C., Angelica, Allegany Co. Original.
Wales, Theron A., Elmira, Chemung Co. Original.
Wall, Charles A., 306 Hudson St., Buffalo, Erie Co.
Wallace, Edwin E., Jasper, Steuben Co.
Wallach, Joseph G., 7 W. 82d St., New York, New York Co. Original.
Walser, William C., West New Brighton, Richmond Co.
Walsh, Simon J., 25 E. 128th St., New York, New York Co.
Ward, Charles S., 30 W. 33d St., New York, New York Co. Founder.
Ward, John J., Ellenville, Ulster Co.
Ward, R. H., 53 4th St., Troy, Rensselaer Co.
Warner, Frederic M., 66 W. 56th St., New York, New York Co.
Warner, John W., 107 E. 72d St., New York, New York Co.
Waterworth, William, 3 Hancock St., Brooklyn, Kings Co.
Webster, W. B., Schuylerville, Saratoga Co.
Weeks, John E., 154 Madison Ave., New York, New York Co.
Welles, S. R., Waterloo, Seneca Co.
Wells, E. H., Binghamton, Broome Co.
Wells, William L., New Rochelle, Westchester Co. Original.
West, Joseph E., 171 Genesee St., Utica, Oneida Co.
Weston, Albert T., 226 Central Park West, bet. 82d and 83d Sts., New
  York, New York Co.
Wheeler, Isaac G., Marilla, Erie Co.
Wheeler, John T., Chatham, Columbia Co.
Whipple, Electa B., 491 Porter Ave., Buffalo, Erie Co.
White, Charles B., 107 W. 72d St., New York, New York Co.
White, J. Blake, 1013 Madison Ave., New York, New York Co.
White, Whitman V., 1024 Park Ave., New York, New York Co. Founder.
*White, William T., 130 E. 30th St., New York, New York Co. Founder.
Whitford, James, Onondaga Valley, Onondaga Co. Original.
Wieber, George, 181 S. 5th St., Brooklyn, Kings Co. Original.
Wiener, Joseph, 1046 5th Ave., New York, New York Co. Founder.
Wiggin, Frederick Holme, 55 W. 36th St., New York, New York Co.
Williams, George O., Greene, Chenango Co.
Williams, Henry Smith, Randall's Island, New York, New York Co.

* Deceased.

Williams, William H., 207 17th St., Brooklyn, Kings Co. Original.
Williamson, Edward A., Westchester Road, Westchester Co.
Willoughby, M., 1335 Main St., Buffalo, Erie Co.
Wilson, Thomas, Claverack, Columbia Co. Founder.
Witbeck, Charles E., Cohoes, Albany Co.
Woodend, William E., 171 E. 116th St., New York, New York Co.
Woodruff, E. Gould, Watkins, Schuyler Co.
Woodruff, R. Allen, Philmont, Columbia Co.
Woodworth, T. Floyd, Kinderhook, Columbia Co.
Wright, Theodore Goodell, Plainville, Hartford Co., Conn. (Non-resident.)
Wyckoff, Cornelius C., 482 Delaware Ave., Buffalo, Erie Co. Founder.
Wyckoff, Richard M., 532 Clinton Ave., Brooklyn, Kings Co. Founder.
Wyeth, John A., 27 E. 38th St., New York, New York Co. Original.
Young, Augustus A., Newark, Wayne Co. Original.
*Young, John, Fishkill-on-Hudson, Dutchess Co. Original.
Young, John D., Starkville, Herkimer Co. Original.
Young, William, Cold Spring, Putnam Co. Founder. (Retired list.)
Zeh, Edgar, Waterford, Saratoga Co.
Zeh, Merlin J., 1521 Broadway, West Troy, Albany Co.

Of 164 Founders, 109 remain on the list; of 286 Original Fellows, 217 remain on the list. Total Fellowship, 791.

RETIRED FELLOWS.

Charles G. Bacon, Fulton, Oswego County (1891).
M. M. Bagg, Utica, Oneida County (1891).
George B. Banks, Hartsdale, Westchester County (1892).
Lyman Barton, Willsborough, Essex County (1890).
F. R. Bentley, Cheshire, Ontario County (1891).
William N. Bonesteel, Troy, Rensselaer County (1890).
Alonzo Churchill, Utica, Oneida County (1890).
C. L. Dayton, Buffalo, Erie County (1891).
Philip DuB. HoornBeek, Wawarsing, Ulster County (1891).
Samuel Ingraham, Palmyra, Wayne County (1890).
Jonathan S. Kneeland, Onondaga County (1890).
H. W. Nichols, Canandaigua, Ontario County (1893).
H. A. Pooler, 84 Gramercy Park, New York, New York County (1892).
H. N. Porter, Washington, D. C. (1891).
Avery Segur, 281 Henry St., Brooklyn, Kings County (1893).
E. W. Simmons, Canandaigua, Ontario County (1892).
L. S. Sprague, Williamson, Wayne County (1891).
H. C. Tompkins, Knowlesville, Orleans County (1893).
William Young, Cold Spring, Putnam County (1891).

* Deceased.

NON-RESIDENT FELLOWS.

N. P. Dandridge, 148 Broadway, Cincinnati, Ohio.
Stuart Eldridge, Yokohama, Japan.
Alfred C. McDaniel, San Antonio, Texas.
Donald Maclean, 652 Mission St., Detroit, Mich.
James Bissett Murdoch, 4232 Fifth Ave., Pittsburgh, Pa.
E. T. Sabal, 45 W. Monroe St., Jacksonville, Fla.
David St. John, Hackensack, N. J.
Theodore Goodell Wright, Plainville, Hartford Co., Conn.

HONORARY FELLOWS.

Sir John Simon, 40 Kensington Square, London, England (1890).

CORRESPONDING FELLOWS.

William Goodell, 1418 Spruce St., Philadelphia, Pa. (1890).
Henry O. Marcey, 116 Boylston St., Boston, Mass. (1890).

DECEASED FELLOWS.

DECEASED FELLOWS.

NAME	AGE	COUNTY	PLACE OF BIRTH	DATE OF DEATH	MEDICAL COLLEGE	YEAR OF GRADUATION
dns, John G. (F)¹	77	New York	New York City	June 19, 384	Coll. Phys. and Surg., N. Y.	1880
Fdn, O. M. (O)²	83	Delaware	Delaware Co., N. Y.	Nov. 27, 1891.	...ik, Vt.	1881
Andrews, John S. (O)	61	Kings	Bristol, Conn.	Jan. 8, 1889.	Univ. City of New York	1849
Ashton, Isaiah H.	39	Westchester	Philadelphia, Pa.	Feb. 16, 899.	University of Pennsylvania	1870
vary, George W. (F)	61	Chenango	Earlville, N. Y.	Nov. 1, 98.	Albany Medical College	1860
rxsder (F)	74	Montgomery	Oppenheim, N. Y.	Aug. 27, 1886.	...en, Vt.	1842
Bsk, Myron N. (F)	73	S atoga	West Berkshire, Vt.	May 21, 99.	Vermont Medical College	1842
Ballou, William R.	29	New York	Bath, Me.	March 9, 803.	Bellevue Hosp. Med. Coll.	1886
Bsker, A. M. (O)	37	Erie	Kendall, Orleans Co., N. Y.	Dec. 6, 1887.	University of Buffalo	1877
Bsyte, ines (O)	65	New York	New York	March 27, 1891.	Coll. Phys. and Surg., N. Y.	1846
Baynes, William T. (O)	48	Rensselaer	England	Jan. 22, 1892.	Albany dal llege	1871
Bemus, William P.	68	Chautauqua	Chautauqua Co.	Sept. 19, 1890.	Berkshire Medical College	1847
Fbn, Wm N. (O).	85	New York	Roxbury, Conn.	Aug. 10, 1890.	Yale	1882
Buckley, adfes (O)	:	Monroe	....		University of Pennsylvania	1870
Bsdn, Dsiel D. (O)	70	Rensselaer	Brunswick, N. Y.	April 19, 1890.	Albany Medical College	1846
usBd, J. Henry (O)	45	Ontario	United States	Feb. 25, 1890.	Buffalo Medical College	1875
Burwell, George N. (O)	72	Erie	Norway, Herkimer Co.	May 15, 1891.	University of Pennsylvania	1848
Carroll, lsd Ludlow (F)	60	New York	New York City	Oct. 30, 1898.	Univ. City of New York	1855
Case, Mary W.	33	Rensselaer	New York State	Aug. 19, 1889.	Women's Med. Coll., Phila.	1882
Chace, Wm (F)	58	Chautauqua	St. Catharine's, Canada	Dec. 27, 1891.	Coll. Phys. and Surg., N. Y.	1858
Cdlh, Allen S. (F)	62	New York	Great Barrington, Mass.	Oct. 24, 1884.	...tdn, Vt., .	1848
Gsk, Alonzo	80	New York	Chester, Mass.	Sept. 18, 1887.	Coll. Phys. and Surg., N. Y.	1885

¹ (F) Founder.   ² (O) Original Fellow.

Name	No.	County	Place	Date	Medical College	Year
Clark, Simeon T. (O)	55	Niagara	Canton, Mass.	Dec. 24, 1891.	Berkshire Med. Coll.	1860
Coit, William N. (F)	52	Clinton	Plattsburgh, N. Y.	Aug. 4, 1886.	University of Pennsylvania	1856
Collins, Isaac G. (F)	53	Westchester	Granville, N. Y.	Dec. 18, 1885.	Albany Medical College	1858
Collins, Thomas B. (O)	61	Monroe	Mendon, N. Y.	Feb. 17, 1888.	Jefferson Med. Coll., Phila.	1851
Cooper, William S. (F)	70	Rensselaer	Scotland	May 26, 1890.	Albany Medical College	1860
Cornell, F. O. (O)	29	Montgomery	Glenville, N. Y.	Dec. 3, 1884.	Albany Medical College	1890
Cotes, J. R.	54	Genesee	Batavia, N. Y.	March 20, 1884.	Med. Dep. Univ. Buffalo	1852
Creamer, Joseph	63	Kings	Halifax, Nova Scotia	Jan. 6, 1883.	Coll. Phys. and Surg., N. Y.	1850
Crutenden, Albert G.	75	Ontario	Covington, N. Y.	June 7, 1890.	Willoughby Univ., Ohio	1840
Damainville, Lucien	52	New York	Erie, Pa.	Dec. 15, 1891.	Long Island Coll. Hosp.	1860
Davidson, John (F)	91	Queens	New York City	Dec. 26, 1884.	Lic. N. Y. St. Med. Soc.	1829
De La Mater, S. G. (F)	73	Schenectady	Bethlehem, Alb. Co., N. Y.	June 23, 1888.	Albany Medical College	1842
Du Bois, Abram (F)	81	New York	Red Hook, N. Y.	Aug. 29, 1891.	Coll. Phys. and Surg., N. Y.	1835
Eager, William B. (O)	65	Orange	Orange Co.	Jan. 18, 1890.	Coll. Phys. and Surg., N. Y.	1848
Earll, George W. (F)	53	Onondaga	Mottville, N. Y.	July 8, 1890.	Buffalo Medical College	1858
Edgerly, Edward F. (F)	50	Essex	Moriah, Essex Co.	June 23, 1889.	Albany Medical College	1864
Elder, Jennie S.	32	Onondaga	Syracuse, N. Y.	Feb. 2, 1889.	Med. Dep. Syracuse Univ.	1878
Ferguson, James (O)	74	Warren	Kortwright, N. Y.	Oct. 27, 1892.	Castleton, Vt.	1841
Fitch, William (F)	70	Tompkins	Franklin, N. Y.	Sept. 14, 1893.	Albany Medical College	1846
Flint, Austin (F)	73	New York	Petersham, Mass.	March 13, 1886.	Harvard Medical College	1833
Flood, Patrick Henry (O)	72	Chemung	Pennsylvania	March 12, 1886.	Geneva Medical College	1845
Fox, Ell	57	Herkimer	Columbia, N. Y.	Oct. 13, 1890.	Med. Dep. Univ. City N. Y.	1855
Fuller, Winfield S. (O)	48	Monroe	Walworth, N. Y.	Jan. 13, 1888.	Coll. Phys. and Surg., N. Y.	1861
Garrish, John P. (O)	76	New York	New Brunswick, N. J.	April 1, 1891.	Jefferson Med. Coll., Phila.	1896
Gay, Charles C. F. (F)	66	Erie	Pittsfield, Mass.	March 27, 1886.	Berkshire Medical College	1846
Gray, John Perdue (F)	61	Oneida	Half Moon, Pa.	Nov. 29, 1886.	University of Pennsylvania	1849
Gray, John W. (F)	58	Livingston	America	April 17, 1886.	University of New York	1856
Green, Caleb (F)	73	Cortland	La Fayette, N. Y.	May 10, 1893.	Geneva Medical College	1844

NAME.	AGE.	COUNTY.	PLACE OF BIRTH.	DATE OF DEATH.	MEDICAL COLLEGE.	
Griswold, Gaspar (O)	29	New York	New York City	March 4, 1886.	Bellevue Hosp. Med. Coll.	1878
Guernsey, Dessault (F)	55	Dutchess	Wilton, N. Y.	Dec. 9, 1885.	Coll. Phys. and Surg., N. Y.	1850
Hall, H. C. (O)	41	Broome	America	June 1, 1887.	University of New York	1869
Hall, John E. (O)	38	Albany	New Marlboro', Mass.	Nov. 3, 1888.	Albany Medical College	1877
Hamilton, Frank H. (F)	73	New York	Wilmington, Vt.	Aug. 11, 1886.	University of Pennsylvania	1835
Higgins, Seabury M. (O)	67	Onondaga	Brewster, Mass.	Dec. 9, 1889.	University City of N. Y.	1848
Hinds, Frederic J. (O)	32	Washington	East Greenwich, N. Y.	April 26, 1887.	Bellevue Hosp. Med. Coll.	1876
Hollister, Edwin O. (O)	41	Ontario	Batavia, N. Y.	Oct. 8, 1887.	Bellevue Hosp. Med. Coll.	1874
Hunt, James H. (O)	44	Orange	Centreville, Sullivan Co.	Dec. 20, 1892.	Bellevue Hosp. Med. Coll.	1872
Husted, N. C. (F)	66	Westchester	Round Hill, Conn.	Nov. 19, 1891.	University City of N. Y.	1850
Hutchison, Joseph C. (F)	60	Kings	Old Franklin, Mo.	July 17, 1887.	University of Pennsylvania	1848
Hyde, Frederick (F)	80	Cortland	Whitney Point, N. Y.	Oct. 15, 1887.	Fairfield Medical College	1836
Johnston, Francis U. (F)	66	Richmond	New York City	Nov. 20, 1892.	Coll. Phys. and Surg., N. Y.	1852
King, James E. (O)	66	Erie	Warren, Pa.	Jan. 21, 1888.	Buffalo Medical College	1848
Knapp, Edwin A. (O)	67	Onondaga	New York State	Dec. 7, 1890.	Geneva Med. Coll.	1851
Knapp, John H. (O)	67	Cortland	New Fairfield, Conn.	April 30, 1886.	{ Chenango Co. Med. Soc. / Geneva Med. Coll.	1843 / 1861
Lamb, Milton M.	66	Rensselaer	Verona, N. Y.	April 10, 1892.	Castleton, Vt.	1856
Lamont, John Campbell	47	Wayne	Edinburgh, Scotland	Dec. 13, 1887.	Med. Dep. Univ. City N. Y.	1862
Lauer, Eugene (O)	40	New York	Germany	Oct. 31, 1886.	Giessen and Marburg	1866
Lester, Sullivan W. (O)	40	Rensselaer	Niantic, Conn.	Jan. 5, 1890.	Med. Dep. Univ. City N. Y.	1881
Linsly, Jared (F)	84	New York	Northfield, Conn.	July 12, 1887,	Coll. Phys. and Surg., N, Y.	1820

Name		County	Birthplace	Date	College	Year
Lyman, E. S. (O)	80	Chenango	Torrington, Conn.	Nov. 20, 1892.	Regents Univ. N. Y.	1870
Matthews, David	60	New York	Sullivan County	July 9, 1891.	Coll. Phys. and Surg., N. Y.	1860
Maury, Rutson	27	New York	North Carolina	May 5, 1892.	Bellevue Hosp. Med. Coll.	1887
McClellan, Christopher R.	73	Kings	Maryland	Jan. 13, 1887.	University of Maryland	1835
McEwen, Robert C. (F)	60	Saratoga	Bainbridge, N. Y.	Dec. 26, 1888.	Coll. Phys. and Surg., N. Y.	1856
McTammany, George H.	31	Rensselaer	Troy, N. Y.	April 12, 1891.	Albany Medical College	1884
McTammany, Wm. F. (O)	36	Rensselaer	Troy, N. Y.	July 21, 1888.	Bellevue Hosp. Med. Coll.	1880
Moore, Joseph W. (F)	47	Albany	Troy, N. Y.	Sept. 9, 1880.	Castleton, Vt.	1859
Morrell, Isaac	79	Chemung	Cornish, Me.	Sept. 8, 1887.	Bowdoin Medical College	1832
Pask, William (O)	55	Erie	England	Aug. 24, 1884.	Med. Dep. Univ. Buffalo	1884
Peck, M. R. (O)	62	Warren	Sand Lake, N. Y.	April 4, 1884.	Albany Medical College	1851
Pollard, Abiathar	90	Essex	Bridgewater, Vt	April 15, 1893.	Castleton, Vt.	1836
Pomeroy, Charles G. (F)	71	Wayne	New York.	Dec. 14, 1887.	{ Ontario Co. Med. Soc.	1837
					Jefferson Medical Coll.	1850
Pryer, W. Chardavoyne (F)	54	Westchester	New York City	Sept. 24, 1888.	Coll. Phys. and Surg., N. Y.	1862
Purdy, Isaac (O)	57	Sullivan	Walkill, N. Y.	Dec. 6, 1885.	Castleton, Vt.	1851
Reynolds, Rufus C. (F)	70	Monroe	Columbia, Herkimer Co.	Dec. 22, 1886.	Fairfield Med. Coll., N. Y.	1830
Ring, William (F)	63	Erie	United States	April 20, 1887.	University of Buffalo	1848
Robinson, Joseph W.	49	Steuben	Angelica, N. Y.	Jan. 4, 1887.	Buffalo Medical College	1862
Rochester, Thomas F. (F)	63	Erie	Rochester, N. Y.	May 24, 1887.	University of Pennsylvania	1848
Sabin, Robert Hall (F)	56	Albany	Saxton's River, Vt	Dec. 4, 1888.	Albany Medical College	1856
Sayre, Lewis Hall (F)	38	New York	New York City	Jan. 2, 1890.	Bellevue Hosp. Med. Coll.	1876
Schoonmaker, E. J. (F)	65	Seneca	Ulster Co., N. Y.	Aug. 19, 1889.	Geneva Medical College	1848
Skiff, George V. (O)	53	New York	Pike, N. Y.	Jan. 28, 1890.	Univ. City of New York	1860
Slack, Henry (F)	57	Dutchess	Albany, N. Y.	Dec. 10, 1888.	Albany Medical College	1852
Slocum, J. O. (F)	65	Onondaga	Pompey, N. Y.	Mar. 3, 1885.	Castleton, Vt.	1846
Smith, David M.	35	Yates	New York City	Mar. 19, 1891.	Bellevue Hosp. Med. Coll.	1877
Smith, Joseph T. (F)	60	Ontario	Farmington, N. Y.	Dec. 9, 1890.	Jefferson Med. Coll., Phila.	1854

NAME.	AGE.	COUNTY.	PLACE OF BIRTH.	DATE OF DEATH.	MEDICAL COLLEGE.	
Smith, Marcellus R. (O)	74	Cortland	Taylor, N. Y.	Dec. 11, 1890.	Geneva Medical College	1847
Sprague, William B. (F)	55	Genesee	Pavilion, N. Y.	Mar. 16, 1891.	University of Buffalo	1857
Squire, Truman Hoffman	66	Chemung	Russia, Herkimer Co.	Nov. 27, 1889.	Coll. Phys. and Surg., N. Y.	1848
Steele, Charles G.	27	Erie	Buffalo. N. Y.	Feb. 12, 1888.	University of Buffalo	1886
Steinführer, Gustavus A. (F)	37	Schenectady	Germany	July 2, 1890.	Coll. Phys. and Surg., N. Y.	1874
Stevens, Frederick P. (O)	31	New York	Ithaca, N. Y.	Dec. 4, 1884.	Bellevue Hosp. Med. Coll.	1877
Stevenson, William G.	44	Rockland	Troy, Ohio	Feb. 3, 1888.	Bellevue Hosp. Med. Coll.	1864
Sutton, George Samuel	63	Dutchess	Louisville, N. Y.	Sept. 6, 1888.	Coll. Phys. and Surg., N. Y.	1859
Taylor, Isaac E. (F)	79	New York	Philadelphia, Pa.	Oct. 30, 1889.	University of Pennsylvania	1834
Van Dusen, Melville E.	38	Steuben	Wheeler, N. Y.	June 15, 1891.	Med. Dep. Univ. Mich.	1879
Vaughn, Frank O. (O)	44	Erie	Buffalo, N. Y.	Mar. 18, 1891.	Med. Dep. Buffalo Univ.	1880
Webb, Edwin (O)	85	Queens	Devonport, England	Jan. 29, 1890.	Coll. Phys. and Surg., N. Y.	1825
West, M. Calvin	58	Oneida	Rome, N. Y.	Oct. 20, 1891.	Michigan University	1860
White, Francis V.	56	New York	New York City	Oct. 9, 1889.	Univ. City of New York	1855
White, William T. (F)	64	New York	Richmond, Me.	Sept. 17, 1893.	New York Med. Coll.	1865
Willis, A. B.	43	Schenectady	Coeymans, N. Y.	May 10, 1891.	Albany Medical College	1870
Winship, Cornelius A. (O)	62	Rensselaer	Litchfield, Conn.	Feb. 14, 1888.	Albany Medical College	1858
Wood, Charles S. (F)	65	New York	Litchfield, Conn.	Feb. 1, 1890.	Jefferson Med. Coll., Phila.	1851
Woodend, William D. (F)	61	Suffolk	Portsmouth, Va.	Mar. 8, 1893.	University of Pennsylvania	1855
Woodruff, William D. (F)	60	Suffolk	Portsmouth, Va.	Mar. 10, 1893.	University of Pennsylvania	1855
Young, John (O)	71	Dutchess	Ireland	Sept. 2, 1893.	Coll. Phys. and Surg., N. Y.	1844
Young, Oscar H. (O)	43	Delaware	Pennsylvania	Jan. 21, 1880.	Jefferson Med. Coll. Phila.	1876

Total Deceased Fellows, 120.

INDEX.

536

INDEX.

DAYTON, Hon. CHARLES W., response to toast, 447.
Deceased Fellows, list of, 530.
Delegates, list of, 17.
DENNIS, F. S., appendicitis, 235.
Discussion on lesions of the pleura, 84.
Dr. JOHN SHRADY, 84.
Dr. WILLIAM McCOLLOM, 95.
Dr. J. B. WHITE, 101.
Dr. J. G. TRUAX, 111.
Dr. C. A. LEALE, 116.
Discussion on the treatment of appendicitis, 235.
Dr. F. S. DENNIS, 235.
Dr. J. W. S. GOULEY, 242.
Dr. DONALD MACLEAN, 243.
Dr. J. D. BRYANT, 245.
Dr. J. A. WYETH, 246.
Dr. E. D. FERGUSON, 247.
Dr. W. T. LUSK, 247.
Dr. J. CRONYN, 248.
District branches. See Branches.
DOUGLAS, GEORGE, discussion on voluntary commitments to asylums for the insane, 202.
enteric fever, 218.
DUDLEY, A. PALMER, discussion on treatment after trachelorrhaphy, 191.
Dysmenorrhoea, pelvic inflammation, and pelvic abscess, a new and non-operative method of treating, Dr. T. J. McGILLICUDDY, 288.
ELIOT, GUSTAVUS, treatment of enteric fever, 204.
Enteric fever, treatment of, Dr. GUSTAVUS ELIOT, 204.
Epithelioma and cancroid ulcers, treatment of, Dr. N. L. NORTH, 71.
Executive committee, Third branch, 462.
Fifth branch, 468.
Fellows registered at the 10th annual meeting, 13.
lists of, 486.
FERGUSON, E. D., nephrotomy and nephrectomy, 62.
discussion on lesions of the pleura, 121.
treatment after trachelorrhaphy, 193.
voluntary commitments to asylums for the insane, 203.
remarks on appendicitis, 247.
remarks as toast-master, 437, etc.
Fermentative dyspepsia, remarks on, Dr. AUSTIN FLINT, 141.

Festivities of the first decennial meeting, 437.
FINDER, WILLIAM, Jr., discussion on enteric fever, 218.
vaccinia after typhoid fever, 264.
FLINT, AUSTIN, remarks on fermentative dyspepsia, 141.
response to toast, 437.
GOULEY, JOHN W. S., discussion on nephrotomy and nephrectomy, 70.
remarks on appendicitis, 242.
memoir of ALFRED L. CARROLL, M. D., 402.
Gout and rheumatism, rare forms of, SIR JAMES A. GRANT, 220.
GRANGER, WILLIAM D., voluntary commitments to asylums for the insane, 194.
GRANT, SIR JAMES A., rare forms of gout and rheumatism, 220.
letter from, 441.
GREEN, CALEB, memoir of, 423.
HARRISON, GEORGE T., obstetrical and gynaecological work of the association, 385.
HART, Mr. ERNEST, response to toast, 441.
HARVIE, JOHN B., fifty operations on uterine cervix, 297.
Honorary Fellows, list of, 528.
HUNT, JAMES HALSEY, memoir of, 427.
Invited guests, 17.
JOHNSTON, FRANCIS UPTON, memoir of, 430.
JOHNSTONE, Mr. L. M., memoir of FRANCIS U. JOHNSTON, M. D., 430.
Kings County Medical Association, annual report, 476.
LEALE, CHARLES A., discussion on lesions of the pleura, 116.
cure of consumption and empyema, 313.
response to toast, 450.
LESTER, ELIAS, discussion on voluntary commitments to asylums for the insane, 202.
enteric fever, 218.
Library committee, report of, 483.
List of presidents and vice-presidents, 9.
Fellows registered at the 10th annual meeting, 13.
delegates, 17.
invited guests, 17.
Fellows by district and county, 486.
alphabetically, 510.

FIRST DECENNIAL INDEX.

36

37

[NOTE.—The editor asks indulgence for errors resulting from his inability to give the time which would be required to verify the references while reading the proof.]